BIOLOGICAL AND CHEMICAL TERRORISM:

A PHARMACY PREPAREDNESS GUIDE

Written, compiled, and edited by
Edward P. Krenzelok, Pharm.D., FAACT, DABAT
Director
Pittsburgh Poison Center
Children's Hospital of Pittsburgh
Professor of Pharmacy and Pediatrics
University of Pittsburgh

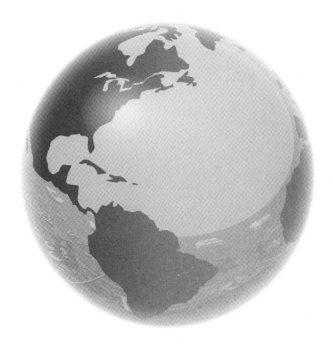

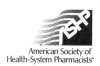

American Society of
Health-System Pharmacists®

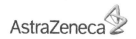

Made possible through a grant from AstraZeneca

Acquisitions Editor
Cynthia Reilly

Development Editor/Project Manager
Cynthia Reilly

Production Manager
Johnna Hershey

Production and Cover Design Services
York Graphic Services, York, Pennsylvania

Any correspondence regarding this publication should be sent to the publisher, American Society of Health-System Pharmacists®, 7272 Wisconsin Avenue, Bethesda, MD 20814, Special Publishing. Produced in conjunction with the ASHP Publications Production Center.

The information presented herein reflects the opinions of the editor. It should not be interpreted as an official policy of ASHP or as an endorsement of any product.

Drug information and its applications are constantly evolving because of ongoing research and clinical experience and are often subject to professional judgment and interpretation by the practitioner and to the uniqueness of a clinical situation. The author and ASHP have made every effort to ensure the accuracy and completeness of the information presented in this book. However, the reader is advised that the publisher, author, contributors, editors, and reviewers cannot be responsible for the continued currency of the information, for any errors or omissions, and/or for any consequences arising from the use of the information in the clinical setting.

©2003, American Society of Health-System Pharmacists, Inc. All rights reserved.

No part of this publication may be reproduced or transmitted in any form or by any means, electronic or mechanical, including photocopying, microfilming, and recording, or by any information storage and retrieval system, without written permission from the American Society of Health-System Pharmacists.

ASHP® is a service mark of the American Society of Health-System Pharmacists, Inc.; registered in the U.S. Patent and Trademark Office.

ISBN: 1-58528-048-8

TABLE OF **CONTENTS**

ABOUT THE EDITOR

Edward P. Krenzelok, Pharm.D., FAACT, DABAT

Dr. Krenzelok is the Director of the Pittsburgh Poison Center at Children's Hospital of Pittsburgh and a Professor of Pharmacy and Pediatrics at the University of Pittsburgh. He received his Bachelor of Science degree in pharmacy from the University of Wisconsin in 1971 and his Doctor of Pharmacy degree from the University of Minnesota in 1974. Dr. Krenzelok is active in several professional toxicology and medically related societies and associations and is a past President of the American Academy of Clinical Toxicology. He is certified in clinical toxicology by the American Board of Applied Toxicology and has been awarded the distinction of being a Fellow in the American Academy of Clinical Toxicology. He is Chair of the United States Pharmacopeia Clinical Toxicology and Drug Expert Committee, is a former member of the Food and Drug Administration Non-prescription Drug Advisory Committee, serves on the editorial boards and review panels of numerous medical journals, and is the author of several hundred scientific publications and book chapters.

Dr. Krenzelok has been active in biological and chemical terrorism preparedness activities locally, regionally, and in the Commonwealth of Pennsylvania since 1995. He has published papers on the role of poison centers and terrorism, innovative real-time surveillance for biological and chemical terrorism, and the development of a regional pharmaceutical cache to respond to a terrorism event. Dr. Krenzelok is a frequent guest lecturer on the topics of biological and chemical terrorism.

DEDICATION

This book is dedicated to those who have been the unfortunate victims of any type of terrorism. It is also dedicated to health-system pharmacists, health care providers, poison information specialists, and public health officials who have the daunting responsibility of preparing to care for the victims of future biological and chemical terrorism events.

I am indebted to my wife, Nancy, and daughters, Ann and Elizabeth, for the support and love they provided to me during the production of this work and to my mother, Marie, and late father, Paul, who always supported and encouraged my educational endeavors.

REVIEWERS AND ACKNOWLEDGMENTS

ASHP would like to thank the following reviewers who contributed to the development of this book:

Victor Cohen, B.S., Pharm.D.
Assistant Professor of Pharmacy Practice
Arnold & Marie Schwartz College of Pharmacy
    Practice
Long Island University
Clinical Pharmacy Manager of the Department
    of Emergency Medicine
Maimonides Medical Center, New York

Craig Davenport, Pharm.D.
Director of Pharmacy
Soldiers & Sailors Memorial Hospital
Penn Yan, New York

Robert V. DiGregorio, Pharm.D.
Associate Professor
Arnold & Marie Schwartz College of Pharmacy
    Practice
Long Island University
Clinical Coordinator for Pharmacy and
    Emergency Services
Brookdale Hospital Medical Center, New York

John Grabenstein, J.D.
Anthrax Vaccine Immunization Program Agency
U.S. Army Medical Command
Falls Church, Virginia

David Hardy, M.S., R.Ph.
Director of Pharmacy
Health Resource Services
Seattle, Washington

Curtis Kellner, Pharm.D.
Director of Pharmacy and Corporate Director
St. Vincent's Hospital
New York, New York

Cdr. Michael J. Montello, M.S.
Deputy-Chief Pharmacy Officer
Disaster Medical Assistance Team-1
U.S. Public Health Service
Bethesda, Maryland

Cliff Moore, R.Ph.
Director of Pharmacy, Respiratory and
    Cardiology Services
St. Clare's Hospital
Denville, New Jersey

Barbara M. Poe, R.Ph., M.B.A.
Director of Pharmacy Services
Norman Regional Hospital
Norman, Oklahoma

David S. Teeter, Pharm.D.
Department of Veterans Affairs
Office of Operations, Security and
    Preparedness
Indianapolis, Indiana

ASHP would also like to thank Eleanor O'Rangers and Harvey Maldow at AstraZeneca for bringing this project to our attention and for their generous funding. Thanks also to ASHP staff Colleen O'Malley, Joseph Deffenbaugh, and Daniel J. Cobaugh for their guidance and input.

INTRODUCTION

Terrorism is no longer a hypothetical issue in the United States. It is reality! This became abundantly apparent when the tragic events of September 11, 2001, shocked America. Soon thereafter, anthrax cases surfaced in October 2001, sending a shocked nation into near panic. Government, law enforcement, and public health officials were consumed with the reality of biological terrorism, attempting to anticipate what terroristic challenge would appear next. Every aspect of health care delivery was forced to mobilize its resources to prepare for the next wave of terrorism. The stark reality that most health care professionals and their institutions were unprepared was amplified by the media.

The public and health care providers alike were uncomfortably anxious about the medical community's ill preparedness. Hospitals became consumed with assessing their preparedness and developing plans to deal with the mysterious and unknown. Weren't anthrax, plague, tularemia, and viral hemorrhagic fever exotic diseases endemic only to developing nations? How contagious were the infectious diseases? Hadn't smallpox been eradicated? What antidotes were necessary to treat the unthinkable—nerve and mustard gas exposures? What antibiotics would be effective? Did the hospital pharmacy stock an adequate supply of antidotes and antibiotics? How many patients could the hospital manage? Who would pay for the preparedness? These and dozens of other questions were posed and solutions sought. Every department in a hospital was faced with developing plans to prepare for new types of disasters—mass casualties caused by weapons of mass destruction (WMD), or nuclear, biological, or chemical (NBC) terrorism events.

Because radiology and nuclear medicine are common to hospitals, radiation disaster preparedness policies may need merely to be updated to address the threat of nuclear (radiation) terrorism. However, an estimated 80 percent of U.S. hospitals did not have biological and chemical terrorism preparedness plans. A hospital biological and chemical preparedness plan is the sum of all departmental preparedness plans. A key participant in the successful management of the victims of biological and chemical terrorism is the health-system pharmacy. Pharmaceutical care that involves pharmacological antagonists (antidotes) and antibiotics are critical to favorable patient outcomes. Therefore, the health-system pharmacy must have a comprehensive preparedness plan.

The purpose of this book is to provide the health-system pharmacy with the basic tools with which to develop a biological and chemical terrorism response or preparedness plan. To develop a viable plan that is consistent with the needs of the health-system pharmacy, institution, and community, it is essential to understand the basic elements and possible agents of biological and chemical terrorism.

The first section of the book covers the history of biological and chemical terrorism. The evolution from biological and chemical warfare to biological and chemical terrorism is described. The use of these agents for terrorism is a relatively new phenomenon, and their historical use may provide basic intelligence to guide the anticipation of future use. Biological and chemical warfare agents of past decades form the basis for many of today's educational endeavors.

To develop a sound health-system pharmacy biological and chemical terrorism preparedness plan, pharmacists must have a basic understanding of the anticipated agents of terrorism. The second section of the book is divided into two segments: Biological Terrorism Agents and Chemical Terrorism Agents. Publications from the current literature are presented to provide a comprehensive review of the biological and chemical agents that are expected to be used and to pose the greatest risk. The *Journal of the American Medical Association's* series on biological terrorism agents provides an excellent foundation for understanding diseases such as anthrax, smallpox, plague, tularemia, botulism, and the hemorrhagic viral fevers. Medical journals have not addressed preparedness for chemical agent terrorism as comprehensively as they have the biological agents. The U.S. military has developed extensive information resources on the pathophysiology and treatment of victims of chemical warfare, and this information can be applied directly to the use of the same agents for terroristic purposes. Descriptions of chemical agents from the *Medical Management of Chemical*

Casualties Handbook, from the U.S. Army Medical Research Institute of Chemical Defense–Chemical Casualty Care Division, provide an excellent discussion of pulmonary agents, cyanide, vesicants, and nerve agents. To facilitate a rapid review of each biological or chemical terrorism agent, the biologicals and chemicals are summarized at the beginning of each segment. These summaries provide an overview of the relevant aspects of each entity and may be useful reviews in a time of crisis.

Section three, Reference Resources on Biological and Chemical Terrorism, serves as an extensive, but by no means exhaustive, compilation of reference resources that may assist the health-system pharmacist in developing a biological and chemical terrorism preparedness plan. Additionally, it can assist the health-system pharmacist in identifying important papers for the pharmacy's biological and chemical terrorism reference library and file. Efforts should be made to develop and maintain an up-to-date reference library on biological and chemical terrorism. The day when a crisis occurs is not the appropriate time to begin this process. Preparedness is key!

Once aware of the potential biological and chemical threats, the health-system pharmacist should develop a preparedness plan. Section four, Hospital Pharmacy Preparedness, includes an extensive review of the pharmacy literature regarding general disaster planning and specific suggestions about how to prepare for biological and chemical terrorism. The literature review is followed by a selection of papers on disaster and preparedness planning that were published in the *American Journal of Health-System Pharmacy* that address specific aspects of bioterrorism preparedness planning. This series of papers provides an excellent foundation upon which to build a biological and chemical preparedness plan for the health-system pharmacy.

Use this book as a foundation or starting point. It is intended to provide direction and guidance. Every health-system pharmacy (e.g., community, university) will have different needs, and it is hoped that this book will assist health-system pharmacies in addressing some of the challenges that they face in the development and implementation of a biological and chemical terrorism preparedness plan.

SECTION **ONE**

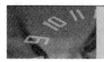
History of Biological and Chemical Terrorism

INTRODUCTION

The tragic events of September 11, 2001, when commercial jets crashed into the twin towers of the World Trade Center in New York City and into the Pentagon and a field in western Pennsylvania, have changed our lives dramatically. Tens of thousands of lives were affected by the deaths of nearly 3;000 innocent victims who perished on 9/11. A new era emerged, and the Americans' vulnerability to terrorism became a stark reality. A common theme was "I can't believe that this happened to us." Human resilience prevented those terrorist acts from disrupting the core of American life. However, just as people began to cope with the tragedy of 9/11, yet another act of terrorism challenged America—the diagnosis of inhalational anthrax on October 4, 2001,[1] and the subsequent anthrax-related deaths of five individuals. *Bioterrorism* became a household word and instilled in Americans the fear of a new unknown. However, this is not the first time that Americans have faced the challenges associated with weapons of mass casualty, which include explosive, biological, and chemical terrorism.

Biological and Chemical Warfare

Biological and chemical terrorism evolved from the battle-field. Early attempts to use biological and chemical warfare were crude and focused on the use of smoke, filth, human cadavers, and decaying animal carcasses. In antiquity, attempts were often made to poison or contaminate water sources such as wells and reservoirs. The earliest description of chemical warfare occurred during the feud between Athens and Sparta in 423 BC.[2] The Spartans used sulfur and tree pitch to create an intensely irritating smoke that forced the Athenian defenders to flee. In the seventh century AD a Greek alchemist developed Greek fire, which contained a mixture of flammable substances (i.e., resin, pitch, sulfur, naphtha, lime, salt peter).[2] This floating concoction would be ignited and then set afire to destroy wooden boats.

In the fourteenth century, the Tartars experienced a plague epidemic and attempted to turn their misfortune into a tactical offensive weapon by catapulting the cadavers of plague victims into their adversary's city.[3] Plague is transmitted by fleas that carry the bacteria *Yersinia pestis*.[4] It is more likely that flea-infested rats served as the vector instead of the cadavers, since fleas require living tissue to survive.[3] However, it has been suggested that plague-infected refugees from this conflict may have been responsible for the second continental pandemic as they traveled to Mediterranean port cities.[3]

During the French and Indian War (1754-1763) in North America, the British conceived a plan to destroy the Native Americans who were sympathetic to the French by introducing smallpox to this smallpox-naïve population.[2, 3, 5] An outbreak of smallpox at Fort Pitt provided the opportunity to contaminate blankets that were distributed to the Indians. While a devastating outbreak of smallpox did occur, it is questionable whether the blankets were responsible, since smallpox is generally transmitted via droplet transmission.[6] These are some of the earliest examples of the use of biological and chemical agents in tactical warfare.

The agents of biological and chemical warfare are not new. As noted in Tables 1.1 and 1.2, some have been recognized for centuries.[5]

The modern use of unconventional warfare began tragically on April 22, 1915, near Ypres, Belgium, when German soldiers released 150 tons of chlorine gas.[2] This horrific event killed approximately 5,000 and injured an additional 10,000 Allied troops. Thus the era of chemical warfare began, and during the course of the war chemical use expanded, incorporating the use of chloropicrin, mustard,

Table 1.1 Biological Agents

Agent	Year Identified
Plague	3,000 years ago
Smallpox	1122 BC
Anthrax	1863 AD
Cholera	1883
Typhus	1909
Glanders	1882
Brucellosis	1887
Ricin	1889
Tularemia	1911

TABLE 1.2 Chemical Agents

Agent	Year Identified
Chlorine	1774
Cyanogen chloride	1802
Phosgene	1812
Mustard	1822

and phosgene, which wreaked havoc on unprepared soldiers and their horses (used for transport). The accounts vary but an estimated 90,000 soldiers were killed and a million more were injured.[2, 7]

Contemporary biological warfare also has its roots in World War I (WWI) and the postwar era. There is evidence that Germany developed an aggressive covert plan to infect the Allies' livestock and animal feed with bacterial pathogens such as pseudomonas.[3, 5] The operations occurred in Europe and the United States by German saboteurs in an attempt to infect horses the U.S. cavalry would use in their fight against the German army. The world was shocked by the use of these unconventional tactics, which led to the 1925 Geneva Protocol for the Prohibition of the Use in War of Asphyxiating, Poisonous or other Gases and of Bacteriological Methods of Warfare.[3, 5] This treaty prohibited the deployment of biological and chemical weapons, but it was weak, lacked enforcement, and failed to prohibit further research or production of these weapons. Consequently, many countries, including the United States, began to develop offensive biological and chemical warfare programs.

Prior to and during World War II (WWII) the Japanese pursued an aggressive biological warfare development program. Their research center was located in Manchuria and was ultimately known as the infamous Unit, or Detachment, 731.[3,5] With a staff of approximately 3,000, Unit 731 exposed prisoners to infectious agents such as *Neisseria meningitidis* (meningitis), *Shigella* (shigellosis), *Salmonella* (cholera), and *Yersinia pestis* (plague). An estimated 10,000 prisoners perished. The program went beyond Unit 731, and the Japanese acknowledged that they conducted field trials in which they attacked Chinese cities in efforts to inflict disease and contaminate food. For example, they released fleas with *Yersinia pestis* from aircraft to introduce the plague. There is some evidence to suggest that the Japanese used the alkylating agents mustard and Lewisite in 1939 in China.[5] However, they did not incorporate these agents into their general warfare tactics.

The Germans developed sophisticated chemical warfare capabilities and performed inhumane biological experimentation on concentration camp prisoners.[3] The prisoners were infected with highly contagious agents and then subjected to the use of medications and vaccines that were designed to treat the inflicted disease. Biological warfare is not known to have been used by Hitler's Germany. However, in anticipation of biological warfare by the Nazis, the Allies developed weaponized anthrax to retaliate against a potential German biological attack. Considerable chemical warfare research was conducted in Germany both before and during WWII. German scientists developed the highly toxic cholinesterase inhibitors that were designated as the "G" (for German) agents: GA-tabun, GB-sarin, and GD-soman.[5] Devastating losses would have occurred to Allied troops if the G agents had been used. However, these agents were never used offensively. It is surmised that Hitler forbade it as he himself had been a chemical warfare victim during WWI.

In 1942 the United States began an offensive biological warfare development program, choosing anthrax as its weaponized biological.[3] However, the United States did not use biological agents. With the advent of the Korean War the U.S. program underwent significant expansion. The program included the use of human volunteers and even the dispersal of aerosolized simulated bacterial agents over a number of U.S. cities.[3] The actual U.S. arsenal of biological agents included some of the very agents that are of concern today as weapons of terrorism:[3]

- *Bacillis anthracis*
- *Botulinum toxin*
- *Francisella tularensis*
- *Brucella suis*

- *Coxiella burnetii*
- Staphylococcal enterotoxin B
- Venezuelan equine encephalitis virus

The American program even included the development of agents that would destroy crops and wreak famine and economic chaos. Ultimately, these agents were destroyed in accordance with the 1972 Convention on the Prohibition of the Development, Production and Stockpiling of Bacteriological (Biological) and Toxin Weapons and Their Destruction.[3] However, this convention did not apply to the destruction of chemical weapons, and the United States still maintains supplies of weaponized chemical agents.[8] It is quite apparent that not all countries have complied with the edicts of the 1972 convention nor destroyed their chemical weapons.

There are numerous contemporary examples that profile the continued development of biological and chemical warfare agents. The infamous use of ricin (the highly toxic component of castor beans) to assassinate the Bulgarian dissident Georgi Markov is legendary.[3,5] Markov was injected from a spring-loaded umbrella with a diminutive ricin-containing pellet. Therefore, ricin is often discussed as a potential weapon of mass casualty. While ricin is one of the most poisonous agents known, it has little application on the battlefield or as a successful biological terrorism agent since it is not volatile and would be difficult to aerosolize. Egypt is said to have used mustard in its 1967 war against Yemen.[5] The Soviets may have been signatories on the 1972 convention but that did not stifle their biological warfare program. In April 1979 the unintentional release of a small quantity of anthrax spores from a secret research complex in Sverdlovsk, Russia, resulted in the development of 77 cases of human anthrax and the fatalities of 66 individuals and countless animals that were in the downwind distribution path of the anthrax spores.[3,5,9]

Other notable uses of recent biological and chemical warfare include the alleged use of mycotoxins the North Vietnamese used against Laotians who were sympathetic to the United States during the Vietnam conflict; the confirmed use of mustard against the Kurds and Iranians by Iraq during conflicts in the 1980s; and the alleged use of chemical agents by the Russians in their war against Afghanistan rebels in the 1980s.[10]

During the Persian Gulf War, American troops expected the Iraqi army to use both biological and chemical agents against them. While no such agents were known to have been used, there was evidence of weaponized biological and chemical agents and confirmation that by 1991 the

Iraqis had investigated five different bacterial pathogens, one fungal strain, five viruses, and four different toxins.[11]

Terrorism

It should be apparent that the domestic terrorism that now faces the world is not new and evolved from use on the battlefield. In contrast to battlefield warfare, terrorism introduces these agents in a new context and not one developed solely to kill adversaries. The Federal Bureau of Investigation (FBI) defines terrorism as "the unlawful use of force and violence against persons or property to intimidate or coerce a government, the civilian population, or any segment thereof, in furtherance of political or social objectives."[12] Terrorism has three goals:[13]

- Demonstrate that a government cannot protect its people (September 11, 2001)
- Evoke an extreme response (the war on terrorism)
- Use the extreme response as a recruitment tool (new cells of Al Qaeda)

Terrorism can take on the persona of physical threat and intimidation, but it most frequently involves four types of destructive action:

- Explosive (Murrah Federal Building, Oklahoma City; World Trade Center)
- Nuclear (radioactive contamination or explosion)
- Biological (anthrax, smallpox, botulism toxin)
- Chemical (GB-sarin, mustard)

Bioterrorism is often used—inappropriately—as a generic term that refers to all forms of terrorism. The word *bioterrorism* is derived from *bio*, which means that the agent is derived from something that is living.[10] Therefore, a bioterrorism agent may be a bacteria, such as *Bacillus anthracis* (anthrax); a virus, like smallpox; or a chemical derived from a botanical, like ricin.

Terrorism, especially biological and chemical, has produced a new and often invisible enemy that creates fear of the unknown. Following the identification of the first anthrax case in Florida, on October 4, 2001, 22 cases were identified nationwide, and five fatalities resulted.[11] Most Americans were unfamiliar with anthrax, and the fear of the unknown resulted in anxiety, panic, and even mass sociogenic illness.[7, 14] This demonstrates the effectiveness of the mere threat of biological and chemical terrorism. The lives of those who perished from anthrax should not be diminished. However, it is important to place other events associated with morbidity and mortality in perspective. For example:

- The homicide rate in the United States for 2000 was approximately 11 murders/100,000 people.[15]
- The flu inflicts approximately 20,000 fatalities in the United States every year.[16]
- Drunk drivers are responsible for over 17,000 deaths each year.[17]
- Food poisoning sickens tens of thousands each year, and an estimated 5,200 die from food-borne disease on an annual basis.[18]
- Carbon monoxide poisoning kills over 5,000 people annually.[19]

That these statistics fail to make the headlines may demonstrate a degree of complacency with the known. The unknown factor creates exactly the terrorists desire—fear, panic, disruption, chaos.

Domestic terrorism is a complex problem that may be state sponsored ("axis of evil" countries), group initiated (Ku Klux Klan), or individually motivated (Timothy McVey—Murrah Federal Building). A number of motivational factors may lead to an act of terrorism:[20, 21]

- Attention-seeking behavior
- Copy-cat phenomenon
- Ecological
- Economic
- Nationalism
- Political
- Religious
- Revenge

While Americans may think that biological and chemical terrorism are new to the United States, there are a multitude of incidents that have occurred over the last three decades.[20] In 1970 the Weather Underground planned to incapacitate U.S. cities by poisoning water supplies in order to exemplify the impotence of the U.S. government. A group known as RISE was working on a plan to attack civilian populations and water supplies with a variety of pathogens in 1972. Their goal was to destroy most of mankind and prevent further destruction of nature. The Rajneeshee cult, followers of Bhagan Shree Rajneesh, contaminated the salad bars of numerous restaurants in an Oregon community with salmonella in 1984 in an attempt to seize control of municipal government by sickening voters.[20, 22] The plot failed to achieve its goal, but 751 cases of salmonella gastroenteritis were reported. In 1991 the Minnesota Patriots Council, an anti-federal tax group, plotted to harm U.S. government officials with a ricin-based poison.

Two incidents that occurred in Japan in 1994 and 1995 prompted the aggressive antiterrorism preparedness efforts that have been ongoing in the United States. In 1994 the Aum Shinrikyo cult released sarin, the toxic anticholinesterase nerve agent, in a residential neighborhood near Tokyo, resulting in approximately 200 casualties, including several fatalities.[23] Even more devastating was the March 20, 1995, sarin gas attack in the Tokyo subway system. The terrorist attack was timed to occur at a convergence point under government buildings as revenge and as part of an antigovernment plot. A dozen people perished, over 1,000 casualties occurred, and over 5,000 individuals utilized emergency medical services.[9, 22] The incident illustrated how a terrorist event could inflict panic, incapacitate a city, overwhelm an emergency medical response system, and spread fear throughout the world. In 1998 scores of abortion clinics in the United States received hoax anthrax letters, and white supremacist Larry Wayne Harris allegedly threatened to release anthrax in Las Vegas.[20]

Biological and chemical terrorism is a contemporary problem to which Americans are vulnerable due to the nature of our society. The risk of terrorism is comparatively low, as are the associated morbidity and mortality. However, preparedness is the key to minimizing the adverse outcomes associated with biological and chemical terrorism. If a biological or chemical terrorism event occurs, pharmacists must be prepared to answer the challenge by understanding these forms of terrorism and how to mitigate their effects, being fully aware of the appropriate pharmaceutical care, and having ample supplies of critical pharmaceuticals to respond to the emergent terrorist event.

REFERENCES

1. Lane HC, Fauci AS. Bioterrorism on the home front: A new challenge for American medicine. *JAMA* 2001;286:2595-2597.

2. Joy RJT. Historical aspects of medical defense against chemical warfare. In: Sidell FR, Takafuji ET, Franz DR, eds. *Textbook of military medicine: Medical aspects of chemical and biological warfare.* Washington, DC: Office of the Surgeon General, 1997:87-109.

3. Christopher GW, Cieslak TJ, Pavlin JA, et al. Biological warfare: A historical perspective. *JAMA* 1997;278:412-417.

4. Inglesby TV, Dennis DT, Henderson DA, et al. Plague as a biological weapon: Medical and public health management. *JAMA* 2000;283:2281-2290.

5. Smart JK. History of chemical and biological warfare: An American perspective. In: Sidell FR, Takafuji ET, Franz DR, eds. *Textbook of military medicine: Medical aspects of chemical and biological warfare.* Washington, DC: Office of the Surgeon General, 1997:9-86.

6. Henderson DA, Inglesby TV, Bartland JG, et al. Smallpox as a biological weapon: Medical and public health management. *JAMA* 1999;281:2127-2137.

7. Bartholomew RE, Wessely S. Protean nature of mass sociogenic illness: From possessed nuns to chemical and biological terrorism fears. *Br J Psych* 2002;180:300-306.

8. Crouch BI. Role of poison control centers in disaster response planning. *Am J Health-Syst Pharm* 2002;59:1159-1163.

9. Guillemin MM, Hugh-Jones M, Langmuir A, et al. The Sverdlovsk anthrax outbreak of 1979. *Science* 1994;18:1202-1208.

10. Sidell FR, Franz DR. Overview: Defense against the effects of chemical and biological weapons. In: Sidell FR, Takafuji ET, Franz DR, eds. *Textbook of military medicine: Medical aspects of chemical and biological warfare.* Washington, DC: Office of the Surgeon General, 1997:9-86.

11. Zilinskas RA. Iraq's biological weapons: The past as future? *JAMA* 1997;278:418-424.

12. Gregory ER, Cruther JM, Shadel B, et al. Terrorism from a public health perspective. *Am J Med Sci* 2002;323:291-298.

13. Coates JF. What's next? Foreseeable terrorist's acts. *Innovative Times* 2002;10:1-4.

14. Blendon RJ, Benson JM, DesRoches CM, et al. The impact of anthrax attacks on the American public. *Medscape Gen Med* 2002;4:1-9.

15. U.S. Department of Justice. Bureau of Justice Statistics. http://www.ojp.usdoj.gov/bjs/glance/homage.htm (accessed September 11, 2002).

16. Myers DG. Do we fear the right things? http://www.davidmyers.org/fears/ (accessed September 11, 2002).

17. Mothers Against Drunk Driving (MADD) Website. http://www.madd.org/stats/0,1056,1112,00.html (accessed September 11, 2002).

18. Mead PS, Slutsker L, Dietz V, et al. Food-related illness and death in the United States. *Emerging Infect Dis* 1999;5:607-625.

19. Cobb N, Etzel RA. Unintentional carbon monoxide-related deaths in the United States, 1979-1988. *JAMA* 1991;266:659-663.

20. Stern J. The prospect of domestic terrorism. *Emerging Infect Dis* 1999;5:517-522.

21. Tucker JB. Historical trends related to bioterrorism: An empirical analysis. *Emerging Infect Dis* 1999;5:498-504.

22. Török TJ, Tauxe RV, Wise RP, et al. A large community outbreak of salmonellosis caused by intentional contamination of restaurant salad bars. *JAMA* 1997;278:389-395.

23. Tetsu O, Takasu N, Ishimatsu S, et al. Report on 640 victims of the Tokyo subway sarin attack. *Ann Emerg Med* 1996;28:129-135.

SUGGESTED READINGS

Pavlin JA. Epidemiology of bioterrorism. *Emerging Infect Dis* 1999;5:528-530.

Henderson DA. Bioterrorism as a public health threat. *Emerging Infect Dis* 1998;4:488-492.

Eitzen EM. Education is the key to defense against bioterrorism. *Ann Emerg Med* 1999;34:221-223.

Alexander D. Nature's impartiality, man's inhumanity: Reflections on terrorism and world crisis in a context of historical disaster. *Disasters* 2002;26:1-9.

McDade JE, Franz D. Bioterrorism as a public health threat. *Emerging Infect Dis* 1998;4:493-494.

Noah DL, Huebner KD, Darling RG, et al. The history and threat of biological warfare and terrorism. *Emerg Med Clin N Am* 2002;20:255-271.

SECTION TWO, **SEGMENT ONE**

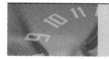

Biological Terrorism Agents

INTRODUCTION

As the United States was recovering from the shock of the events of September 11, 2001, a subsequent event stunned the country on October 4, 2001, when the first anthrax terrorism case was diagnosed. Prior to this date, there had been anthrax hoaxes and a number of nonfatal incidents of illness that were perpetrated illegally, but these had not been considered acts of biological terrorism. However, actual anthrax cases, 22 in total; quarantine of government office buildings and post offices; and contaminated American mail confirmed that biological terrorism was no longer a hypothetical. While anthrax was the focus of attention, "What is next?" became the focus of preparedness planning.

Before preparedness planning is effective, the agents of biological terrorism and their methods of dissemination must be understood. Biological terrorism is analogous to carbon monoxide poisoning—it is silent, colorless, odorless, and not apparent until the signs of illness appear. Biological agents, especially those that are communicable, are ideal terrorism agents because each infected individual serves as a vector to spread the disease. Meteorological conditions may allow the widespread dissemination of infectious agents. The public is vulnerable because illness does not occur until the bacteria or virus has an opportunity to incubate and replicate in the human host. The initial presentation of the disease may be flulike and minimized by the ill person. Treatment may be sought only after the disease is fully manifest.

The anticipated biological terrorism diseases are not household maladies like influenza, chickenpox, and tonsillitis. The lack of familiarity with the diseases prompts many questions: Should smallpox vaccination be reinstituted? Is the plague a reality? What about tularemia and botulism? Are we vulnerable to the exotic viral hemorrhagic fevers?

These questions and more are answered in an accompanying series of papers that were published previously in the *Journal of the American Medical Association*. Every health-system pharmacist should acquaint him- or herself with the features of the diseases that may be a consequence of biological terrorist activities. Each agent is summarized in the following sections and presented in detail in the reprinted articles following this summary. In developing guidelines or policies and in directing patient care, it is important to be aware of the contemporary literature and standards of care and not to rely solely on this work to make those decisions.

Anthrax

Anthrax is a disease caused by the bacteria *Bacillus anthracis*. Concern about the use of *Bacillus anthracis* as a bioterrorism agent arose as the world learned of the potential use of anthrax by Iraq during the Gulf War and Iraq's links to terrorist activities. In 1998 scores of abortion clinics received hoax anthrax letters, and white supremacist Larry Wayne Harris allegedly threatened to release anthrax in Las Vegas, which further heightened the awareness of anthrax as a potential bioterrorism agent. The 22 cases in the fall of 2001 brought anthrax from the realm of possibility to that lethal reality when five individuals perished from inhalational anthrax.

Anthrax is a Gram-positive, spore-forming *Bacillus* bacteria. While the bacteria are highly infectious (but not contagious) and produce lethal toxins that are responsible for the pathology associated with anthrax, exposure to the spores usually initializes the disease process. The spores are stable for decades and, when introduced into the human body, germinate in the presence of nutrients found in blood and tissue. The resulting *Bacillus anthracis* bacteria proliferate and infect their host. The spores are very small (invisible without microscopic enhancement) and enter their host via the lungs (inhalational anthrax), a break in the skin (dermal, or cutaneous, anthrax) or via the gastrointestinal tract. From a bioterrorism perspective, inhalational and cutaneous anthrax are the most likely forms of the disease that will be encountered, as confirmed by the 2001 anthrax cases in the United States.

The small size of *Bacillus anthracis* spores and the ease of dispersing an aerosol of spores make them an ideal inhalational bioterrorism agent. After the spores are inhaled, they are absorbed from the respiratory tract and transported to regional lymph nodes by macrophages, spreading from node to node. After germination occurs, *Bacillus anthracis* bacteria release toxins that produce hemorrhagic necrosis within the nodes. Subsequently, the necrotic process extends into the mediastinum (cavity between the lungs). Additional dissemination occurs via the lymphatic system, which results in systemic disease.

The classical presentation of inhalational anthrax resembles flu. Symptom presentation and disease course may be related to the size of the exposure inoculum and the patient's vulnerability. Fever, malaise, and fatigue occur and confuse the early diagnosis of anthrax with a cold. This is followed by the precipitous onset of respiratory distress and septicemia. Approximately 50 percent of patients develop meningitis.

Cutaneous anthrax is characterized by the development of vesicles that evolve into a black scab, or eschar. Cutaneous anthrax, if untreated, may progress to the systemic disease described with inhalational anthrax. Gastrointestinal anthrax is unlikely to be related to a bioterrorism event, because it is usually contracted from eating the undercooked meat of infected animals.

The general treatment of anthrax involves antibiotic prophylaxis for exposed but asymptomatic individuals and aggressive antibiotic therapy and supportive care for symptomatic patients. Specific therapy will depend on the type of anthrax and patient severity. Early antibiotic administration prior to the development of symptoms is very successful. While the antibiotics are ineffective against the spores, *Bacillus anthracis* bacteria are sensitive to a large number of antibiotics. Ciprofloxacin and doxycycline are recommended most routinely because of their effectiveness and twice-a-day dosing, thereby enhancing compliance. The length of antibiotic therapy may be extended to 60 days to insure that the presence of circulating spores does not exceed the course of antibiotic therapy.

Selection of the appropriate antibiotic depends on the known antibiotic sensitivity of the *Bacillus anthracis* strain, the presence of an antibiotic allergy, age contraindications, pregnancy, antibiotic availability, and so forth. In general, ciprofloxacin and other fluoroquinolones are not advised in children less than 16–18 years old due to the link with arthropathy. Doxycycline is not recommended in children less than 9 years of age, because it may cause retarded skeletal growth and dental enamel staining. If the risk of infection is high and ciprofloxacin and doxycycline are the only available choices, doxycycline is recommended over ciprofloxacin in children. Ciprofloxacin is the preferred antibiotic during pregnancy, with doxycycline as the alternative agent.

Anthrax vaccine is not available universally, but it may be appropriate for prolonged protection, especially following exposure to large numbers of spores, and is available from the Centers for Disease Control.

The pharmacy stock of antibiotics should be adequate to treat the anticipated inpatient and outpatient volume, as well as the staff and their family members in the immediate time period following the decision to provide prophylaxis. The National Pharmaceutical Stockpile (NPS) should be available within approximately 24 hours to provide sustained dosing for outpatients.

Summarized in part from Inglesby TV, O'Toole T, Henderson DA, et al. Anthrax as a biological weapon, 2002: Updated recommendations for management. JAMA 2002;287:2236-2252.

Smallpox

Unlike anthrax, which is a bacterial disease, smallpox is caused by an Orthopoxvirus, variola. Like anthrax, smallpox is a highly infectious and devastating disease. In contrast to anthrax, it is also highly contagious, which makes smallpox a feared bioterrorism weapon. Other features that make smallpox an attractive bioterrorism agent are its stability, ability to be aerosolized, and the vulnerability of the world's population since smallpox was eradicated in 1977 and, with a few exceptions, worldwide general vaccination programs ceased in about 1980.

Allegedly, only two reference laboratories in the world maintain virus stocks—the Institute of Virus Preparations in Moscow and the Centers for Disease Control and Prevention in Atlanta, Georgia. If these two laboratories are secure and are the sole repositories of variola virus, the risk of smallpox bioterrorism is low. However, there are significant concerns that Russia may have continued research into the warfare applications of smallpox and that dissident and disgruntled scientists may market their expertise to rogue nations. For this reason, the U.S. Department of Health and Human Services has embarked on an ambitious program to produce sufficient smallpox vaccine for all U.S. residents by the end of 2002. Questions remain about the dormant immunity of individuals who

were vaccinated prior to 1972, when routine U.S. smallpox vaccination ceased. Current plans (Centers for Disease Control, September 16, 2002) in case an outbreak of smallpox is confirmed in the United States call for rapid voluntary vaccination of the affected or potentially affected populations. By the conclusion of 2002, there will be sufficient smallpox vaccine to vaccinate the entire population of the United States, and it is estimated that 280 million doses will be distributed to predesignated clinics within five to seven days.

Most U.S. health care providers have never diagnosed or observed a patient with smallpox. There is validated concern that an index case of smallpox might be misdiagnosed. A full-blown case of smallpox has a classical presentation that should raise suspicion in even the most naïve of health care providers. The early stages of smallpox will challenge even the most astute clinicians, however, since the symptoms are vague constitutional manifestations, such as malaise, fever, vomiting, headache, and backache. These symptoms occur at the end of the incubation period, which is approximately 12 days but may vary from 7 to 17 days. Within 1 to 3 days after the initial symptoms occur, a maculopapular rash appears on the oral mucosa, face, hands, and forearms. The rash spreads in dramatic fashion and becomes vesicular and then pustular. Scabbing begins after approximately one week and persists for about two weeks, leaving the patient with deep scars. The fatality rate approximates 30 percent in unvaccinated individuals, and some malignant forms of smallpox have even higher fatality rates.

Smallpox is spread through droplets that are expelled by infected individuals or through direct contact. Virus titers in the oral cavity and thus the saliva may be very high before the disease is overtly obvious—making the smallpox highly contagious. An infected individual, such as a terrorist, could walk freely throughout public venues, spreading the disease prior to developing the fulminant stigmata of smallpox.

Quarantine, vaccination, and supportive care form the cornerstone of treating smallpox patients. Vaccination within four days of exposure has been demonstrated to confer some protection against the development of the actual disease and to reduce the associated morbidity and mortality. While the risks associated with vaccination are low as compared to the sequelae associated with smallpox, vaccination is not without the risk of serious complications. Groups at special risk, such as patients with eczema, malignancy, HIV, immune disorders, and pregnancy, present special challenges. Even patients with these conditions should be vaccinated if they have been exposed to the smallpox virus. Those who have not been exposed to smallpox should consider not being vaccinated until they have discussed their condition with a physician. Pharmacists with clinical responsibilities should take special precautions to minimize or avoid exposure.

Summarized in part from Henderson DA, Inglesby TV, Bartlett JG, et al. Smallpox as a biological weapon: Medical and public health management. JAMA 1999;281:2127-2137.

Plague

The pestilence of plague is well-known. The black, or bubonic, plague was responsible for the death of an estimated 25 million individuals during the Middle Ages in Europe. The horrors of the plague have been embellished in fairy tales, and outbreaks continue to occur. The English lexicon uses the word *plague* to suggest dire consequences (e.g., "This decision will continue to *plague* us"). The use of plague as a warfare agent has a sordid history, and contemporary militaries have identified means of weaponizing the bacteria responsible for plague and to aerosolize it to maximize its devastating effects.

Plague is a contagious disease that is caused by the bacteria *Yersinia pestis,* which is a Gram-negative nonsporulating bacillus. Two primary types of plague occur: bubonic and pneumonic. Bubonic plague is the naturally occurring variety that utilizes the common flea as the vector. As the fleas harboring *Yersinia pestis* bite a human they inoculate the victim with *Yersinia pestis* bacteria, which migrate to lymph nodes, proliferate, and cause necrosis of the nodes, which leads to systemic dissemination of the bacteria and profound illness. Within two to seven days of being bitten, the human host becomes symptomatic with fever, chills, weakness, and swelling of affected lymph nodes. The swollen nodes are referred to as "bubos." Patients can develop secondary septicemia or even pneumonic plague.

Pneumonic plague is the variant of the plague most likely to follow its use as a bioterrorism agent. Like anthrax and smallpox, *Yersinia pestis* can be aerosolized easily and inhaled by unsuspecting victims and thus produce devastating disease. Following the inhalation of the bacteria, symptoms most often appear within two to four days, and like anthrax, the onset is probably dose-dependent— the higher the inoculum, the more rapid the onset of clinical disease. The early presentation includes fever, cough, and dyspnea. Gastrointestinal symptoms are common. If the patient is untreated, the profound respiratory insult may produce death within two to four days. In contrast to

anthrax, in which pneumonia is not a feature of the respiratory compromise, pneumonic plague does commonly manifest in pneumonia.

Currently a plague vaccine is not available commercially, and aggressive supportive care and early intervention with antibiotics are critical to a favorable outcome. Patients with pneumonic plague should be treated, preferably with parenteral streptomycin or gentamicin. Alternative choices include parenteral doxycycline, ciprofloxacin, and chloramphenicol. The preferred choices for postexposure prophylaxis are doxycycline and ciprofloxacin, which are included in the NPS. In selecting the most appropriate antibiotic, consideration should be given to the age of the patient and whether the patient is pregnant or immunosuppressed. It is customary to administer seven days of postexposure antibiotic prophylaxis. Plague is highly contagious, and pharmacists with clinical responsibilities should take appropriate precautions.

Summarized in part from Inglesby TV, Dennis DT, Henderson DA, et al. Plague as a biological weapon: Medical and public health management. JAMA 2000;283:2281-2290.

Tularemia

Despite the fact that tularemia is endemic to the United States, neither health care professionals nor the general public are familiar generally with the disease. Yet, due to the extensive military research and weaponization of *Francisella tularensis,* which is the causative bacteria of tularemia, it is one of the principle bioterrorism diseases that merit preparedness.

Francisella tularensis is an aerobic, nonmotile, Gram-negative coccobacillus that produces tularemia, an infectious but not contagious disease. From a bioterrorism perspective, aerosolized *Francisella tularensis* can produce inhalational or pneumonic tularemia. However, inhalational tularemia can also occur naturally, especially in rural settings, when contaminated animal carcasses are moved or when rodent-infested hay is disturbed. Therefore, the diagnosis of tularemia in an urban population should create a high index of suspicion that it may be secondary to bioterrorism.

Francisella tularensis aerosolization and dispersion in a densely populated urban setting would result in the presentation of patients within 1 to 14 days, but primarily in the first 3 to 5 days after exposure. The abrupt onset of fever, headache, chills, weakness, and upper-respiratory symptoms that progress to pneumonia would be a classical presentation for tularemia. However, the vagueness of the presentation and its similarity to influenza poses a diagnostic challenge unless bioterrorism is suspected. Both plague and anthrax progress in a more fulminant fashion, and their presence can be confirmed serologically more rapidly than tularemia. The presentation may also be varied in that some forms of the disease produce significant lymphadenopathy or oropharyngeal symptoms. The diagnosis is challenging.

A commercially available vaccine is not available in the United States, and as with anthrax and plague, the treatment of tularemia centers on early intervention with the appropriate antimicrobial. The approach to antibiotic therapy is similar to the treatment of plague. Aminoglycosides are preferred in patients with active tularemia. Postexposure oral prophylaxis with doxycycline or ciprofloxacin for 14 days (tularemia has a longer incubation period) is recommended. In selecting the most appropriate antibiotic, consideration should be given to the age of the patient and whether the patient is pregnant or immunosuppressed.

Summarized in part from Dennis DT, Inglesby TV, Henderson DA, et al. Tularemia as a biological weapon: Medical and public health management. JAMA 2001;285:2763-2773.

Botulism

Anthrax, plague, smallpox, and tularemia are bioterrorism diseases that require bacteria or a virus to produce a pathological condition. Under natural circumstances, botulism is a disease that is caused by the bacterium *Clostridium botulinum*. However, in the bioterrorism arena botulism would be caused by exposure to the actual botulinum toxin that was cultivated and prepared as a bioterrorism agent rather than by aerosolization and inhalation of *Clostridium botulinum*.

Clostridium botulinum is ubiquitous and found in the soil throughout the world, making it easily accessible to terrorists. Most people are familiar with botulism as a potentially fatal type of food poisoning. Most recently botulinum toxin has received Food and Drug Administration approval for the cosmetic treatment of facial wrinkles and is known commercially as "botox." There are a number of other medical applications for the use of botulinum toxin. Botulinum toxin's appeal as a biological terrorism weapon rests with the fact that it is the most toxic substance known to humanity. It is estimated that one gram has the potential to kill at least one million individuals.

Clinical botulism occurs because the toxin binds at peripheral nerve cholinergic synapses and prevents the release of acetylcholine, which is responsible for muscle contraction. Consequently, flaccid muscle paralysis occurs. The classical presentation is a descending bilateral paralysis that affects vision (e.g., diplopia, ptosis, blurred vision), facial muscle control, dysphagia, respiratory failure, and the like. As with any toxin, the severity of the pathophysiology will depend on the amount of toxin that is delivered to the patient.

The time to onset of symptoms will range from 10 to 72 hours. It is much less likely that large quantities of botulinum toxin would be aerosolized than that terrorists would attempt to poison a food source and inflict a limited number of casualties. Botulism is not infectious or contagious, and person-to-person transmission cannot occur.

The diagnosis of botulism may challenge the unsuspecting clinician, who may confuse it with Gillain-Barré syndrome, myasthenia gravis, stroke, or another neurologic disorder. However, botulism produces a bilateral descending paralysis that should help to differentiate it from other neurological disorders.

Because botulism is caused by an exogenous toxin, not a bacterial infection, antimicrobial therapy is not indicated. The management of botulism is intensive and requires aggressive supportive care and the use of mechanical ventilators, which could overwhelm the capabilities of a hospital if there are a large number of victims. Patients may require lengthy hospitalization, which would further tax a hospital's resources. The early use of equine antitoxin can neutralize botulinum toxin types A, B, and E, but it does not reverse preexisting paralysis. The Centers for Disease Control (CDC) is the sole source of botulism antitoxin, and the acquisition delay further complicates the effective treatment of botulism.

Summarized in part from Arnon SS, Schechter R, Inglesby TV, et al. Botulinum toxin as a biological weapon: Medical and public health management. JAMA 2001;285:1059-1070.

Hemorrhagic Fever Viruses

The Ebola and Marburg viruses and Lassa, dengue, and Rift Valley fevers conjure images of exotic, incurable diseases from Africa and developing nations. In fact, the hemorrhagic fever viruses have been weaponized by Russia and the United States and possibly other nations. The viruses are feared because they are highly virulent and there are no effective countermeasures to treat the associated illnesses.

A number of viruses are responsible for the disease entities, which are often difficult to differentiate. The fact that
these diseases are not indigenous to the United States
would further complicate the diagnosis of a hemorrhagic
fever virus. The clinical presentation may be consistent
with an influenza-like malady. The diseases require an
incubation period of 2 to 21 days, and patients late in the
course of their disease may experience hemorrhagic
problems. The fatality index may be as high as 90 percent
with Ebola but much lower with other varieties.

The suspicion or confirmation of hemorrhagic fever virus
in the United States would strongly suggest a bioterrorism motivation. An isolated case in a patient who has
traveled recently from endemic areas reduces the likelihood of bioterrorism but still mandates an extensive epidemiological and law enforcement investigation.

Supportive care is the foundation of therapeutic intervention since vaccines and specific pharmacological antagonists
are unavailable. Ribavirin antiviral therapy provides some
effectiveness against a limited number of the hemorrhagic
fever viruses. Pharmacists who practice in patient care
areas must be fastidious about using personal protective
equipment when providing pharmaceutical care to a
patient with a suspected or confirmed hemorrhagic fever
virus.

*Summarized in part from Borio L, Inglesby T, Peters CJ,
et al. Hemorrhagic fever viruses as biological weapons:
Medical and public health management. JAMA
2002;287:2391-2405.*

READINGS

Anthrax as a Biological Weapon, 2002
Updated Recommendations for Management

Thomas V. Inglesby, MD

Tara O'Toole, MD, MPH

Donald A. Henderson, MD, MPH

John G. Bartlett, MD

Michael S. Ascher, MD

Edward Eitzen, MD, MPH

Arthur M. Friedlander, MD

Julie Gerberding, MD, MPH

Jerome Hauer, MPH

James Hughes, MD

Joseph McDade, PhD

Michael T. Osterholm, PhD, MPH

Gerald Parker, PhD, DVM

Trish M. Perl, MD, MSc

Philip K. Russell, MD

Kevin Tonat, DrPH, MPH

for the Working Group on Civilian Biodefense

Objective To review and update consensus-based recommendations for medical and public health professionals following a *Bacillus anthracis* attack against a civilian population.

Participants The working group included 23 experts from academic medical centers, research organizations, and governmental, military, public health, and emergency management institutions and agencies.

Evidence MEDLINE databases were searched from January 1966 to January 2002, using the Medical Subject Headings *anthrax*, *Bacillus anthracis*, *biological weapon*, *biological terrorism*, *biological warfare*, and *biowarfare*. Reference review identified work published before 1966. Participants identified unpublished sources.

Consensus Process The first draft synthesized the gathered information. Written comments were incorporated into subsequent drafts. The final statement incorporated all relevant evidence from the search along with consensus recommendations.

Conclusions Specific recommendations include diagnosis of anthrax infection, indications for vaccination, therapy, postexposure prophylaxis, decontamination of the environment, and suggested research. This revised consensus statement presents new information based on the analysis of the anthrax attacks of 2001, including developments in the investigation of the anthrax attacks of 2001; important symptoms, signs, and laboratory studies; new diagnostic clues that may help future recognition of this disease; current anthrax vaccine information; updated antibiotic therapeutic considerations; and judgments about environmental surveillance and decontamination.

JAMA. 2002;287:2236-2252   www.jama.com

O F THE BIOLOGICAL AGENTS that may be used as weapons, the Working Group on Civilian Biodefense identified a limited number of organisms that, in worst case scenarios, could cause disease and deaths in sufficient numbers to gravely impact a city or region. *Bacillus anthracis*, the bacterium that causes anthrax, is one of the most serious of these.

Several countries are believed to have offensive biological weapons programs, and some independent terrorist groups have suggested their intent to use biological weapons. Because the possibility of a terrorist attack using bioweapons is especially difficult to predict, detect, or prevent, it is among the most feared terrorism scenarios.[1] In September 2001, *B anthracis* spores were sent to several locations via the US Postal Service. Twenty-two confirmed or suspect cases of anthrax infection resulted. Eleven of these were inhalational cases, of whom 5 died; 11 were cutaneous cases (7 confirmed, 4 suspected).[2] In this article, these attacks are termed *the anthrax attacks of 2001*. The consequences of these attacks substantiated many findings and recommendations in the Working Group on Civilian Biodefense's previous consensus statement published in 1999[3]; however, the new information from these attacks warrant updating the previous statement.

Before the anthrax attacks in 2001, modern experience with inhalational anthrax was limited to an epidemic in Sverdlovsk, Russia, in 1979 following an unintentional release of *B anthracis* spores from a Soviet bioweapons factory and to 18 occupational exposure cases in the United States during the 20th century. Information about the potential impact of a large, covert attack using *B anthracis* or the possible effi-

Author Affiliations: The Center for Civilian Biodefense Strategies (Drs Inglesby, O'Toole, Henderson, Bartlett, and Perl) and the Schools of Medicine (Drs Inglesby, Bartlett, and Perl) and Public Health (Drs O'Toole and Henderson), Johns Hopkins University, Department of Health and Human Services (Drs Ascher, and Russell and Mr Hauer), Baltimore, and US Army Medical Research Institute of Infectious Diseases, (Drs Eitzen, Friedlander, and Parker), Frederick, Md; Centers for Disease Control and Prevention, Atlanta, Ga (Drs Hughes, McDade, and Gerberding); Center for Infectious Disease Research and Policy, University of Minnesota School of Public Health, Minneapolis (Dr Osterholm); and the Office of Emergency Preparedness, Department of Health and Human Services, Rockville, Md (Dr Tonat).
Corresponding Author and Reprints: Thomas V. Inglesby, MD, Johns Hopkins Center for Civilian Biodefense Strategies, Johns Hopkins University, Candler Bldg, Suite 830, 111 Market Pl, Baltimore, MD 21202 (e-mail: tvi@jhsph.edu).

©2002 American Medical Association. All rights reserved.

Reprinted with permission from *JAMA*; May 1, 2002, Vol 287, No. 17

cacy of postattack vaccination or therapeutic measures remains limited. Policies and strategies continue to rely partially on interpretation and extrapolation from an incomplete and evolving knowledge base.

CONSENSUS METHODS

The working group comprised 23 representatives from academic medical centers; research organizations; and government, military, public health, and emergency management institutions and agencies. For the original consensus statement,[3] we searched MEDLINE databases from January 1966 to April 1998 using Medical Subject Headings of *anthrax*, *Bacillus anthracis*, *biological weapon*, *biological terrorism*, *biological warfare*, and *biowarfare*. Reference review identified work published before 1966. Working group members identified unpublished sources.

The first consensus statement, published in 1999,[3] followed a synthesis of the information and revision of 3 drafts. We reviewed anthrax literature again in January 2002, with special attention to articles following the anthrax attacks of 2001. Members commented on a revised document; proposed revisions were incorporated with the working group's support for the final consensus document.

The assessment and recommendations provided herein represent our best professional judgment based on current data and expertise. The conclusions and recommendations need to be regularly reassessed as new information develops.

HISTORY OF CURRENT THREAT

For centuries, *B anthracis* has caused disease in animals and serious illness in humans.[4] Research on anthrax as a biological weapon began more than 80 years ago.[5] Most national offensive bioweapons programs were terminated following widespread ratification or signing of the Biological Weapons Convention (BWC) in the early 1970s[6]; the US offensive bioweapons program was terminated after President Nixon's 1969 and 1970 executive

orders. However, some nations continued offensive bioweapons development programs despite ratification of the BWC. In 1995, Iraq acknowledged producing and weaponizing *B anthracis* to the United Nations Special Commission.[7] The former Soviet Union is also known to have had a large *B anthracis* production program as part of its offensive bioweapons program.[8] A recent analysis reports that there is clear evidence of or widespread assertions from nongovernmental sources alleging the existence of offensive biological weapons programs in at least 13 countries.[6]

The anthrax attacks of 2001 have heightened concern about the feasibility of large-scale aerosol bioweapons attacks by terrorist groups. It has been feared that independent, well-funded groups could obtain a manufactured weapons product or acquire the expertise and resources to produce the materials for an attack. However, some analysts have questioned whether "weapons grade" material such as that used in the 2001 attacks (ie, powders of *B anthracis* with characteristics such as high spore concentration, uniform particle size, low electrostatic charge, treated to reduce clumping) could be produced by those not supported by the resources of a nation-state. The US Department of Defense recently reported that 3 defense employees with some technical skills but without expert knowledge of bioweapons manufactured a simulant of *B anthracis* in less than a month for $1 million.[9] It is reported that Aum Shinrikyo, the cult responsible for the 1995 release of sarin nerve gas in a Tokyo subway station,[10] dispersed aerosols of anthrax and botulism throughout Tokyo at least 8 times.[11] Forensic analysis of the *B anthracis* strain used in these attacks revealed that this isolate most closely matched the Sterne 34F2 strain, which is used for animal vaccination programs and is not a significant risk to humans.[12] It is probable that the cult attacks produced no illnesses for this and other technical reasons. Al Quaeda also has sought to acquire bioweapons in its terrorist planning efforts although the ex-

tent to which they have been successful is not reported.[13]

In the anthrax attacks of 2001, *B anthracis* spores were sent in at least 5 letters to Florida, New York City, and Washington, DC. Twenty-two confirmed or suspected cases resulted. All of the identified letters were mailed from Trenton, NJ. The *B anthracis* spores in all the letters were identified as the Ames strain. The specific source (provenance) of *B anthracis* cultures used to create the spore-containing powder remains unknown at time of this publication.

It is now recognized that the original Ames strain of *B anthracis* did not come from a laboratory in Ames, Iowa, rather from a laboratory in College Station, Tex. Several distinct Ames strains have been recognized by investigating scientists, which are being compared with the Ames strain used in the attack. At least 1 of these comparison Ames strains was recovered from a goat that died in Texas in 1997.[14]

Sen Daschle's letter reportedly had 2 g of *B anthracis* containing powder; the quantity in the other envelopes has not been disclosed. The powder has been reported to contain between 100 billion to 1 trillion spores per gram[15] although no official analysis of the concentration of spores or the chemical composition of the powder has been published.

The anthrax attacks of 2001 used 1 of many possible methods of attack. The use of aerosol-delivery technologies inside buildings or over large outdoor areas is another method of attack that has been studied. In 1970, the World Health Organization[16] and in 1993 the Office of Technology Assessment[17] analyzed the potential scope of larger attacks. The 1979 Sverdlovsk accident provides data on the only known aerosol release of *B anthracis* spores resulting in an epidemic.[18]

An aerosol release of *B anthracis* would be odorless and invisible and would have the potential to travel many kilometers before dissipating.[16,19] Aerosol technologies for large-scale dissemination have been developed and tested

©2002 American Medical Association. All rights reserved.

Reprinted with permission from *JAMA*; May 1, 2002, Vol 287, No. 17

Figure 1. Gram Stain of Blood in Culture Media

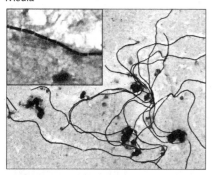

Gram-positive bacilli in long chains (original magnification ×20). Enlargement shows typical "jointed bamboo-rod" appearance of *Bacillus anthracis* (original magnification ×100). Reprinted from Borio et al.[36]

by Iraq[7] and the former Soviet Union[8] Few details of those tests are available. The US military also conducted such trials over the Pacific Ocean in the 1960s. A US study near Johnston Atoll in the South Pacific reported a plane "sprayed a 32-mile long line of agent that traveled for more then 60 miles before it lost its infectiousness."[20]

In 1970, the World Health Organization estimated that 50 kg of *B anthracis* released over an urban population of 5 million would sicken 250 000 and kill 100 000.[16] A US Congressional Office of Technology assessment analysis from 1993 estimated that between 130 000 and 3 million deaths would follow the release of 100 kg of *B anthracis*, a lethality matching that of a hydrogen bomb.[17]

EPIDEMIOLOGY OF ANTHRAX

Naturally occurring anthrax in humans is a disease acquired from contact with anthrax-infected animals or anthrax-contaminated animal products. The disease most commonly occurs in herbivores, which are infected after ingesting spores from the soil. Large anthrax epizootics in herbivores have been reported.[21] A published report states that anthrax killed 1 million sheep in Iran in 1945[22]; this number is supported by an unpublished Iranian governmental document.[23] Animal vaccination programs

have reduced drastically the animal mortality from the disease.[24] However, *B anthracis* spores remain prevalent in soil samples throughout the world and cause anthrax cases among herbivores annually.[22,25,26]

Anthrax infection occurs in humans by 3 major routes: inhalational, cutaneous, and gastrointestinal. Naturally occurring inhalational anthrax is now rare. Eighteen cases of inhalational anthrax were reported in the United States from 1900 to 1976; none were identified or reported thereafter. Most of these cases occurred in special-risk groups, including goat hair mill or wool or tannery workers; 2 of them were laboratory associated.[27]

Cutaneous anthrax is the most common naturally occurring form, with an estimated 2000 cases reported annually worldwide.[26] The disease typically follows exposure to anthrax-infected animals. In the United States, 224 cases of cutaneous anthrax were reported between 1944 and 1994.[28] One case was reported in 2000.[29] The largest reported epidemic occurred in Zimbabwe between 1979 and 1985, when more than 10 000 human cases of anthrax were reported, nearly all of them cutaneous.[30]

Although gastrointestinal anthrax is uncommon, outbreaks are continually reported in Africa and Asia[26,31,32] following ingestion of insufficiently cooked contaminated meat. Two distinct syndromes are oral-pharyngeal and abdominal.[31,33,34] Little information is available about the risks of direct contamination of food or water with *B anthracis* spores. Experimental efforts to infect primates by direct gastrointestinal instillation of *B anthracis* spores have not been successful.[35] Gastrointestinal infection could occur only after consumption of large numbers of vegetative cells, such as what might be found in raw or undercooked meat from an infected herbivore, but experimental data is lacking.

Inhalational anthrax is expected to account for most serious morbidity and most mortality following the use of *B anthracis* as an aerosolized biological weapon. Given the absence of natu-

rally occurring cases of inhalational anthrax in the United States since 1976, the occurrence of a single case is now cause for alarm.

MICROBIOLOGY

B anthracis derives from the Greek word for coal, *anthrakis*, because of the black skin lesions it causes. *B anthracis* is an aerobic, gram-positive, spore-forming, nonmotile *Bacillus* species. The nonflagellated vegetative cell is large (1-8 μm long, 1-1.5 μm wide). Spore size is approximately 1 μm. Spores grow readily on all ordinary laboratory media at 37°C, with a "jointed bamboo-rod" cellular appearance (**FIGURE 1**) and a unique "curled-hair" colonial appearance. Experienced microbiologists should be able to identify this cellular and colonial morphology; however, few practicing microbiologists outside the veterinary community have seen *B anthracis* colonies beyond what they may have seen in published material.[37] *B anthracis* spores germinate when they enter an environment rich in amino acids, nucleosides, and glucose, such as that found in the blood or tissues of an animal or human host. The rapidly multiplying vegetative *B anthracis* bacilli, on the contrary, will only form spores after local nutrients are exhausted, such as when anthrax-infected body fluids are exposed to ambient air.[22] Vegetative bacteria have poor survival outside of an animal or human host; colony counts decline to being undetectable within 24 hours following inoculation into water.[22] This contrasts with the environmentally hardy properties of the *B anthracis* spore, which can survive for decades in ambient conditions.[37]

PATHOGENESIS AND CLINICAL MANIFESTATIONS
Inhalational Anthrax

Inhalational anthrax follows deposition into alveolar spaces of spore-bearing particles in the 1- to 5-μm range.[38,39] Macrophages then ingest the spores, some of which are lysed and destroyed. Surviving spores are transported via lymphatics to mediastinal lymph nodes, where germination oc-

©2002 American Medical Association. All rights reserved.

Reprinted with permission from *JAMA*; May 1, 2002, Vol 287, No. 17

curs after a period of spore dormancy of variable and possibly extended duration.[35,40,41] The trigger(s) responsible for the transformation of *B anthracis* spores to vegetative cells is not fully understood.[42] In Sverdlovsk, cases occurred from 2 to 43 days after exposure.[18] In experimental infection of monkeys, fatal disease occurred up to 58 days[40] and 98 days[43] after exposure. Viable spores were demonstrated in the mediastinal lymph nodes of 1 monkey 100 days after exposure.[44]

Once germination occurs, clinical symptoms follow rapidly. Replicating *B anthracis* bacilli release toxins that lead to hemorrhage, edema, and necrosis.[32,45] In experimental animals, once toxin production has reached a critical threshold, death occurs even if sterility of the bloodstream is achieved with antibiotics.[27] Extrapolations from animal data suggest that the human LD_{50} (ie, dose sufficient to kill 50% of persons exposed to it) is 2500 to 55000 inhaled *B anthracis* spores.[46] The LD_{10} was as low as 100 spores in 1 series of monkeys.[43] Recently published extrapolations from primate data suggest that as few as 1 to 3 spores may be sufficient to cause infection.[47] The dose of spores that caused infection in any of the 11 patients with inhalational anthrax in 2001 could not be estimated although the 2 cases of fatal inhalational anthrax in New York City and Connecticut provoked speculation that the fatal dose, at least in some individuals, may be quite low.

A number of factors contribute to the pathogenesis of *B anthracis*, which makes 3 toxins— *protective antigen, lethal factor,* and *edema factor*—that combine to form 2 toxins: lethal toxin and edema toxin (**FIGURE 2**). The protective antigen allows the binding of lethal and edema factors to the affected cell membrane and facilitates their subsequent transport across the cell membrane. Edema toxin impairs neutrophil function in vivo and affects water homeostasis leading to edema, and lethal toxin causes release of tumor necrosis factor α and interleukin 1 β, factors that are believed to be linked to the

sudden death in severe anthrax infection.[48] The molecular target of lethal and edema factors within the affected cell is not yet elucidated.[49] In addition to these virulence factors, *B anthracis* has a capsule that prevents phagocytosis. Full virulence requires the presence of both an antiphagocytic capsule and the

Figure 2. Pathogenesis of *Bacillus anthracis*

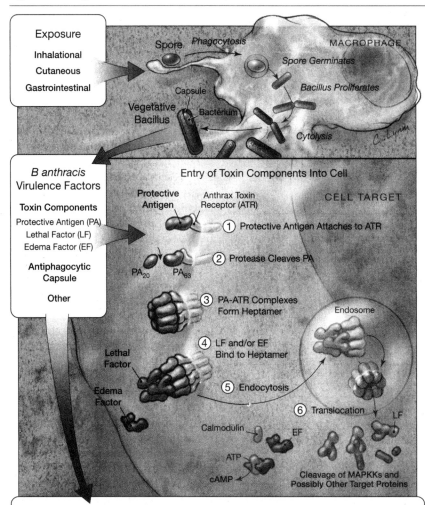

The major known virulence factors of *B anthracis* include the exotoxins edema toxin (PA and EF) and lethal toxin (PA and LF) and the antiphagocytic capsule. Although many exact molecular mechanisms involved in the pathogenicity of the anthrax toxins are uncertain, they appear to inhibit immune function, interrupt intracellular signaling pathways, and lyse cell targets causing massive release of proinflammatory mediators. ATP indicates adenosine triphosphate; cAMP, cyclic adenosine monophosphate; MAPKK, mitogen-activated protein kinase kinase; and MAPK, mitogen-activated protein kinase.

©2002 American Medical Association. All rights reserved.

Reprinted with permission from *JAMA*; May 1, 2002, Vol 287, No. 17

Table 1. Initial Symptoms, Physical Findings, and Test Results in Patients With Inhalational Anthrax Following US Anthrax Attacks in October and November 2001*

Symptoms (N = 10)	
Fever and chills	10
Sweats, often drenching	7
Fatigue, malaise, lethargy	10
Cough, minimal or nonproductive	9
Nausea or vomiting	9
Dyspnea	8
Chest discomfort or pleuritic pain	7
Myalgias	6
Headache	5
Confusion	4
Abdominal pain	3
Sore throat	2
Rhinorrhea	1

Physical Findings	
Fever >37.8°C	7
Tachycardia, heart rate >100/min	8
Hypotension, <110 mm Hg	1

Laboratory Results	
White blood cell count, median	9800 × 10³/μL
Differential neutrophilia, >70%	7
Neutrophil band forms, >5%	4†
Elevated transaminases, SGOT or SPGT >40 U/L‡	9
Hypoxemia, alveolar-arterial oxygen gradient >30 mm Hg on room air oxygen saturation <94%	6
Metabolic acidosis	2
Elevated creatinine, >1.5 mg/dL (132.6 μmol/L)	1

Chest X-ray Film Findings	
Any abnormality	10
Mediastinal widening	7
Infiltrates or consolidation	7
Pleural effusion	8

Chest Computed Tomographic Findings§	
Any abnormality	8
Mediastinal lymphadenopathy, widening	7
Pleural effusion	8
Infiltrates or consolidation	6

*This table was adapted with permission from Jernigan, et al.[61]
†Five persons had laboratory results measuring neutrophil band forms.
‡SGOT indicates serum glutamic oxalacetic transaminase; SGPT, serum glutamic pyruvic transaminase.
§Eight persons had computed tomographic scan results.

3 toxin components.[37] An additional factor contributing to *B anthracis* pathogenesis is the high concentration of bacteria occurring in affected hosts.[49]

Inhalational anthrax reflects the nature of acquisition of the disease. The term *anthrax pneumonia* is misleading because typical bronchopneumonia does not occur. Postmortem pathological studies of patients from Sverdlovsk showed that all patients had hemorrhagic thoracic lymphadenitis, hemorrhagic mediastinitis, and pleural effusions. About half had hemorrhagic meningitis. None of these autopsies showed evidence of a bronchoalveolar pneumonic process although 11 of 42 patient autopsies had evidence of a focal, hemorrhagic, necrotizing pneumonic lesion analogous to the Ghon complex associated with tuberculosis.[50] These findings are consistent with other human case series and experimentally induced inhalational anthrax in animals.[40,51,52] A recent reanalysis of pathology specimens from 41 of the Sverdlovsk patients was notable primarily for the presence of necrotizing hemorrhagic mediastinitis; pleural effusions averaging 1700 mL in quantity; meningitis in 50%; arteritis and arterial rupture in many; and the lack of prominent pneumonitis. *B anthracis* was recovered in concentrations of up to 100 million colony-forming units per milliliter in blood and spinal fluid.[53]

In animal models, physiological sequelae of severe anthrax infection have included hypocalcemia, profound hypoglycemia, hyperkalemia, depression and paralysis of respiratory center, hypotension, anoxia, respiratory alkalosis, and terminal acidosis,[54,55] suggesting that besides the rapid administration of antibiotics, survival might improve with vigilant correction of electrolyte disturbances and acid-based imbalance, glucose infusion, and early mechanical ventilation and vasopressor administration.

Historical Data. Early diagnosis of inhalational anthrax is difficult and requires a high index of suspicion. Prior to the 2001 attacks, clinical information was limited to a series of 18 cases reported in the 20th century and the limited data from Sverdlovsk. The clinical presentation of inhalational anthrax had been described as a 2-stage illness. Patients reportedly first developed a spectrum of nonspecific symptoms, including fever, dyspnea, cough, headache, vomiting, chills, weakness, abdominal pain, and chest pain.[18,27] Signs of illness and laboratory studies were nonspecific. This stage of illness lasted from hours to a few days. In some patients, a brief period of apparent recovery followed. Other patients progressed directly to the second, fulminant stage of illness.[4,27,56]

This second stage was reported to have developed abruptly, with sudden fever, dyspnea, diaphoresis, and shock. Massive lymphadenopathy and expansion of the mediastinum led to stridor in some cases.[57,58] A chest radiograph most often showed a widened mediastinum consistent with lymphadenopathy.[57] Up to half of patients developed hemorrhagic meningitis with concomitant meningismus, delirium, and obtundation. In this second stage, cyanosis and hypotension progressed rapidly; death sometimes occurred within hours.[4,27,56]

In the 20th-century series of US cases, the mortality rate of occupationally acquired inhalational anthrax was 89%, but the majority of these cases occurred before the development of critical care units and, in most cases, before the advent of antibiotics.[27] At Sverdlovsk, it had been reported that 68 of the 79 patients with inhalational anthrax died.[18] However a separate report from a hospital physician recorded 358 ill with 45 dead; another recorded 48 deaths among 110 patients.[59] A recent analysis of available Sverdlovsk data suggests there may have been as many as 250 cases with 100 deaths.[60] Sverdlovsk patients who had onset of disease 30 or more days after release of organisms had a higher reported survival rate than those with earlier disease onset. Antibiotics, antianthrax globulin, corticosteroids, mechanical ventilation, and vaccine were used to treat some residents in the affected area after the accident, but how many were given vaccine and antibiotics is unknown, nor is it known which patients received these interventions or when. It is also uncertain if the *B anthracis* strain (or strains) to which patients was exposed were susceptible to the antibiotics used during the outbreak. However, a community-wide intervention about the 15th day after exposure did appear to diminish the projected attack rate.[60] In fatal cases, the

©2002 American Medical Association. All rights reserved.

Reprinted with permission from *JAMA*; May 1, 2002, Vol 287, No. 17

interval between onset of symptoms and death averaged 3 days. This is similar to the disease course and case fatality rate in untreated experimental monkeys, which have developed rapidly fatal disease even after a latency as long as 58 days.[40]

2001 Attacks Data. The anthrax attacks of 2001 resulted in 11 cases of inhalational anthrax, 5 of whom died. Symptoms, signs, and important laboratory data from these patients are listed in TABLE 1. Several clinical findings from the first 10 patients with inhalational anthrax deserve emphasis.[36,61-66] Malaise and fever were presenting symptoms in all 10 cases. Cough, nausea, and vomiting were also prominent. Drenching sweats, dyspnea, chest pain, and headache were also seen in a majority of patients. Fever and tachycardia were seen in the majority of patients at presentation, as were hypoxemia and elevations in transaminases.

Importantly, all 10 patients had abnormal chest x-ray film results: 7 had mediastinal widening; 7 had infiltrates; and 8 had pleural effusions. Chest computed tomographic (CT) scans showed abnormal results in all 8 patients who had this test: 7 had mediastinal widening; 6, infiltrates; 8, pleural effusions.

Data are insufficient to identify factors associated with survival although early recognition and initiation of treatment and use of more than 1 antibiotic have been suggested as possible factors.[61] For the 6 patients for whom such information is known, the median period from presumed time of exposure to the onset of symptoms was 4 days (range, 4-6 days). Patients sought care a median of 3.5 days after symptom onset. All 4 patients exhibiting signs of fulminant illness prior to antibiotic administration died.[61] Of note, the incubation period of the 2 fatal cases from New York City and Connecticut is not known.

Cutaneous Anthrax

Historically, cutaneous anthrax has been known to occur following the deposition of the organism into skin;

previous cuts or abrasions made one especially susceptible to infection.[30,67] Areas of exposed skin, such as arms, hands, face, and neck, were the most frequently affected. In Sverdlovsk, cutaneous cases occurred only as late as 12 days after the original aerosol release; no reports of cutaneous cases appeared after prolonged latency.[18]

After the spore germinates in skin tissues, toxin production results in local edema. An initially pruritic macule or papule enlarges into a round ulcer by the second day. Subsequently, 1- to 3-mm vesicles may appear that discharge clear or serosanguinous fluid containing numerous organisms on Gram stain. As shown in FIGURE 3, development of a painless, depressed, black eschar follows, often associated with extensive local edema. The anthrax eschar dries, loosens, and falls off in the next 1 to 2 weeks. Lymphangitis and painful lymphadenopathy can occur with associated systemic symptoms. Differential diagnosis of eschars includes tularemia, scrub typhus, rickettsial spotted fevers, rat bite fever, and ecthyma gangrenosum.[68] Noninfectious causes of eschars include arachnid bites[63] and vasculitides. Although antibiotic therapy does not appear to change the course of eschar formation and healing, it does decrease the likelihood of systemic disease. Without antibiotic therapy, the mortality rate has been reported to be as high as 20%; with appropriate antibiotic treatment, death due to cutaneous anthrax has been reported to be rare.[4]

Following the anthrax attacks of 2001, there have been 11 confirmed or probable cases of cutaneous anthrax. One case report of cutaneous anthrax resulting from these attacks has been published (Figure 3).[63] This child had no reported evidence of prior visible cuts, abrasions, or lesions at the site of the cutaneous lesion that developed. The mean incubation period for cutaneous anthrax cases diagnosed in 2001 was 5 days, with a range of 1 to 10 days, based on estimated dates of exposure to *B anthracis*–contaminated letters. Cutaneous lesions occurred on the forearm, neck, chest, and fingers.[69]

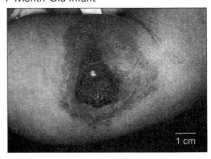

Figure 3. Lesion of Cutaneous Anthrax Associated With Microangiopathic Hemolytic Anemia and Coagulopathy in a 7-Month-Old Infant

By hospital day 12, a 2-cm black eschar was present in the center of the cutaneous lesion. Reprinted from Freedman et al.[63]

The only published case report of cutaneous anthrax from the attacks of 2001 is notable for the difficulty in recognition of the disease in a previously healthy 7-month-old, the rapid progression to severe systemic illness despite hospitalization, and clinical manifestations that included microangiopathic hemolytic anemia with renal involvement, coagulopathy, and hyponatremia.[63] Fortunately, this child recovered, and none of the cutaneous cases of anthrax diagnosed after the 2001 attacks were fatal.

Gastrointestinal Anthrax

Some think gastrointestinal anthrax occurs after deposition and germination of spores in the upper or lower gastrointestinal tract. However, considering the rapid transit time in the gastrointestinal tract, it seems more likely that many such cases must result from the ingestion of large numbers of vegetative bacilli from poorly cooked infected meat rather than from spores. In any event, the oral-pharyngeal form of disease results in an oral or esophageal ulcer and leads to the development of regional lymphadenopathy, edema, and sepsis.[31,33] Disease in the lower gastrointestinal tract manifests as primary intestinal lesions occurring predominantly in the terminal ileum or cecum,[50] presenting initially with nausea, vomiting, and malaise and progressing rapidly to bloody diarrhea, acute abdomen, or sep-

©2002 American Medical Association. All rights reserved.

Reprinted with permission from *JAMA*; May 1, 2002, Vol 287, No. 17

Table 2. Diagnosis of Inhalational Anthrax Infection*

Category	Findings
Epidemiology	Sudden appearance of several cases of severe acute febrile illness with fulminant course and death or Acute febrile illness in persons identified as being at risk following a specific attack (eg, those in the 2001attacks: postal workers, members of the news media, and politicians and their staff)
Diagnostic tests	Chest radiograph: widened mediastinum, infiltrates, pleural effusion Chest computed tomographic scan: hyperdense hilar and mediastinal nodes, mediastinal edema, infiltrates, pleural effusion Thoracentesis: hemorrhagic pleural effusions
Microbiology	Peripheral blood smear: gram-positive bacilli on blood smear Blood culture growth of large gram-positive bacilli with preliminary identification of *Bacillus* species†
Pathology	Hemorrhagic mediastinitis, hemorrhagic thoracic lymphadenitis, hemorrhagic meningitis; DFA stain of infected tissues

*See Table 1 for list of febrile illness symptoms and signs.
†Most rapid assays are available only at laboratories participating in the Laboratory Response Network.

Figure 4. Chest Radiograph and Computed Tomography (CT) Image

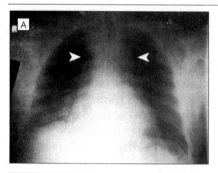 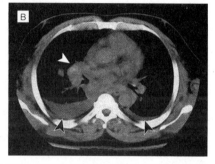

A, Portable chest radiograph of 56-year-old man with inhalational anthrax depicts a widened mediastinum (white arrowheads), bilateral hilar fullness, a right pleural effusion, and bilateral perihilar air-space disease. B, Noncontrast spiral CT scan depicts an enlarged and hyperdense right hilar lymph node (white arrowhead), bilateral pleural effusions (black arrowheads), and edema of the mediastinal fat. Reprinted from Mayer et al.[66]

sis. Massive ascites has occurred in some cases of gastrointestinal anthrax.[34] Advanced infection may appear similar to the sepsis syndrome occurring in either inhalational or cutaneous anthrax.[4] Some authors suggest that aggressive medical intervention as would be recommended for inhalational anthrax may reduce mortality. Given the difficulty of early diagnosis of gastrointestinal anthrax, however, mortality may be high.[4] Postmortem examinations in Sverdlovsk showed gastrointestinal submucosal lesions in 39 of 42 patients,[50] but all of these patients were also found to have definitive pathologic evidence of an inhalational source of infection. There were no gastrointestinal cases of anthrax diagnosed in either the Sverdlovsk series or following the anthrax attacks of 2001.

DIAGNOSIS

TABLE 2 lists the epidemiology, diagnostic tests, microbiology, and pathology for a diagnosis of inhalational anthrax infection. Given the rarity of anthrax infection, the first clinical or laboratory suspicion of an anthrax illness must lead to early initiation of antibiotic treatment pending confirmed diagnosis and should provoke immediate notification of the local or state public health department, local hospital epidemiologist, and local or state public health laboratory. In the United States, a Laboratory Response Network (LRN) has been established through a collaboration of the Association of Public Health Laboratories and the CDC (details are available at: http://www.bt.cdc.gov/LabIssues/index .asp). Currently 81 clinical laborato-

ries in the LRN can diagnose bioweapons pathogens. Several preliminary diagnostic tests for *B anthracis* can be performed in hospital laboratories using routine procedures. *B anthracis* is a gram-positive, nonhemolytic, encapsulated, penicillin-sensitive, spore-forming bacillus. Confirmatory tests such as immuno-histochemical staining, gamma phage, and polymerase chain reaction assays must still be performed by special reference laboratories in the LRN.

The determination of individual patient exposure to *B anthracis* on the basis of environmental testing is complex due to the uncertain specificity and sensitivity of rapid field tests and the difficulty of assessing individual risks of exposure. A patient (or patients) seeking medical treatment for symptoms of inhalational anthrax will likely be the first evidence of a clandestine release of *B anthracis* as a biological weapon. The appearance of even a single previously healthy patient who becomes acutely ill with nonspecific febrile illness and symptoms and signs consistent with those listed in Table 1 and whose condition rapidly deteriorates should receive prompt consideration for a diagnosis of anthrax infection. The recognition of cutaneous cases of anthrax may also be the first evidence of an anthrax attack.[70]

The likely presence of abnormal findings on either chest x-ray film or chest CT scan is diagnostically important. Although anthrax does not cause a classic bronchopneumonia pathologically, it can cause widened mediastinum, massive pleural effusions, air bronchograms, necrotizing pneumonic lesions, and/or consolidation, as has been noted above.[36,55,56,61,64-66] The result can be hypoxemia and chest imaging abnormalities that may or may not be clinically distinguishable from pneumonia. In the anthrax attacks of 2001, each of the first 10 patients had abnormal chest x-ray film results and each of 8 patients for whom CT scans were obtained had abnormal results. These included widened mediastinum on chest radiograph and effusions on chest CT scan (FIGURE 4). Such findings in a previ-

©2002 American Medical Association. All rights reserved.

Reprinted with permission from *JAMA*; May 1, 2002, Vol 287, No. 17

ously healthy patient with evidence of overwhelming febrile illness or sepsis would be highly suggestive of advanced inhalational anthrax.

The bacterial burden may be so great in advanced inhalational anthrax infection that bacilli are visible on Gram stain of peripheral blood, as was seen following the 2001 attacks. The most useful microbiologic test is the standard blood culture, which should show growth in 6 to 24 hours. Each of the 8 patients who had blood cultures obtained prior to initiation of antibiotics had positive blood cultures.[61] However, blood cultures appear to be sterilized after even 1 or 2 doses of antibiotics, underscoring the importance of obtaining cultures prior to initiation of antibiotic therapy (J. Gerberding, oral communication, March 7, 2002). If the laboratory has been alerted to the possibility of anthrax, biochemical testing and review of colonial morphology could provide a preliminary diagnosis 12 to 24 hours after inoculation of the cultures. Definitive diagnosis could be promptly confirmed by an LRN laboratory. However, if the clinical laboratory has not been alerted to the possibility of anthrax, *B anthracis* may not be correctly identified. Routine procedures customarily identify a *Bacillus* species in a blood culture approximately 24 hours after growth, but some laboratories do not further identify *Bacillus* species unless specifically requested. This is because the isolation of *Bacillus* species most often represents growth of the common contaminant *Bacillus cereus*.[71] Given the possibility of future anthrax attacks, it is recommended that routine clinical laboratory procedures be modified, so *B anthracis* is specifically excluded after identification of a *Bacillus* species bacteremia unless there are compelling reasons not to do so. If it cannot be excluded then the isolate should be transferred to an LRN laboratory.

Sputum culture and Gram stain are unlikely to be diagnostic of inhalational anthrax, given the frequent lack of a pneumonic process.[37] Gram stain of sputum was reported positive in only 1 case

of inhalational anthrax in the 2001 series. If cutaneous anthrax is suspected, a Gram stain and culture of vesicular fluid should be obtained. If the Gram stain is negative or the patient is taking antibiotics already, punch biopsy should be performed, and specimens sent to a laboratory with the ability to perform immunohistochemical staining or polymerase chain reaction assays.[69,70] Blood cultures should be obtained and antibiotics should be initiated pending confirmation of the diagnosis of inhalational or cutaneous anthrax.

Nasal swabs were obtained in some persons believed to be at risk of inhalational anthrax following the anthrax attacks of 2001. Although a study has shown the presence of *B anthracis* spores in nares of some monkeys following experimental exposure to *B anthracis* spores for some time after exposure,[72] the predictive value of the nasal swab test for diagnosing inhalational anthrax in humans is unknown and untested. It is not known how quickly antibiotics make spore recovery on nasal swab tests impossible. One patient who died from inhalational anthrax had a negative nasal swab.[36] Thus, the CDC advised in the fall of 2001 that the nasal swab should not be used as a clinical diagnostic test. If obtained for an epidemiological purpose, nasal swab results should not be used to rule out infection in a patient. Persons who have positive nasal swab results for *B anthracis* should receive a course of postexposure antibiotic prophylaxis since a positive swab would indicate that the individual had been exposed to aerosolized *B anthracis*.

Antibodies to the protective antigen (PA) of *B anthracis*, termed *anti-PA IgG*, have been shown to confer immunity in animal models following anthrax vaccination.[73,74] Anti-PA IgG serologies have been obtained from several of those involved in the 2001 anthrax attacks, but the results of these assays are not yet published. Given the lack of data in humans and the expected period required to develop an anti-PA IgG response, this test should not be used as a diagnostic test for anthrax infection in the acutely

ill patient but may be useful for epidemiologic purposes.

Postmortem findings are especially important following an unexplained death. Thoracic hemorrhagic necrotizing lymphadenitis and hemorrhagic necrotizing mediastinitis in a previously healthy adult are essentially pathognomonic of inhalational anthrax.[50,58] Hemorrhagic meningitis should also raise strong suspicion of anthrax infection.[32,50,58,75] However, given the rarity of anthrax, a pathologist might not identify these findings as caused by anthrax unless previously alerted to this possibility.

If only a few patients present contemporaneously, the clinical similarity of early inhalational anthrax infection to other acute febrile respiratory infections may delay initial diagnosis although probably not for long. The severity of the illness and its rapid progression, coupled with unusual radiological findings, possible identification of *B anthracis* in blood or cerebrospinal fluid, and the unique pathologic findings should serve as an early alarm. The index case of inhalational anthrax in the 2001 attacks was identified because of an alert clinician who suspected the disease on the basis of large gram-positive bacilli in cerebrospinal fluid in a patient with a compatible clinical illness, and as a result of the subsequent analysis by laboratory staff who had recently undergone bioterrorism preparedness training.[65]

VACCINATION

The US anthrax vaccine, named anthrax vaccine adsorbed (AVA), is an inactivated cell-free product, licensed in 1970, and produced by Bioport Corp, Lansing, Mich. The vaccine is licensed to be given in a 6-dose series. In 1997, it was mandated that all US military active- and reserve-duty personnel receive it.[76] The vaccine is made from the cell-free filtrate of a nonencapsulated attenuated strain of *B anthracis*.[77] The principal antigen responsible for inducing immunity is the PA.[26,32] In the rabbit model, the quantity of antibody to PA has been corre-

©2002 American Medical Association. All rights reserved.

Reprinted with permission from *JAMA*; May 1, 2002, Vol 287, No. 17

lated with the level of protection against experimental anthrax infection.[78]

Preexposure vaccination with AVA has been shown to be efficacious against experimental challenge in a number of animal studies.[78-80] A similar vaccine was shown in a placebo-controlled human trial to be efficacious against cutaneous anthrax.[81] The efficacy of postexposure vaccination with AVA has been studied in monkeys.[40] Among 60 monkeys exposed to 8 LD_{50} of B anthracis spores at baseline, 9 of 10 control animals died, and 8 of 10 animals treated with vaccine alone died. None of 29 animals died while receiving doxycycline, ciprofloxacin, or penicillin for 30 days; 5 developed anthrax once treatment ceased. The remaining 24 all died when rechallenged. The 9 receiving doxycycline for 30 days plus vaccine at baseline and day 14 after exposure did not die from anthrax infection even after being rechallenged.[40]

The safety of the anthrax vaccine has been the subject of much study. A recent report reviewed the results of surveillance for adverse events in the Department of Defense program of 1998-2000.[82] At the time of that report, 425 976 service members had received 1 620 793 doses of AVA. There were higher rates of local reactions to the vaccine in women than men, but "no patterns of unexpected local or systemic adverse events" were identified.[82] A recent review of safety of AVA anthrax vaccination in employees of the United States Army Medical Research Institute of Infectious Diseases (USAMRIID) over the past 25 years reported that 1583 persons had received 10 722 doses of AVA.[83] One percent of these inoculations (101/10 722) were associated with 1 or more systemic events (defined as headache, malaise, myalgia, fever, nausea, vomiting, dizziness, chills, diarrhea, hives, anorexia, arthralgias, diaphoresis, blurred vision, generalized itching, or sore throat). The most frequently reported systemic adverse event was headache (0.4% of doses). Local or injection site reactions were reported in 3.6%. No long-term sequelae were reported in this series.

The Institute of Medicine (IOM) recently published a report on the safety and efficacy of AVA,[84] which concluded that AVA is effective against inhalational anthrax and concluded that if given with appropriate antibiotic therapy, it may help prevent the development of disease after exposure. The IOM committee also concluded that AVA was acceptably safe. Committee recommendations for new research include studies to describe the relationship between immunity and quantitative antibody levels; further studies to test the efficacy of AVA in combination with antibiotics in preventing inhalational anthrax infection; studies of alternative routes and schedules of administration of AVA; and continued monitoring of reported adverse events following vaccination. The committee did not evaluate the production process used by the manufacturer.

A recently published report[85] analyzed a cohort of 4092 women at 2 military bases from January 1999 to March 2000. The study compared pregnancy rates and adverse birth outcomes between groups of women who had been vaccinated with women who had not been vaccinated and the study found that anthrax vaccination with AVA had no effect on pregnancy or adverse birth outcomes.

A human live attenuated vaccine has been produced and used in countries of the former Soviet Union.[86] In the Western world, live attenuated vaccines have been considered unsuitable for use in humans because of safety concerns.[86]

Current vaccine supplies are limited, and the US production capacity remains modest. Bioport is the single US manufacturing facility for the licensed anthrax vaccine. Production has only recently resumed after a halt required the company to alter production methods so that it conformed to the US Food and Drug Administration (FDA) Good Manufacturing Practice standard. Bioport has a contract to produce 4.6 million doses of vaccine for the US Department of Defense that cannot be met until at least 2003 (D.

A. Henderson, oral communication, February 2002).

The use of AVA was not initiated immediately in persons believed to have been exposed to B anthracis during the 2001 anthrax attacks for a variety of reasons, including the unavailability of vaccine supplies. Subsequently, near the end of the 60-day period of antibiotic prophylaxis, persons deemed by investigating public health authorities to have been at high risk for exposure were offered postexposure AVA series (3 inoculations at 2-week intervals, given on days 1, 14, and 28) as an adjunct to prolonged postexposure antibiotic prophylaxis. This group of affected persons was also offered the alternatives of continuing a prolonged course of antibiotics or of receiving close medical follow-up without vaccination or additional antibiotics.[87] This vaccine is licensed for use in the preexposure setting, but because it had not been licensed for use in the postexposure context, it was given under investigational new drug procedures.

The working group continues to conclude that vaccination of exposed persons following a biological attack in conjunction with antibiotic administration for 60 days following exposure provide optimal protection to those exposed. However, until ample reserve stockpiles of vaccine are available, reliance must be placed on antibiotic administration. To date, there have been no reported cases of anthrax infection among those exposed in the 2001 anthrax attacks who took prophylactic antibiotics, even in those persons not complying with the complete 60-day course of therapy.

Preexposure vaccination of some persons deemed to be in high-risk groups should be considered when substantial supplies of vaccine become available. A fast-track program to develop recombinant anthrax vaccine is now under way. This may lead to more plentiful vaccine stocks as well as a product that requires fewer inoculations.[88] Studies to evaluate intramuscular vs subcutaneous routes of administration and less frequent dosing of AVA are also under way. (J. Hughes, oral communication, February 2002.)

©2002 American Medical Association. All rights reserved.

Reprinted with permission from *JAMA*; May 1, 2002, Vol 287, No. 17

THERAPY

Recommendations for antibiotic and vaccine use in the setting of an aerosolized *B anthracis* attack are conditioned by a very small series of cases in humans, a limited number of studies in experimental animals, and the possible necessity of treating large numbers of casualties. A number of possible therapeutic strategies have yet to be explored experimentally or to be submitted for approval to the FDA. For these reasons, the working group offers consensus recommendations based on the best available evidence. The recommendations do not necessarily represent uses currently approved by the FDA or an official position on the part of any of the federal agencies whose scientists participated in these discussions and will need to be revised as further relevant information becomes available.

Given the rapid course of symptomatic inhalational anthrax, early antibiotic administration is essential. A delay of antibiotic treatment for patients with anthrax infection may substantially lessen chances for survival.[89,90] Given the difficulty in achieving rapid microbiologic diagnosis of anthrax, all persons in high-risk groups who develop fever or evidence of systemic disease should start receiving therapy for possible anthrax infection as soon as possible while awaiting the results of laboratory studies.

There are no controlled clinical studies for the treatment of inhalational anthrax in humans. Thus, antibiotic regimens commonly recommended for empirical treatment of sepsis have not been studied. In fact, natural strains of *B anthracis* are resistant to many of the antibiotics used in empirical regimens for sepsis treatment, such as those regimens based on the extended-spectrum cephalosporins.[91,92] Most naturally occurring *B anthracis* strains are sensitive to penicillin, which historically has been the preferred anthrax therapy. Doxycycline is the preferred option among the tetracycline class because of its proven efficacy in monkey studies[56] and its ease of administration. Other members of this class of antibiotics are suitable alternatives. Although treatment of anthrax in-

fection with ciprofloxacin has not been studied in humans, animal models suggest excellent efficacy.[40,56,93] In vitro data suggest that other fluoroquinolone antibiotics would have equivalent efficacy although no animal data using a primate model of inhalational anthrax are available.[92] Penicillin, doxycycline, and ciprofloxacin are approved by the FDA for the treatment of inhalational anthrax infection,[56,89,90,94] and other antibiotics are under study. Other drugs that are usually active in vitro include clindamycin, rifampin, imipenem, aminoglycosides, chloramphenicol, vancomycin, cefazolin, tetracycline, linezolid, and the macrolides.

Reports have been published of a *B anthracis* strain that was engineered to resist the tetracycline and penicillin classes of antibiotics.[95] Balancing considerations of treatment efficacy with concerns regarding resistance, the working group in 1999 recommended that ciprofloxacin or other fluoroquinolone therapy be initiated in adults with presumed inhalational anthrax infection.[3] It was advised that antibiotic resistance to penicillin- and tetracycline-class antibiotics should be assumed following a terrorist attack until laboratory testing demonstrated otherwise. Once the antibiotic susceptibility of the *B anthracis* strain of the index case had been determined, the most widely available, efficacious, and least toxic antibiotic was recommended for patients requiring treatment and persons requiring postexposure prophylaxis. Since the 1999 consensus statement publication, a study[96] demonstrated the development of in vitro resistance of an isolate of the Sterne strain of *B anthracis* to ofloxacin (a fluoroquinolone closely related to ciprofloxacin) following subculturing and multiple cell passage.

Following the anthrax attacks of 2001, the CDC[97] offered guidelines advocating use of 2 or 3 antibiotics in combination in persons with inhalational anthrax based on susceptibility testing with epidemic strains. Limited early information following the attacks suggested that persons with inhalational anthrax treated

intravenously with 2 or more antibiotics active against *B anthracis* had a greater chance of survival.[61] Given the limited number of persons who developed inhalational anthrax, the paucity of comparative data, and other uncertainties, it remains unclear whether the use of 2 or more antibiotics confers a survival advantage, but combination therapy is a reasonable therapeutic approach in the face of life-threatening illness. Another factor supporting the initiation of combination antibiotic therapy for treatment of inhalational anthrax is the possibility that an engineered strain of *B anthracis* resistant to 1 or more antibiotics might be used in a future attack. Some infectious disease experts have also advocated the use of clindamycin, citing the theoretical benefit of diminishing bacterial toxin production, a strategy used in some toxin-mediated streptococcal infections.[98] There are no data as yet that bear specifically on this question. Central nervous system penetration is another consideration; doxycycline or fluoroquinolone may not reach therapeutic levels in the cerebrospinal fluid. Thus, in the aftermath of the anthrax attacks, some infectious disease authorities recommended preferential use of ciprofloxacin over doxycycline, plus augmentation with chloramphenicol, rifampin, or penicillin when meningitis is established or suspected.

The *B anthracis* isolate recovered from patients with inhalational anthrax was susceptible to all of the antibiotics expected in a naturally occurring strain.[97] This isolate showed an inducible β-lactamase in addition to a constitutive cephalosporinase. The importance of the inducible β-lactamase is unknown; these strains are highly susceptible to penicillin in vitro, with minimum inhibiting concentrations less than .06 µg/mL. A theoretical concern is that this sensitivity could be overcome with a large bacterial burden. For this reason, the CDC advised that patients with inhalational anthrax should not be treated with penicillin or amoxicillin as monotherapy and that ciprofloxacin or doxycycline be considered the standards based on in vitro activ-

©2002 American Medical Association. All rights reserved.

Table 3. Recommended Therapy for Inhalational Anthrax Infection in the Contained Casualty Setting[a,b]

Category	Initial IV Therapy [c,d]	Duration
Adults	Ciprofloxacin, 400 mg every 12 h or Doxycycline, 100 mg every 12 h[f] and 1 or 2 Additional antimicrobials[d]	IV treatment initially[e] before switching to oral antimicrobial therapy when clinically appropriate: Ciprofloxacin 500 mg twice daily or Doxycycline 100 mg twice daily Continue oral and IV treatment for 60 d[j]
Children	Ciprofloxacin, 10-15 mg/kg every 12 h[g,h] or Doxycycline[f,i] for those aged >8 y and weight >45 kg: 100 mg every 12 h; >8 y and weight ≤45 kg: 2.2 mg/kg every 12 h; ≤8 y: 2.2 mg/kg every 12 h and 1 or 2 Additional antimicrobials[d]	IV treatment initially[e] before switching to oral antimicrobial therapy when clinically appropriate: Ciprofloxacin 10-15 mg/kg every 12 h[h] or Doxycycline[i] for those aged >8 y and weight >45 kg: 100 mg twice daily >8 y and weight ≤45 kg: 2.2 mg/kg twice daily ≤8 y: 2.2 mg/kg 2 daily Continue oral and IV treatment for 60 d[j]
Pregnant women[k]	Same for nonpregnant adults	IV treatment initially before switching to oral antimicrobial therapy when clinically appropriate[b]; oral therapy regimens are the same for nonpregnant adults
Immunocompromised persons	Same for nonimmunocompromised adults and children	

[a]This table is adapted with permission from *Morbidity and Mortality Weekly Report*.[97] For gastrointestinal and oropharyngeal anthrax, use regimens recommended for inhalational anthrax.

[b]Ciprofloxacin or doxycycline should be considered an essential part of first-line therapy for inhalational anthrax.

[c]Steroids may be considered as an adjunct therapy for patients with severe edema and for meningitis based on experience with bacterial meningitis of other etiologies.

[d]Other agents with in vitro activity include rifampin, vancomycin, penicillin, ampicillin, chloramphenicol, imipenem, clindamycin, and clarithromycin. Because of concerns of constitutive and inducible β-lactamases in *Bacillus anthracis*, penicillin and ampicillin should not be used alone. Consultation with an infectious disease specialist is advised.

[e]Initial therapy may be altered based on clinical course of the patient; 1 or 2 antimicrobial agents may be adequate as the patient improves.

[f]If meningitis is suspected, doxycycline may be less optimal because of poor central nervous system penetration.

[g]If intravenous (IV) ciprofloxacin is not available, oral ciprofloxacin may be acceptable because it is rapidly and well absorbed from the gastrointestinal tract with no substantial loss by first-pass metabolism. Maximum serum concentrations are attained 1 to 2 hours after oral dosing but may not be achieved if vomiting or ileus is present.

[h]In children, ciprofloxacin dosage should not exceed 1 g/d.

[i]The American Academy of Pediatrics recommends treatment of young children with tetracyclines for serious infections (ie, Rocky Mountain spotted fever).

[j]Because of the potential persistence of spores after an aerosol exposure, antimicrobial therapy should be continued for 60 days.

[k]Although tetracyclines are not recommended during pregnancy, their use may be indicated for life-threatening illness. Adverse effects on developing teeth and bones of fetus are dose related; therefore, doxycycline might be used for a short time (7-14 days) before 6 months of gestation. The high death rate from the infection outweighs the risk posed by the antimicrobial agent.

ity, efficacy in the monkey model, and FDA approval.

In the contained casualty setting (a situation in which a modest number of patients require therapy), the working group supports these new CDC antibiotic recommendations[97] (TABLE 3) and advises the use of intravenous antibiotic administration. These recommendations will need to be revised as new data become available.

If the number of persons requiring therapy following a bioterrorist attack with anthrax is sufficiently high (ie, a mass casualty setting), the working group recognizes that combination drug therapy and intravenous therapy may no longer be possible for reasons of logistics and/or exhaustion of equipment and antibiotic supplies. In such circumstances, oral therapy may be the only feasible option (TABLE 4). The threshold number of cases at which combination and parenteral therapy become impossible depends on a variety of factors, including local and regional health care resources.

In experimental animals, antibiotic therapy during anthrax infection has prevented development of an immune response.[40,95] This suggests that even if the antibiotic-treated patient survives anthrax infection, the risk of recurring disease may persist for a prolonged period because of the possibility of delayed germination of spores. Therefore, we recommend that antibiotic therapy be continued for at least 60 days postexposure, with oral therapy replacing intravenous therapy when the patient is clinically stable enough to take oral medication.

Cutaneous anthrax historically has been treated with oral penicillin. For reasons articulated above, the working group recommends that oral fluoroquinolone or doxycycline in the adult dosage schedules described in TABLE 5 be used to treat cutaneous anthrax until antibiotic susceptibility is proven. Amoxicillin is a suitable alternative if there are contraindications to fluoroquinolones or doxycycline such as pregnancy, lactating mother, age younger than 18 years,

or antibiotic intolerance. For cutaneous lesions associated with extensive edema or for cutaneous lesions of the head and neck, clinical management should be conservative as per inhalational anthrax treatment guidelines in Table 3. Although previous guidelines have suggested treating cutaneous anthrax for 7 to 10 days,[32,71] the working group recommends treatment for 60 days postexposure in the setting of bioterrorism, given the presumed concomitant inhalational exposure to the primary aerosol. Treatment of cutaneous anthrax generally prevents progression to systemic disease although it does not prevent the formation and evolution of the eschar. Topical therapy is not useful.[4]

In addition to penicillin, the fluoroquinolones and the tetracycline class of antibiotics, other antibiotics effective in vitro include chloramphenicol, clindamycin, extended-spectrum penicillins, macrolides, aminoglycosides, vancomycin, cefazolin, and other first-generation cephalosporins.[91,99] The efficacy of these antibiotics has not yet been tested

©2002 American Medical Association. All rights reserved.

Reprinted with permission from *JAMA*; May 1, 2002, Vol 287, No. 17

Table 4. Recommended Therapy for Inhalational Anthrax Infection in the Mass Casualty Setting or for Postexposure Prophylaxis*

Category	Initial Oral Therapy†	Alternative Therapy if Strain Is Proved Susceptible	Duration After Exposure, d
Adults	Ciprofloxacin, 500 mg orally every 12 h	Doxycycline, 100 mg orally every 12 h‡ Amoxicillin, 500 mg orally every 8 h§	60
Children	Ciprofloxacin, 20-30 mg/kg per d orally taken in 2 daily doses, not to exceed 1 g/d‖	Weight ≥20 kg: amoxicillin, 500 mg orally every 8 h§ Weight <20 kg: amoxicillin, 40 mg/kg taken orally in 3 doses every 8 h§	60
Pregnant women¶	Ciprofloxacin, 500 mg orally every 12 h	Amoxicillin, 500 mg orally every 8 h§	60
Immunosuppressed persons	Same as for nonimmunosuppressed adults and children		

*Some of these recommendations are based on animal studies or in vitro studies and are not approved by the US Food and Drug Administration.
†In vitro studies suggest ofloxacin (400 mg orally every 12 hours, or levofloxacin, 500 mg orally every 24 hours) could be substituted for ciprofloxacin.
‡In vitro studies suggest that 500 mg of tetracycline orally every 6 hours could be substituted for doxycycline. In addition, 400 mg of gatifloxacin or monifloxacin, both fluoroquinolones with mechanisms of action consistent with ciprofloxacin, taken orally daily could be substituted.
§According to the Centers for Disease Control and Prevention recommendations, amoxicillin is suitable for postexposure prophylaxis only after 10 to 14 days of fluoroquinolones or doxycycline treatment and then only if there are contraindications to these 2 classes of medications (eg, pregnancy, lactating mother, age <18 years, or intolerance of other antibiotics).
‖Doxycycline could also be used if antibiotic susceptibility testing, exhaustion of drug supplies, adverse reactions preclude use of ciprofloxacin. For children heavier than 45 kg, adult dosage should be used. For children lighter than 45 kg, 2.5 mg/kg of doxycycline orally every 12 hours should be used.
¶See "Management of Pregnant Population" for details.

in humans or animal studies. The working group recommends the use of these antibiotics only to augment fluoroquinolones or tetracyclines or if the preferred drugs are contraindicated, not available, or inactive in vitro in susceptibility testing. *B anthracis* strains exhibit natural resistance to sulfamethoxazole, trimethoprim, cefuroxime, cefotaxime sodium, aztreonam, and ceftazidime.[91,92,99] Therefore, these antibiotics should not be used.

Pleural effusions were present in all of the first 10 patients with inhalational anthrax in 2001. Seven needed drainage of their pleural effusions, 3 required chest tubes.[69] Future patients with inhalational anthrax should be expected to have pleural effusions that will likely require drainage.

Postexposure Prophylaxis

Guidelines for which populations would require postexposure prophylaxis to prevent inhalational anthrax following the release of a *B anthracis* aerosol as a biological weapon will need to be developed by public health officials depending on epidemiological circumstances. These decisions would require estimates of the timing, location, and conditions of the exposure.[100] Ongoing case monitoring would be needed to define the high-risk groups, to direct follow-up, and to guide the addition or deletion of groups requiring postexposure prophylaxis.

There are no FDA-approved postexposure antibiotic regimens following ex-

Table 5. Recommended Therapy for Cutaneous Anthrax Infection Associated With a Bioterrorism Attack*

Category	Initial Oral Therapy†	Duration, d‡
Adults	Ciprofloxacin, 500 mg twice daily† or Doxycycline, 100 mg twice daily†	60
Children§	Ciprofloxacin, 10-15 mg/kg every 12 h (not to exceed 1 g/d)† or Doxycycline for those aged§ >8 y and weight >45 kg: 100 mg every 12 h >8 y and weight ≤45 kg: 2.2 mg/kg every 12 h ≤8 y: 2.2 mg/kg every 12 h	60
Pregnant women‖	Ciprofloxacin, 500 mg twice daily or Doxycycline, 100 mg twice daily	60
Immunocompromised persons	Same for nonimmunocompromised adults and children	

*This table is adapted with permission from the *Morbidity and Mortality Weekly Report*.[98] Cutaneous anthrax with signs of systemic involvement, extensive edema, or lesions on the head or neck require intravenous therapy, and a multidrug approach is recommended (Table 3).
†Ciprofloxacin or doxycycline should be considered first-line therapy. Amoxicillin can be substituted if a patient cannot take a fluoroquinolone or tetracycline class drug. Adults are recommended to take 500 mg of amoxicillin orally 3 times a day. For children, 80 mg/kg of amoxicillin to be divided into 3 doses in 8-hour increments is an option for completion of therapy after clinical improvement. Oral amoxicillin dose is based on the need to achieve appropriate minimum inhibitory concentration levels.
‡Previous guidelines have suggested treating cutaneous anthrax for 7 to 10 days, but 60 days is recommended for bioterrorism attacks, given the likelihood of exposure to aerosolized *Bacillus anthracis*.
§The American Academy of Pediatrics recommends treatment of young children with tetracyclines for serious infections (eg, Rocky Mountain spotted fever).
‖Although tetracyclines or ciprofloxacin is not recommended during pregnancy, their use may be indicated for life-threatening illness. Adverse effects on developing teeth and bones of a fetus are dose related; therefore, doxycycline might be used for a short time (7-14 days) before 6 months of gestation.

posure to a *B anthracis* aerosol. Therefore, for postexposure prophylaxis, we recommend the same antibiotic regimen as that recommended for treatment of mass casualties; prophylaxis should be continued for at least 60 days postexposure (Table 4). Preliminary analysis of US postal workers who were advised to take 60 days of antibiotic prophylaxis for exposure to *B anthracis* spores following the anthrax attacks of 2001 showed that 2% sought medical attention because of concern of possible

severe allergic reactions related to the medications, but no persons required hospitalization because of an adverse drug reaction.[101] Many persons did not begin or complete their recommended antibiotic course for a variety of reasons, including gastrointestinal tract intolerance, underscoring the need for careful medical follow-up during the period of prophylaxis.[101] In addition, given the uncertainties regarding how many weeks or months spores may remain latent in the period following discontinu-

©2002 American Medical Association. All rights reserved.

Reprinted with permission from *JAMA*; May 1, 2002, Vol 287, No. 17

ation of postexposure prophylaxis, persons should be instructed to report immediately flulike symptoms or febrile illness to their physicians who should then evaluate the need to initiate treatment for possible inhalational anthrax. As noted above, postexposure vaccination is recommended as an adjunct to postexposure antibiotic prophylaxis if vaccine is available.

Management of Special Groups

Consensus recommendations for special groups as set forth herein reflect the clinical and evidence-based judgments of the working group and at this time do not necessarily correspond with FDA-approved use, indications, or labeling.

Children. It has been recommended that ciprofloxacin and other fluoroquinolones should not be used in children younger than 16 to 18 years because of a link to permanent arthropathy in adolescent animals and transient arthropathy in a small number of children.[94] However, balancing these risks against the risks of anthrax infections caused by an engineered antibiotic-resistant strain, the working group recommends that ciprofloxacin be used as a component of combination therapy for children with inhalational anthrax. For postexposure prophylaxis or following a mass casualty attack, monotherapy with fluoroquinolones is recommended by the working group[97] (Table 4).

The American Academy of Pediatrics has recommended that doxycycline not be used in children younger than 9 years because the drug has resulted in retarded skeletal growth in infants and discolored teeth in infants and children.[94] However, the serious risk of infection following an anthrax attack supports the consensus recommendation that doxycycline, instead of ciprofloxacin, be used in children if antibiotic susceptibility testing, exhaustion of drug supplies, or adverse reactions preclude use of ciprofloxacin.

According to CDC recommendations, amoxicillin was suitable for treatment or postexposure prophylaxis of possible anthrax infection following the anthrax attacks of 2001 only after 14

to 21 days of fluoroquinolone or doxycycline administration because of the concern about the presence of a β-lactamase.[102] In a contained casualty setting, the working group recommends that children with inhalational anthrax receive intravenous antibiotics (Table 3). In a mass casualty setting and as postexposure prophylaxis, the working group recommends that children receive oral antibiotics (Table 4).

The US anthrax vaccine is licensed for use only in persons aged 18 to 65 years because studies to date have been conducted exclusively in this group.[77] No data exist for children, but based on experience with other inactivated vaccines, it is likely that the vaccine would be safe and effective.

Pregnant Women. Fluoroquinolones are not generally recommended during pregnancy because of their known association with arthropathy in adolescent animals and small numbers of children. Animal studies have discovered no evidence of teratogenicity related to ciprofloxacin, but no controlled studies of ciprofloxacin in pregnant women have been conducted. Balancing these possible risks against the concerns of anthrax due to engineered antibiotic-resistant strains, the working group recommends that pregnant women receive ciprofloxacin as part of combination therapy for treatment of inhalational anthrax (Table 3). We also recommend that pregnant women receive fluoroquinolones in the usual adult dosages for postexposure prophylaxis or monotherapy treatment in the mass casualty setting (Table 4). The tetracycline class of antibiotics has been associated with both toxic effects in the liver in pregnant women and fetal toxic effects, including retarded skeletal growth.[94]

Balancing the risks of anthrax infection with those associated with doxycycline use in pregnancy, the working group recommends that doxycycline can be used as an alternative to ciprofloxacin as part of combination therapy in pregnant women for treatment of inhalational anthrax. For postexposure prophylaxis or in mass casualty settings, doxycycline can also be used as

an alternate to ciprofloxacin in pregnant women. If doxycycline is used in pregnant women, periodic liver function testing should be performed. No adequate controlled trials of penicillin or amoxicillin administration during pregnancy exist. However, the CDC recommends penicillin for the treatment of syphilis during pregnancy and amoxicillin as a treatment alternative for chlamydial infections during pregnancy.[94] According to CDC recommendations, amoxicillin is suitable postexposure prophylaxis or treatment of inhalational anthrax in pregnancy only after 14 to 21 days of fluoroquinolone or doxycycline administration.[102]

Ciprofloxacin (and other fluoroquinolones), penicillin, and doxycycline (and other tetracyclines) are each excreted in breast milk. Therefore, a breastfeeding woman should be treated or given prophylaxis with the same antibiotic as her infant based on what is most safe and effective for the infant.

Immunosuppressed Persons. The antibiotic treatment or postexposure prophylaxis for anthrax among those who are immunosuppressed has not been studied in human or animal models of anthrax infection. Therefore, the working group consensus recommends administering antibiotics in the same regimens recommended for immunocompetent adults and children.

INFECTION CONTROL

There are no data to suggest that patient-to-patient transmission of anthrax occurs and no person-to-person transmission occurred following the anthrax attacks of 2001.[18,67] Standard barrier isolation precautions are recommended for hospitalized patients with all forms of anthrax infection, but the use of high-efficiency particulate air filter masks or other measures for airborne protection are not indicated.[103] There is no need to immunize or provide prophylaxis to patient contacts (eg, household contacts, friends, coworkers) unless a determination is made that they, like the patient, were exposed to the aerosol or surface contamination at the time of the attack.

©2002 American Medical Association. All rights reserved.

Reprinted with permission from *JAMA*; May 1, 2002, Vol 287, No. 17

In addition to immediate notification of the hospital epidemiologist and state health department, the local hospital microbiology laboratories should be notified at the first indication of anthrax so that safe specimen processing under biosafety level 2 conditions can be undertaken as is customary in most hospital laboratories.[56] A number of disinfectants used for standard hospital infection control, such as hypochlorite, are effective in cleaning environmental surfaces contaminated with infected bodily fluids.[22,103]

Proper burial or cremation of humans and animals who have died because of anthrax infection is important in preventing further transmission of the disease. Serious consideration should be given to cremation. Embalming of bodies could be associated with special risks.[103] If autopsies are performed, all related instruments and materials should be autoclaved or incinerated.[103] The CDC can provide advice on postmortem procedures in anthrax cases.

DECONTAMINATION

Recommendations for decontamination in the event of an intentional aerosolization of *B anthracis* spores are based on evidence concerning aerosolization techniques, predicted spore survival, environmental exposures at Sverdlovsk and among goat hair mill workers, and environmental data collected following the anthrax attacks of 2001. The greatest risk to humans exposed to an aerosol of *B anthracis* spores occurs when spores first are made airborne, the period called *primary aerosolization*. The aerobiological factors that affect how long spores remain airborne include the size of the dispersed particles and their hydrostatic properties.[100] Technologically sophisticated dispersal methods, such as aerosol release from military aircraft of large quantities of *B anthracis* spores manipulated for use in a weapon, are potentially capable of exposing high numbers of victims over large areas. Recent research by Canadian investigators has demonstrated that even "low-tech" delivery systems, such as the opening of envelopes containing powdered spores in indoor environments, can rapidly deliver high concentrations of spores to persons in the vicinity.[104] In some circumstances, indoor airflows, activity patterns, and heating, ventilation, and air conditioning systems may transport spores to others parts of the building.

Following the period of primary aerosolization, *B anthracis* spores may settle on surfaces, possibly in high concentrations. The risk that *B anthracis* spores might pose by a process of secondary aerosolization (resuspension of spores into the air) is uncertain and is likely dependent on many variables, including the quantity of spores on a surface; the physical characteristics of the powder used in the attack; the type of surface; the nature of the human or mechanical activity that occurs in the affected area and host factors.

A variety of rapid assay kits are available to detect *B anthracis* spores on environmental surfaces. None of these kits has been independently evaluated or endorsed by the CDC, FDA, or Environmental Protection Agency, and their functional characteristics are not known.[105] Many false-positive results occurred following the anthrax attacks of 2001. Thus, any result using currently available rapid assay kits does not necessarily signify the presence of *B anthracis*; it is simply an indication that further testing is required by a certified microbiology laboratory. Similarly, the sensitivity and false-negative rate of disease kits are unknown.

At Sverdlovsk, no new cases of inhalational anthrax developed beyond 43 days after the presumed date of release. None were documented during the months and years afterward, despite only limited decontamination and vaccination of 47 000 of the city's 1 million inhabitants.[59] Some have questioned whether any of the cases with onset of disease beyond 7 days after release might have represented illness following *secondary aerosolization* from the ground or other surfaces. It is impossible to state with certainty that secondary aerosolizations did not occur in Sverdlovsk, but it appears unlikely. The epidemic curve reported is typical for a common-source epidemic,[3,60] and it is possible to account for virtually all confirmed cases having occurred within the area of the plume on the day of the accident. Moreover, if secondary aerosolization had been important, new cases would have likely continued well beyond the observed 43 days.

Although persons working with animal hair or hides are known to be at increased risk of developing inhalational or cutaneous anthrax, surprisingly few occupational exposures in the United States have resulted in disease. During the first half of the 20th century, a significant number of goat hair mill workers were heavily exposed to aerosolized spores. Mandatory vaccination became a requirement for working in goat hair mills only in the 1960s. Prior to that, many unvaccinated person-years of high-risk exposure had occurred, but only 13 cases of inhalational anthrax were reported.[27,54] One study of environmental exposure, conducted at a Pennsylvania goat hair mill, showed that workers inhaled up to 510 *B anthracis* particles of at least 5 µm in diameter per person per 8-hour shift.[54] These concentrations of spores were constantly present in the environment during the time of this study, but no cases of inhalational anthrax occurred.

Field studies using *B anthracis*–like surrogates have been carried out by US Army scientists seeking to determine the risk of secondary aerosolization. One study concluded that there was no significant threat to personnel in areas contaminated by 1 million spores per square meter either from traffic on asphalt-paved roads or from a runway used by helicopters or jet aircraft.[106] A separate study showed that in areas of ground contaminated with 20 million *Bacillus subtilis* spores per square meter, a soldier exercising actively for a 3-hour period would inhale between 1000 and 15 000 spores.[107]

Much has been written about the technical difficulty of decontaminating an environment contaminated with *B anthracis* spores. A classic case is the experience at Gruinard Island, Scotland. During World War II, British mili-

©2002 American Medical Association. All rights reserved.

Reprinted with permission from *JAMA*; May 1, 2002, Vol 287, No. 17

tary undertook explosives testing with *B anthracis* spores. Spores persisted and remained viable for 36 years following the conclusion of testing. Decontamination of the island occurred in stages, beginning in 1979 and ending in 1987 when the island was finally declared fully decontaminated. The total cost is unpublished, but materials required included 280 tons of formaldehyde and 2000 tons of seawater.[108]

Following the anthrax attacks of 2001, substantial efforts were undertaken to decontaminate environmental surfaces exposed to *B anthracis* spores. Sections of the Hart Senate office building in Washington, DC, contaminated from opening a letter laden with *B anthracis*, were reopened only after months of decontamination procedures at an estimated cost of $23 million.[109] Decontamination efforts at many other buildings affected by the anthrax attacks of 2001 have not yet been completed.

Prior to the anthrax attacks of 2001, there had been no recognition or scientific study showing that *B anthracis* spores of "weapons grade" quality would be capable of leaking out the edges of envelopes or through the pores of envelopes, with resulting risk to the health of those handling or processing those letters. When it became clear that the Florida case of anthrax was likely caused by a letter contaminated with *B anthracis*, assessment of postal workers who might have handled or processed that letter showed no illness.[69] When the anthrax cases were discovered, each was linked to a letter that had been opened. At first, there was no evidence of illness among persons handling or processing unopened mail. This fact influenced the judgment that persons handling or processing unopened *B anthracis* letters were not at risk. These judgments changed when illness was discovered in persons who had handled or processed unopened letters in Washington, DC. Much remains unknown about the risks to persons handling or processing unopened letters containing *B anthracis* spores. It is not well understood how the me-

chanical systems of mail processing in a specific building would affect the risk of disease acquisition in a worker handling a contaminated letter in that facility. It is still uncertain what the minimum dose of spores would be to cause infection in humans although it may theoretically be as few as 1 to 3 spores.[47] The mechanisms of disease acquisition in the 2 fatal inhalational anthrax cases in New York City and in Connecticut remain unknown although it is speculated that disease in these 2 cases followed the inhalation of small numbers of spores present in some manner in "cross-contaminated" mail.

The discovery of *B anthracis* spores in a contaminated letter in the office of Sen Daschle in the Hart office building led the Environmental Protection Agency to conduct tests in this office to assess the risk of secondary aerosolization of spores. Prior to the initiation of decontamination efforts in the Hart building, 17 blood agar gel plates were placed around the office and normal activity in the office was simulated. Sixteen of the 17 plates yielded *B anthracis*. Although this experiment did not allow conclusions about the specific risk of persons developing anthrax infection in this context, it did demonstrate that routine activity in an environment contaminated with *B anthracis* spores could cause significant spore resuspension.[110]

Given the above considerations, if an environmental surface is proved to be contaminated with *B anthracis* spores in the immediate area of a spill or close proximity to the point of release of *B anthracis* biological weapons, the working group believes that decontamination of that area would likely decrease the risk of acquiring anthrax by secondary aerosolization. However, as has been demonstrated in environmental decontamination efforts following the anthrax attacks of 2001, decontamination of buildings or parts of buildings following an anthrax attack is technically difficult. For these reasons, the working group would advise that decisions about methods for decontamination following an anthrax attack follow

full expert analysis of the contaminated environment and the anthrax weapon used in the attack and be made in consultation with experts on environmental remediation. If vaccines were available, postexposure vaccination might be a useful intervention for those working in highly contaminated areas, because it could further lower the risk of anthrax infection.

In the setting of an announced alleged *B anthracis* release, such as the series of anthrax hoaxes occurring in many areas of the United States in 1998[111] and following the anthrax attacks of 2001, any person coming in direct physical contact with a substance alleged to be containing *B anthracis* should thoroughly wash the exposed skin and articles of clothing with soap and water.[112] In addition, any person in direct physical contact with the alleged substance should receive postexposure antibiotic prophylaxis until the substance is proved not to be *B anthracis*. The anthrax attacks of 2001 and new research[104] have shown that opening letters containing substantial quantities of *B anthracis* spores in certain conditions can confer risk of disease to persons at some distance from the location of where the letter was opened. For this reason, when a letter is suspected of containing (or proved to contain) *B anthracis*, immediate consultation with local and state public health authorities and the CDC for advised medical management is warranted.

Additional Research

Development of a recombinant anthrax vaccine that would be more easily manufactured and would require fewer doses should remain a top priority. Rapid diagnostic assays that could reliably identify early anthrax infection and quickly distinguish from other flulike or febrile illnesses would become critical in the event of a large-scale attack. Simple animal models for use in comparing antibiotic prophylactic and treatment strategies are also needed. Operational research to better characterize risks posed by environmental contamination of spores,

©2002 American Medical Association. All rights reserved.

Reprinted with permission from *JAMA*; May 1, 2002, Vol 287, No. 17

particularly inside buildings, and research on approaches to minimize risk in indoor environments by means of air filters or methods for environmental cleaning following a release are also needed. A better understanding of the genetics and pathogenesis of anthrax, as well as mechanisms of virulence and immunity, will be of importance in the prospective evaluation of new therapeutic and diagnostic strategies. Novel therapeutic approaches with promise, such as the administration of competitors against the protective antigen complex,[113] should also be tested in animals and developed where evidence supports this. Recent developments such as the publishing of the *B anthracis* genome and the discovery of the crystalline structure of the lethal and edema factor could hold great clinical hope for both the prevention and treatment of anthrax infection.[114]

Ex Officio Participants in the Working Group on Civilian Biodefense: George Curlin, MD, National Institutes of Health, Bethesda, Md; Margaret Hamburg, MD, Nuclear Threat Initiative, Washington, DC; Stuart Nightingale, MD, Office of Assistant Secretary for Planning and Evaluation, DHHS, Washington, DC; William Raub, PhD, Office of Public Health Preparedness, DHHS, Washington, DC; Robert Knouss, MD, Office of Emergency Preparedness, DHHS, Rockville, Md; Marcelle Layton, MD, Office of Communicable Disease, New York City Health Department, New York, NY; and Brian Malkin, formerly of FDA, Rockville, Md.
Funding/Support: Funding for this study primarily was provided by each participant's institution or agency.
Disclaimers: In many cases, the indication and dosages and other information are not consistent with current approved labeling by the US Food and Drug Administration (FDA). The recommendations on the use of drugs and vaccine for uses not approved by the FDA do not represent the official views of the FDA or of any of the federal agencies whose scientists participated in these discussions. Unlabeled uses of the products recommended are noted in the sections of this article in which these products are discussed. Where unlabeled uses are indicated, information used as the basis for the recommendation is discussed. The views, opinions, assertions, and findings contained herein are those of the authors and should not be construed as official US Department of Health and Human Services, US Department of Defense, or US Department of Army positions, policies, or decisions unless so designated by other documentation.
Acknowledgment: The working group wishes to thank Jeanne Guillemin, PhD, Matthew Meselson, PhD, Timothy Townsend, MD, Martin Hugh-Jones, MA, VetMB, MPH, PhD, and Philip Brachman, MD, for their review and commentary on the originally published manuscript, and Molly D'Esopo for her efforts in the preparation of the revised manuscript.

REFERENCES

1. Carter A, Deutsch J, Zelicow P. Catastrophic terrorism. *Foreign Aff.* 1998;77:80-95.
2. Investigation of bioterrorism-related anthrax: Con-
necticut, 2001. *MMWR Morb Mortal Wkly Rep.* 2001; 50:1077-1079.
3. Inglesby TV, Henderson DA, Bartlett JG, et al. Anthrax as a biological weapon. *JAMA.* 1999;281:1735-1745.
4. Lew D. *Bacillus anthracis.* In: Mandell GL, Bennett JE, Dolin R, eds. *Principles and Practice of Infectious Disease.* New York, NY: Churchill Livingstone Inc; 1995:1885-1889.
5. Christopher G, Cieslak T, Pavlin J, Eitzen E. Biological warfare: a historical perspective. *JAMA.* 1997; 278:412-417.
6. Monterey Institute for International Studies chemical and biological weapons resource page. *Chemical and Biological Weapons.* Monterey, Calif: Monterey Institute for International Studies; 2001. Available at: http://cns.miis.edu/research/cbw/possess.htm.
7. Zilinskas RA. Iraq's biological weapons. *JAMA.* 1997; 278:418-424.
8. Alibek K, Handelman S. *Biohazard: The Chilling True Story of the Largest Covert Biological Weapons Program in the World.* New York, NY: Random House; 1999.
9. Miller J. A germ-making plant. *New York Times.* September 4, 2001; A1
10. Public Health Service Office of Emergency Preparedness. *Proceedings of the Seminar on Responding to the Consequences of Chemical and Biological Terrorism;* Washington, DC: US Dept of Health and Human Services; 1995.
11. WuDunn S, Miller J, Broad W. How Japan germ terror alerted world. *New York Times.* May 26, 1998; A1, 6.
12. Keim P, Smith K, Keys C, Takahashi H, Kurata T, Kaufmann A. Molecular investigation of the Aum Shinrikyo anthrax release in Kameido, Japan. *J Clin Microbiol.* 2001;39:4566-4567.
13. Washington File. New CIA report documents global weapons proliferation trends. Washington, DC: US Dept of State; February 1, 2002. Available at: http://usinfo.state.gov/products/washfile. Accessed February 1, 2002.
14. Enserink M. Microbial genomics: TIGR begins assault on the anthrax genome. *Science.* 2002;295: 1442-1443.
15. Kennedy H. Daschle letter bombshell billions of anthrax spores. *New York Daily News.* October 31, 2001: 5.
16. *Health Aspects of Chemical and Biological Weapons.* Geneva, Switzerland: World Health Organization; 1970.
17. Office of Technology Assessment, US Congress. *Proliferation of Weapons of Mass Destruction.* Washington, DC: US Government Printing Office; 1993. Publication OTA-ISC-559.
18. Meselson M, Guillemin J, Hugh-Jones M, et al. The Sverdlovsk anthrax outbreak of 1979. *Science.* 1994;266:1202-1208.
19. Simon J. Biological terrorism: preparing to meet the threat. *JAMA.* 1997;278:428-430.
20. Regis E. *The History of America's Secret Germ Warfare Project.* New York, NY: Random House; 1999.
21. Kohout E, Sehat A, Ashraf M. Anthrax: a continuous problem in south west Iran. *Am J Med Sci.* 1964;247:565.
22. Titball R, Turnbull P, Hutson R. The monitoring and detection of *Bacillus anthracis* in the environment. *Soc Appl Bacteriol Symp Ser.* 1991;20:9S-18S.
23. l'agriculture Pdmd. Premiere Partie. I-la fievre charbonneuse en Iran.1-historique—especes atteintes; 1946. Located at: Archives De L'institute D'hessarek, Teheran, Iran.
24. Pienaar U. Epidemiology of anthrax in wild animals and the control on anthrax epizootics in the Kruger National Park, South Africa. *Fed Proc.* 1967;26:1496-1591.
25. Dragon D, Rennie R. The ecology of anthrax spores. *Can Vet J.* 1995;36:295-301.
26. Brachman P, Friedlander A. Anthrax. In: Plotkin S, Orenstein W, eds. *Vaccines.* 3rd ed. Philadelphia, Pa: WB Saunders Co; 1999:629-637.
27. Brachman P, Friedlander A. Inhalation anthrax. *Ann N Y Acad Sci.* 1980;353:83-93.
28. Summary of notifiable diseases, 1945-1994. *MMWR Morb Mortal Wkly Rep.* 1994;43:70-78.
29. Human anthrax associated with an epizootic among livestock. *MMWR Morb Mortal Wkly Rep.* 2001;50:677-680.
30. Myenye K, Siziya S, Peterson D. Factors associated with human anthrax outbreak in the Chikupo and Ngandu villages of Murewa district in Mashonaland East Province, Zimbabwe. *Cent Afr J Med.* 1996;42: 312-315.
31. Sirisanthana T, Nelson K, Ezzell J, Abshire T. Serological studies of patients with cutaneous and oral-pharyngeal anthrax from northern Thailand. *Am J Trop Med Hyg.* 1988;39:575-581.
32. Friedlander A. Anthrax. In: Zajtchuk R, Bellamy R, eds. *Textbook of Military Medicine: Medical Aspects of Chemical and Biological Warfare.* Washington, DC: Office of the Surgeon General, US Dept of the Army; 1997:467-478.
33. Sirisanthana T, Navacharoen N, Tharavichitkul P, Sirisanthana V, Brown AE. Outbreak of oral-pharyngeal anthrax. *Am J Trop Med Hyg.* 1984;33: 144-150.
34. Dutz W, Saidi F, Kouhout E. Gastric anthrax with massive ascites. *Gut.* 1970;11:352-354.
35. Lincoln R, Hodges D, Klein F, et al. Role of the lymphatics in the pathogenesis of anthrax. *J Infect Dis.* 1965;115:481-494.
36. Borio L, Frank D, Mani V, et al. Death due to bioterrorism-related inhalational anthrax. *JAMA.* 2001; 286:2554-2559.
37. Williams R. *Bacillus anthracis* and other spore forming bacilli. In: Braude AI, Davis LE, Fierer J, eds. *Infectious Disease and Medical Microbiology.* Philadelphia, Pa: WB Saunders Co; 1986:270-278.
38. Druett H, Henderson D, Packman L, Peacock S. Studies on respiratory infection. *J Hyg.* 1953;51:359-371.
39. Hatch T. Distribution and deposition of inhaled particles in respiratory tract. *Bacteriol Rev.* 1961;25: 237-240.
40. Friedlander AM, Welkos SL, Pitt ML, et al. Postexposure prophylaxis against experimental inhalation anthrax. *J Infect Dis.* 1993;167:1239-1242.
41. Ross JM. The pathogenesis of anthrax following the administration of spores by the respiratory route. *J Pathol Bacteriol.* 1957;73:485-495.
42. Hanna PC, Ireland JA. Understanding *Bacillus anthracis* pathogenesis. *Trends Microbiol.* 1999;7:180-182.
43. Glassman H. Industrial inhalation anthrax. *Bacteriol Rev.* 1966;30:657-659.
44. Henderson DW, Peacock S, Belton FC. Observations on the prophylaxis of experimental pulmonary anthrax in the monkey. *J Hyg.* 1956;54:28-36.
45. Smith H, Keppie J. Observations on experimental anthrax. *Nature.* 1954;173:869-870.
46. *Soviet Biological Warfare Threat.* Washington, DC: Defense Intelligence Agency, US Dept of Defense; 1986. Publication DST-161OF-057-86.
47. Peters CJ, Hartley DM. Anthrax inhalation and lethal human infection. *Lancet.* 2002;359:710-711.
48. Dixon TC, Meselson M, Guillemin J, Hanna PC. Anthrax. *N Engl J Med.* 1999;341:815-826.
49. Friedlander AM. Microbiology: tackling anthrax. *Nature.* 2001;414:160-161.
50. Abramova FA, Grinberg LM, Yampolskaya O, Walker DH. Pathology of inhalational anthrax in 42 cases from the Sverdlovsk outbreak in 1979. *Proc Natl Acad Sci U S A.* 1993;90:2291-2294.
51. Dalldorf F, Kaufmann AF, Brachman PS. Woolsorters' disease. *Arch Pathol.* 1971;92:418-426.
52. Gleiser CA, Berdjis CC, Harman HA, Gochenour

©2002 American Medical Association. All rights reserved.

WS. Pathology of experimental respiratory anthrax in Macaca Mulatta. *Br J Exp Pathol.* 1963;44:416-426.

53. Grinberg LM, Abramova FA, Yampolskaya OV, et al. Quantitative pathology of inhalational anthrax, I. *Mod Pathol.* 2001;14:482-495.

54. Dahlgren CM, Buchanan LM, Decker HM, et al. *Bacillus anthracis* aerosols in goat hair processing mills. *Am J Hyg.* 1960;72:24-31.

55. Walker JS, Lincoln RE, Klein F. Pathophysiological and biochemical changes in anthrax. *Fed Proc.* 1967; 26:1539-1544.

56. Franz DR, Jahrling PB, Friedlander A, et al. Clinical recognition and management of patients exposed to biological warfare agents. *JAMA.* 1997;278: 399-411.

57. Vessal K, Yeganehdoust J, Dutz W, Kohout E. Radiologic changes in inhalation anthrax. *Clin Radiol.* 1975;26:471-474.

58. Albrink WS, Brooks SM, Biron RE, Kopel M. Human inhalation anthrax. *Am J Pathol.* 1960;36:457-471.

59. Guillemin J. *Anthrax: The Investigation of a Deadly Outbreak.* Berkeley: University of California Press; 1999.

60. Brookmeyer R, Blades N, Hugh-Jones M, Henderson D. The statistical analysis of truncated data: application to the Sverdlovsk anthrax outbreak. *Biostatistics.* 2001;2:233-247.

61. Jernigan J, Stephens D, Ashford D, Omenaca C, et al. Bioterrorism-related inhalation anthrax: the first 10 cases reported in the United States. *Emerg Infect Dis.* 2001;7:933-944.

62. Barakat LA, Quentzel HL, Jernigan JA, et al. Fatal inhalational anthrax in a 94-year-old Connecticut woman. *JAMA.*2002;287:863-868.

63. Freedman A, Afonja O, Chang M, et al. Cutaneous anthrax associated with microangiopathic hemolytic anemia and coagulopathy in a 7-month-old infant. *JAMA.* 2002;287:869-874.

64. Mina B, Dym JP, Kuepper F, et al. Fatal inhalational anthrax with unknown source of exposure in a 61-year-old woman in New York City. *JAMA.* 2002; 287:858-862.

65. Bush LM, Abrams BH, Beall A, Johnson CC. Index case of fatal inhalational anthrax due to bioterrorism in the United States. *N Engl J Med.* 2001;345: 1607-1610.

66. Mayer TA, Bersoff-Matcha S, Murphy C, et al. Clinical presentation of inhalational anthrax following bioterrorism exposure. *JAMA.* 2001;286:2549-2553.

67. Pile JC, Malone JD, Eitzen EM, Friedlander A. Anthrax as a potential biological warfare agent. *Arch Intern Med.* 1998;158:429-434.

68. Kaye E, Kaye K. Fever and rash. In: Eugene Braunwald, Anthony S. Fauci, Kurt J. Isselbacher, et al, eds. *Harrison's Textbook of Medicine.* New York, NY: McGraw-Hill; 2001.

69. Investigation of bioterrorism-related anthrax and interim guidelines for clinical evaluation of persons with possible anthrax. *MMWR Morb Mortal Wkly Rep.* 2001;50:941-948.

70. Carucci JA, McGovern TW, Norton SA, et al. Cutaneous anthrax management algorithm. *J Am Acad Dermatol.* 2001; Nov 21. Available at: http://www.harcourthealth.com/scripts/om.dll/serve?arttype=full&article=a121613.

71. Penn C, Klotz S. Anthrax. In: Gorbach S, Bartlett J, Blacklow N, eds. *Infectious Diseases.* Philadelphia, Pa: WB Saunders Co; 1998:1575-1578.

72. Hail A, Rossi C, Ludwig G, Ivins B, Tammariello R, Henchal E. Comparison of noninvasive sampling sites for early detection of *Bacillus* anthrax spores from rhesus monkeys after aerosol exposure. *Mil Med.* 1999; 164:833-837.

73. Pitt M, Little S, Ivins B, et al. In vitro correlate of immunity in a rabbit model of inhalational anthrax. *Vaccine.* 2001;19:4768-4773.

74. Welkos S, Little S, Friedlander A, Fritz D, Fellows P. The role of antibodies to *Bacillus anthracis* and anthrax toxin components in inhibiting the early stages of infection by anthrax spores. *Microbiology.* 2001; 147(pt 6):1677-1685.

75. Brachman P. Anthrax. In: Hoeprich PD, Jordan MC, Ronald AR, eds. *Infectious Diseases.* Philadelphia, Pa: JB Lippincott; 1994:1003-1008.

76. Anthrax vaccine, military use in Persian Gulf region [press release]. Washington, DC: US Dept of Defense; September 8, 1998.

77. Michigan Department of Public Health. *Anthrax Vaccine Adsorbed.* Lansing: Michigan Dept of Public Health; 1978.

78. Pitt M, Little S, Ivins B, et al. In vitro correlate of immunity in an animal model of inhalational anthrax. *J Appl Microbiol.* 1999;87:304.

79. Ivins BE, Fellows P, Pitt ML, et al. Efficacy of standard human anthrax vaccine against *Bacillus anthracis* aerosol spore challenge in rhesus monkeys. *Salisbury Med Bull.* 1996;87:125-126.

80. Fellows P, Linscott M, Ivins B, et al. Efficacy of a human anthrax vaccine in guinea pigs, rabbits, and rhesus macaques against challenge by *Bacillus anthracis* isolates of diverse geographical origin. *Vaccine.* 2001;20:635.

81. Brachman PS, Gold H, Plotkin SA, Fekety FR, Werrin M, Ingraham NR. Field evaluation of human anthrax vaccine. *Am J Public Health.* 1962;52:632-645.

82. Surveillance for adverse events associated with anthrax vaccination. *MMWR Morb Mortal Wkly Rep.* 2000;49:341-345.

83. Pittman P, Gibbs P, Cannon T, Friedlander A. Anthrax vaccine. *Vaccine.* 2001;20:972-978.

84. Committee to Assess the Safety and Efficacy of the Anthrax Vaccine, Medical Follow-Up Agency. *The Anthrax Vaccine: Is It Safe? Does It Work?* Washington, DC: Institute of Medicine, National Academy Press. March 2002. Available at: http://www.iom.edu/iom/iomhome.nsf/WFiles/Anthrax-8-pager1FINAL/$file/Anthrax-8-pager1FINAL.pdf

85. Wiesen AR, Littell CT. Relationship between prepregnancy anthrax vaccination and pregnancy and birth outcomes among US Army women. *JAMA.* 2002; 287:1556-1560.

86. Turnbull PC. Anthrax vaccines. *Vaccine.* 1991;9: 533-539.

87. Statement by the Department of Health and Human Services regarding additional options for preventive treatment for those exposed to inhalational anthrax [news release]. Washington, DC: US Dept of Health and Human Services; December 18, 2001.

88. The Counter Bioterrorism Research Agenda of the National Institute of Allergy and Infectious Diseases for CDC Category A Agents. Washington, DC: National Institute of Allergy and Infectious Diseases; February 2002. Available at: http://www.niaid.nih.gov/dmid/pdf/biotresearchagenda.pdf.

89. Barnes J. Penicillin and *B anthracis.* *J Pathol Bacteriol.* 1947;194:113-125.

90. Lincoln R, Klein F, Walker J, et al. Successful treatment of monkeys for septicemic anthrax. *Antimicrob Agents and Chemother—1964.* Washington, DC: American Society for Microbiology; 1965:759-763.

91. Odendaal MW, Peterson PM, de Vos V, Botha AD. The antibiotic sensitivity patterns of *Bacillus anthracis* isolated from the Kruger National Park. *Onderstepoort J Vet Res.* 1991;58:17-19.

92. Doganay M, Aydin N. Antimicrobial susceptibility of *Bacillus anthracis.* *Scand J Infect Dis.* 1991;23: 333-335.

93. Kelly D, Chulay JD, Mikesell P, Friedlander A. Serum concentrations of penicillin, doxycycline, and ciprofloxacin during prolonged therapy in rhesus monkeys. *J Infect Dis.* 1992;166:1184-1187.

94. American Hospital Formulary Service. *AHFS Drug Information.* Bethesda, Md: American Society of Health System Pharmacists; 1996.

95. Stepanov AV, Marinin LI, Pomerantsev AP, Staritsin NA. Development of novel vaccines against anthrax in man. *J Biotechnol.* 1966;44:155-160.

96. Choe C, Bouhaouala S, Brook I, Elliott T, Knudson G. In vitro development of resistance to ofloxacin and doxycycline in *Bacillus anthracis* Sterne. *Antimicrob Agents Chemother.* 2000;44:1766.

97. Investigation of bioterrorism-related anthrax and interim guidelines for exposure management and antimicrobial therapy, October 2001. *MMWR Morb Mortal Wkly Rev.* 2001;50:909-919.

98. Stevens DL, Gibbons AE, Bergstron R, Winn V. The Eagle effect revisited. *J Infect Dis.* 1988;158:23-28.

99. Lightfoot NF, Scott RJ, Turnbull PC. Antimicrobial susceptibility of *Bacillus anthracis.* *Salisbury Med Bull.* 1990;68:95-98.

100. Perkins WA. Public health implications of airborne infection. *Bacteriol Rev.* 1961;25:347-355.

101. Update: adverse events associated with anthrax prophylaxis among postal employees: New Jersey, New York City, and the District of Columbia metropolitan area, 2001. *MMWR Morb Mortal Wkly Rep.* 2001;50:1051-1054

102. Interim recommendations for antimicrobial prophylaxis for children and breastfeeding mothers and treatment of children with anthrax. *MMWR Morb Mortal Wkly Rep.* 2001;50:1014-1016.

103. American Public Health Association. Anthrax. In: Benson AS, ed. *Control of Communicable Diseases Manual.* Washington, DC: American Public Health Association; 1995:18-22.

104. Kournikakis B, Armour SJ, Boulet CA, Spence M, Parsons B. Risk assessment of anthrax threat letters. Defence Research Establishment Suffield. September 2001. Available at: http://www.dres.dnd.ca/Meetings/FirstResponders/tr01-048_annex.pdf.

105. Use of onsite technologies for rapidly assessing environmental *Bacillus anthracis* contamination on surfaces in buildings. *MMWR Morb Mortal Wkly Rep.* 2001;50:1087.

106. Chinn KS. *Reaerosolization Hazard Assessment for Biological Agent-Contaminated Hardstand Areas.* Life Sciences Division, Dugway Proving Ground, Utah: US Dept of the Army; 1996. Publication DPG/JCP-96/012.

107. Resnick IG, Martin DD, Larsen LD. *Evaluation of Need for Detection of Surface Biological Agent Contamination*: Dugway Proving Ground, Life Sciences Division, US Dept of the Army; 1990:1-35. Publication DPG-FR-90-711.

108. Manchee RJ, Stewart WD. The decontamination of Gruinard Island. *Chem Br.* July 1988;690-691.

109. Hsu SS, Cost of anthrax cleanup on Hill to top $23 million, EPA says. *Washington Post.* March 7, 2002: A7.

110. Altman L. New tests confirm potency of anthrax in Senate office building. *New York Times.* December 11, 2001:B6.

111. Bioterrorism alleging use of anthrax and interim guidelines for management—United States, 1998. *MMWR Morb Mortal Wkly Rep.* 1999;48: 69-74.

112. *Medical Response to Biological Warfare and Terrorism.* Gaithersburg, Md: US Army Medical Research Institute of Infectious Diseases, Centers for Disease Control and Prevention, and US Food and Drug Administration; 1998.

113. Mourez M, Kane R, Mogridge J, et al. Designing a polyvalent inhibitor of anthrax toxin. *Nat Biotechnol.* 2001;19:958-961.

114. Friedlander AM. Microbiology: tackling anthrax. *Nature.* 2001;414:160-161.

©2002 American Medical Association. All rights reserved.

CORRECTION

Incorrect Wording: Subsequent to the publication of the Original Contribution entitled "Anthrax as a Biological Weapon, 2002: Updated Recommendations for Management," published in the May 1, 2002, issue of THE JOURNAL (2002;287:2236-2252), the authors wish to make available the following updates based on information from the US Food and Drug Administration and the Centers from Disease Control and Prevention (CDC).

In Table 3 on page 27, the pediatric dosage of ciprofloxacin for "Initial IV [intravenous] Therapy" for inhalational anthrax in the contained casualty setting should read, "10 mg/kg every 12 h (maximum of 400 mg per dose)" and subsequent oral therapy under "Duration" should be "15 mg/kg per dose taken orally every 12 h (maximum of 500 mg per dose)." The doxycycline dosages for children should be based on weight (ie, > or ≤ 45 kg) and not on age.

In Table 4 on page 28, the pediatric dosage of ciprofloxacin for "Initial Oral Therapy" of inhalational anthrax infection in the mass casualty setting or for postexposure prophylaxis should read, "15 mg/kg per dose taken orally every 12 h (maximum 500 mg per dose)." The correct dosage of amoxicillin for children who weigh less than 20 kg in a mass casualty setting or for postexposure prophylaxis is "80 mg/kg to be taken orally in 3 divided doses every 8 h."

The footnote marked by a section mark (§) in Table 4 should read as follows: "According to the CDC recommendations for the bioterrorist attacks in 2001, in which *B anthracis* was susceptible to penicillin, amoxicillin was a suitable alternative for postexposure prophylaxis in infants, children, and women who were pregnant or who were breastfeeding. Amoxicillin was also a suitable alternative for completion of 60 days of antibiotic therapy for patients in these groups with cutaneous or inhalational anthrax whose clinical illness had resolved after treatment with a ciprofloxacin- or doxycycline-based regimen (14-21 days for inhalational or complicated cutaneous anthrax; 7-10 days for uncomplicated cutaneous anthrax). Such patients required prolonged therapy because they were presumably exposed to aerosolized *B anthracis*."

In Table 5 on page 28, the pediatric dosage of ciprofloxacin for treatment of cutaneous anthrax infection should be "15 mg/kg per dose taken orally every 12 h (maximum of 500 mg per dose)." Pediatric doxycycline dosage should be based on weight (ie, > or ≤ 45 kg) not age.

The most current versions of Tables 3, 4, and 5 are available online at: http://jama.ama-assn.org/issues/v287n17/ffull/jst20007.html.

The textual changes are as follows: On page 26, the sentence "Penicillin, doxycycline, and ciprofloxacin are approved by the FDA for the treatment of inhalational anthrax infection,[56,89,90,94] and other antibiotics are under study" should read, "Penicillin and doxycycline are approved by the FDA for the treatment of anthrax.[56,89,90,94] Although neither penicillin, doxycycline, nor ciprofloxacin are specifically approved by the FDA for the treatment of inhalational anthrax, these drugs may be useful when given in combination with other antimicrobial drugs."

On page 28, the sentence in the "Postexposure Prophylaxis" section of the text that says, "There are no FDA-approved postexposure antibiotic regimens following exposure to a *B anthracis* aerosol" should read, "Ciprofloxacin, doxycycline, and penicillin G procaine are approved by the FDA for postexposure prophylaxis of inhalational anthrax."

On page 29 in the "Children" subsection, the sentence that begins "According to CDC recommendations . . ." should read "According to the CDC recommendations for the bioterrorist attacks in 2001, in which *B anthracis* was susceptible to penicillin, amoxicillin was a suitable alternative for postexposure prophylaxis in infants and children (Table 4)." In the "Pregnant Women" subsection, the sentence that begins, "According to the CDC recommendations . . ." should read, "According to the CDC recommendations for the bioterrorist attacks in 2001, in which *B anthracis* was susceptible to penicillin, amoxicillin was a suitable alternative for postexposure prophylaxis in women who were pregnant or who were breastfeeding (Table 4)."

©2002 American Medical Association. All rights reserved.

Reprinted with permission from *JAMA*; October 16, 2002, Vol 288, No. 15

Smallpox as a Biological Weapon
Medical and Public Health Management

Donald A. Henderson, MD, MPH

Thomas V. Inglesby, MD

John G. Bartlett, MD

Michael S. Ascher, MD

Edward Eitzen, MD, MPH

Peter B. Jahrling, PhD

Jerome Hauer, MPH

Marcelle Layton, MD

Joseph McDade, PhD

Michael T. Osterholm, PhD, MPH

Tara O'Toole, MD, MPH

Gerald Parker, PhD, DVM

Trish Perl, MD, MSc

Philip K. Russell, MD

Kevin Tonat, PhD

for the Working Group on
Civilian Biodefense

Objective To develop consensus-based recommendations for measures to be taken by medical and public health professionals following the use of smallpox as a biological weapon against a civilian population.

Participants The working group included 21 representatives from staff of major medical centers and research, government, military, public health, and emergency management institutions and agencies.

Evidence The first author (D.A.H.) conducted a literature search in conjunction with the preparation of another publication on smallpox as well as this article. The literature identified was reviewed and opinions were sought from experts in the diagnosis and management of smallpox, including members of the working group.

Consensus Process The first draft of the consensus statement was a synthesis of information obtained in the evidence-gathering process. Members of the working group provided formal written comments that were incorporated into the second draft of the statement. The working group reviewed the second draft on October 30, 1998. No significant disagreements existed and comments were incorporated into a third draft. The fourth and final statement incorporates all relevant evidence obtained by the literature search in conjunction with final consensus recommendations supported by all working group members.

Conclusions Specific recommendations are made regarding smallpox vaccination, therapy, postexposure isolation and infection control, hospital epidemiology and infection control, home care, decontamination of the environment, and additional research needs. In the event of an actual release of smallpox and subsequent epidemic, early detection, isolation of infected individuals, surveillance of contacts, and a focused selective vaccination program will be the essential items of an effective control program.

JAMA. 1999;281:2127-2137   www.jama.com

T HIS IS THE SECOND ARTICLE IN a series entitled *Medical and Public Health Management Following the Use of a Biological Weapon: Consensus Statements of the Working Group on Civilian Biodefense.*[1] The working group has identified a limited number of widely known organisms that could cause disease and deaths in sufficient numbers to cripple a city or region. Smallpox is one of the most serious of these diseases.

If used as a biological weapon, smallpox represents a serious threat to civilian populations because of its case fatality rate of 30% or more among unvaccinated persons and the absence of specific therapy. Although smallpox has long been feared as the most devastating of all infectious diseases,[2] its potential for devastation today is far greater than at any previous time. Rou-

tine vaccination throughout the United States ceased more than 25 years ago. In a now highly susceptible, mobile population, smallpox would be able to spread widely and rapidly throughout this country and the world.

CONSENSUS METHODS

Members of the working group were selected by the chairman in consultation with principal agency heads in the Department of Health and Human Services (DHHS) and the US Army Medical Research Institute of Infectious Diseases (USAMRIID).

The first author (D.A.H.) conducted a literature search in conjunction with the preparation of another

Author Affiliations: The Center for Civilian Biodefense Studies (Drs Henderson, Inglesby, Bartlett, O'Toole, Perl, and Russell), and the Schools of Public Health (Drs Henderson, O'Toole, and Russell) and Medicine (Drs Inglesby, Bartlett, and Perl), Johns Hopkins University, Baltimore, Md; Viral and Rickettsial Diseases, California Department of Health, Berkeley (Dr Ascher); US Army Medical Research Institute of Infectious Diseases, Frederick, Md (Drs Eitzen, Jahrling, and Parker); Office of Emergency Management (Mr Hauer) and Office of Communicable Disease, New York City Health Department (Dr Layton), New York, NY; Centers for Disease Control and Prevention, Atlanta, Ga (Dr McDade); Acute Disease Epidemiology, Minnesota Department of Health, Minneapolis (Dr Osterholm); and Office of Emergency Preparedness, Department of Health and Human Services, Rockville, Md (Dr Tonat).

Corresponding Author and Reprints: Donald A. Henderson, MD, MPH, Johns Hopkins Center for Civilian Biodefense Studies, Johns Hopkins University, Candler Bldg, Suite 850, 111 Market Pl, Baltimore, MD 21202 (e-mail: dahzero@aol.com).

©1999 American Medical Association. All rights reserved.

publication on smallpox[2] as well as this article. The literature was reviewed and opinions were sought from experts in the diagnosis and management of smallpox, including members of the working group.

The first draft of the working group's consensus statement was the result of synthesis of information obtained in the evidence-gathering process. Members of the working group were asked to make written comments on the first draft of the document in September 1998. Suggested revisions were incorporated into the second draft of the statement. The working group was convened to review the second draft of the statement on October 30, 1998. Consensus recommendations were made and no significant disagreements existed at the conclusion of this meeting. The third draft incorporated changes suggested at the conference and working group members had an additional opportunity to suggest final revisions. The final statement incorporates all relevant evidence obtained by the literature search in conjunction with final consensus recommendations supported by all working group members.

This article is intended to provide the scientific foundation and initial framework for the detailed planning that would follow a bioterrorist attack with smallpox. This planning must encompass coordinated systems approaches to bioterrorism, including public policies and consequence management by local and regional public and private institutions. The assessment and recommendations provided herein represent the best professional judgment of the working group at this time based on data and expertise currently available. The conclusions and recommendations need to be regularly reassessed as new information becomes available.

HISTORY AND POTENTIAL AS A BIOWEAPON

Smallpox probably was first used as a biological weapon during the French and Indian Wars (1754-1767) by British forces in North America.[3] Soldiers distributed blankets that had been used by smallpox patients with the intent of initiating outbreaks among American Indians. Epidemics occurred, killing more than 50% of many affected tribes. With Edward Jenner's demonstration in 1796 that an infection caused by cowpox protected against smallpox and the rapid diffusion worldwide of the practice of cowpox inoculation (ie, vaccination),[4] the potential threat of smallpox as a bioweapon was greatly diminished.

A global campaign, begun in 1967 under the aegis of the World Health Organization (WHO), succeeded in eradicating smallpox in 1977.[1] In 1980, the World Health Assembly recommended that all countries cease vaccination.[5] A WHO expert committee recommended that all laboratories destroy their stocks of variola virus or transfer them to 1 of 2 WHO reference laboratories—the Institute of Virus Preparations in Moscow, Russia, or the Centers for Disease Control and Prevention (CDC) in Atlanta, Ga. All countries reported compliance. The WHO committee later recommended that all virus stocks be destroyed in June 1999, and the 1996 World Health Assembly concurred.[6] In 1998, possible research uses for variola virus were reviewed by a committee of the Institute of Medicine (IOM).[7] The IOM committee concluded, as did the preceding WHO committee, that there were research questions that might be addressed if the virus were to be retained. However, the IOM committee did not explore the costs or relative priority to be assigned to such an effort, and that committee was not asked to weigh the possible benefits resulting from such research activities contrasted with the possible benefits resulting from an international decision to destroy all virus stocks. These considerations will be weighed and decided by the 1999 World Health Assembly.

Recent allegations from Ken Alibek, a former deputy director of the Soviet Union's civilian bioweapons program, have heightened concern that smallpox might be used as a bioweapon. Alibek[8] reported that beginning in 1980, the Soviet government embarked on a successful program to produce the smallpox virus in large quantities and adapt it for use in bombs and intercontinental ballistic missiles; the program had an industrial capacity capable of producing many tons of smallpox virus annually. Furthermore, Alibek reports that Russia even now has a research program that seeks to produce more virulent and contagious recombinant strains. Because financial support for laboratories in Russia has sharply declined in recent years, there are increasing concerns that existing expertise and equipment might fall into non-Russian hands.

The deliberate reintroduction of smallpox as an epidemic disease would be an international crime of unprecedented proportions, but it is now regarded as a possibility. An aerosol release of variola virus would disseminate widely, given the considerable stability of the orthopoxviruses in aerosol form[9] and the likelihood that the infectious dose is very small.[10] Moreover, during the 1960s and 1970s in Europe, when smallpox was imported during the December to April period of high transmission, as many as 10 to 20 second-generation cases were often infected from a single case. Widespread concern and, sometimes, panic occurred, even with outbreaks of fewer than 100 cases, resulting in extensive emergency control measures.[2]

EPIDEMIOLOGY

Smallpox was once worldwide in scope, and before vaccination was practiced, almost everyone eventually contracted the disease. There were 2 principal forms of the disease, variola major and a much milder form, variola minor (or alastrim). Before eradication took place, these forms could be differentiated clinically only when occurring in outbreaks; virological differentiation is now possible.[11,12] Through the end of the 19th century, variola major predominated throughout the world. However, at the turn of the century, variola minor was first detected in South Africa and later in Florida, from whence it spread

©1999 American Medical Association. All rights reserved.

Reprinted with permission from *JAMA*; June 9, 1999, Vol 281, No. 22

across the United States and into Latin America and Europe.[13] Typical variola major epidemics such as those that occurred in Asia resulted in case-fatality rates of 30% or higher among the unvaccinated, whereas variola minor case-fatality rates were customarily 1% or less.[2]

Smallpox spreads from person to person,[10,14] primarily by droplet nuclei or aerosols expelled from the oropharynx of infected persons and by direct contact. Contaminated clothing or bed linens can also spread the virus.[15] There are no known animal or insect reservoirs or vectors.

Historically, the rapidity of smallpox transmission throughout the population was generally slower than for such diseases as measles or chickenpox. Patients spread smallpox primarily to household members and friends; large outbreaks in schools, for example, were uncommon. This finding was accounted for in part by the fact that transmission of smallpox virus did not occur until onset of rash. By then, many patients had been confined to bed because of the high fever and malaise of the prodromal illness. Secondary cases were thus usually restricted to those who came into contact with patients, usually in the household or hospital.

The seasonal occurrence of smallpox was similar to that of chickenpox and measles—its incidence was highest during winter and early spring.[16] This pattern was consonant with the observation that the duration of survival of orthopoxviruses in the aerosolized form was inversely proportional to both temperature and humidity.[9] Likewise, when imported cases occurred in Europe, large outbreaks sometimes developed during the winter months, rarely during the summer.[17]

The patient was most infectious from onset of rash through the first 7 to 10 days of rash (**Figure 1**).[17,18] As scabs formed, infectivity waned rapidly. Although the scabs contained large amounts of viable virus, epidemiological and laboratory studies indicate that they were not especially infectious, pre-

sumably because the virions were bound tightly in the fibrin matrix.[19]

The age distribution of cases depended primarily on the degree of smallpox susceptibility in the population. In most areas, cases predominated among children because adults were protected by immunity induced by vaccination or previous smallpox infection. In rural areas that had seen little vaccination or smallpox, the age distribution of cases was similar to the age distribution of the population. The age distribution pattern of cases in the United States presumably would be such if smallpox were to occur now because vaccination immunity in the population has waned so substantially.

MICROBIOLOGY

Smallpox, a DNA virus, is a member of the genus orthopoxvirus.[20] The orthopoxviruses are among the largest and most complex of all viruses. The virion is characteristically a brick-shaped structure with a diameter of about 200 nm. Three other members of this genus (monkeypox, vaccinia, and cowpox) can also infect humans, causing cutaneous lesions, but only smallpox is readily transmitted from person to person.[2] Monkeypox, a zoonotic disease, presently is found only in tropical rain forest areas of central and western Africa and is not readily transmitted among hu-

mans.[21] Vaccinia and cowpox seldom spread from person to person.

PATHOGENESIS AND CLINICAL PRESENTATION

Natural infection occurs following implantation of the virus on the oropharyngeal or respiratory mucosa.[2] The infectious dose is unknown but is believed to be only a few virions.[10] After the migration of virus to and multiplication in regional lymph nodes, an asymptomatic viremia develops on about the third or fourth day, followed by multiplication of virus in the spleen, bone marrow, and lymph nodes. A secondary viremia begins on about the eighth day and is followed by fever and toxemia. The virus, contained in leukocytes, then localizes in small blood vessels of the dermis and beneath the oral and pharyngeal mucosa and subsequently infects adjacent cells.

At the end of the 12- to 14-day incubation period (range, 7-17 days), the patient typically experiences high fever, malaise, and prostration with headache and backache.[2] Severe abdominal pain and delirium are sometimes present. A maculopapular rash then appears on the mucosa of the mouth and pharynx, face, and forearms, and spreads to the trunk and legs (**Figure 2**).[2] Within 1 to 2 days, the rash becomes vesicular and, later, pustu-

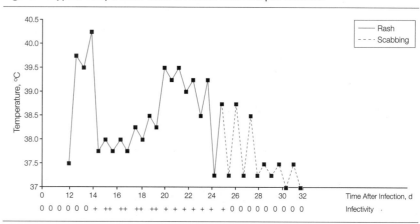

Figure 1. Typical Temperature Chart of Patient With Smallpox Infection

Chart shows approximate time of appearance, evolution of the rash, and magnitude of infectivity relative to the number of days after acquisition of infection.[3,26,29]

©1999 American Medical Association. All rights reserved.

Reprinted with permission from *JAMA*; June 9, 1999, Vol 281, No. 22

lar. The pustules are characteristically round, tense, and deeply embedded in the dermis; crusts begin to form on about the eighth or ninth day of rash. As the patient recovers, the scabs separate and characteristic pitted scarring gradually develops. The scars are most evident on the face and result from the destruction of sebaceous glands followed by shrinking of granulation tissue and fibrosis.[2]

The lesions that first appear in the mouth and pharynx ulcerate quickly because of the absence of a stratum corneum, releasing large amounts of virus into the saliva.[22] Virus titers in saliva are highest during the first week of illness, corresponding with the period during which patients are most infectious. Although the virus in some instances can be detected in swabs taken from the oropharynx as many as 5 to 6 days before the rash develops,[22] transmission does not occur during this period.

Except for the lesions in the skin and mucous membranes and reticulum cell hyperplasia, other organs are seldom involved. Secondary bacterial infection is not common, and death, which usually occurs during the second week of illness, most likely results from the toxemia associated with circulating immune complexes and soluble variola antigens.[2] Encephalitis sometimes ensues that is indistinguishable from the acute perivascular demyelination observed as a complication of infection due to vaccinia, measles, or varicella.[23]

Neutralizing antibodies can be detected by the sixth day of rash and remain at high titers for many years.[24] Hemagglutinin-inhibiting antibodies can be detected on about the sixth day of rash, or about 21 days after infection, and complement-fixing antibodies appear approximately 2 days later. Within 5 years, hemagglutinin-inhibiting antibodies decline to low levels and complement-fixing antibodies rarely persist for longer than 6 months.[2]

Although at least 90% of smallpox cases are clinically characteristic and readily diagnosed in endemic areas, 2 other forms of smallpox are difficult to recognize—hemorrhagic and malignant. Hemorrhagic cases are uniformly fatal and occur among all ages and in both sexes, but pregnant women appear to be unusually susceptible. Illness usually begins with a somewhat shorter incubation period and is characterized by a severely prostrating prodromal illness with high fever and head, back, and abdominal pain. Soon thereafter, a dusky erythema develops, followed by petechiae and frank hemorrhages into the skin and mucous membranes. Death usually occurs by the fifth or sixth day after onset of rash.[23]

In the frequently fatal malignant form, the abrupt onset and prostrating constitutional symptoms are similar. The confluent lesions develop slowly, never progressing to the pustular stage but remaining soft, flattened, and velvety to the touch. The skin has the appearance of a fine-grained, reddish-colored crepe rubber, sometimes with hemorrhages. If the patient survives, the lesions gradually disappear without forming scabs or, in severe cases, large amounts of epidermis might peel away.[23]

The illness associated with variola minor is generally less severe, with fewer constitutional symptoms and a more sparse rash.[25] A milder form of disease is also seen among those who have residual immunity from previous vaccination. In partially immune persons, the rash tends to be atypical and more scant and the evolution of the lesions more rapid.[15]

There is little information about how individuals with different types of immune deficiency responded to natural smallpox infection. Smallpox was eradicated before human immunodeficiency virus (HIV) was identified and

Figure 2. Typical Case of Smallpox Infection in a Child

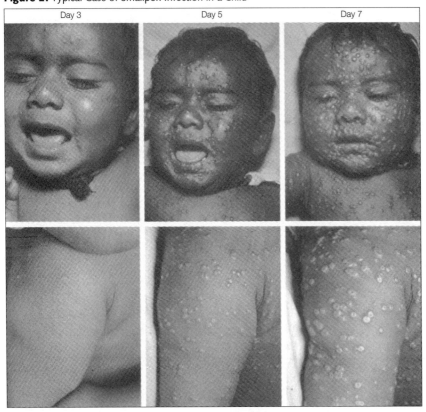

| Day 3 | Day 5 | Day 7 |

Figure shows the appearance of the rash at days 3, 5, and 7 of evolution. Note that lesions are more dense on the face and extremities than on the trunk; that they appear on the palms of the hand; and that they are similar in appearance to each other. If this were a case of chickenpox, one would expect to see, in any area, macules, papules, pustules, and lesions with scabs. Reproduced with permission from the World Health Organization.[2]

©1999 American Medical Association. All rights reserved.

Reprinted with permission from *JAMA*; June 9, 1999, Vol 281, No. 22

before suitable techniques became available for measuring cell-mediated immunity. However, it is probable that the underlying cause of some cases of malignant and hemorrhagic smallpox resulted from defective immune responses. Vaccination of immune-deficient persons sometimes resulted in a continually spreading primary lesion, persistent viremia, and secondary viral infection of many organs. One such case is documented to have occurred in a vaccinated soldier who had HIV infection.[26]

DIAGNOSIS

The discovery of a single suspected case of smallpox must be treated as an international health emergency and be brought immediately to the attention of national officials through local and state health authorities.

The majority of smallpox cases present with a characteristic rash that is centrifugal in distribution, ie, most dense on the face and extremities. The lesions appear during a 1- to 2-day period and evolve at the same rate. On any given part of the body, they are generally at the same stage of development. In varicella (chickenpox), the disease most frequently confused with smallpox, new lesions appear in crops every few days and lesions at very different stages of maturation (ie, vesicles, pustules, and scabs) are found in adjacent areas of skin. Varicella lesions are much more superficial and are almost never found on the palms and soles. The distribution of varicella lesions is centripetal, with a greater concentration of lesions on the trunk than on the face and extremities.

The signs and symptoms of both hemorrhagic and malignant smallpox were such that smallpox was seldom suspected until more typical cases were seen and it was recognized that a smallpox outbreak was in progress. Hemorrhagic cases were most often initially identified as meningococcemia or severe acute leukemia. Malignant cases likewise posed diagnostic problems, most often being mistaken for hemorrhagic chickenpox or prompting surgery because of severe abdominal pain.

Laboratory confirmation of the diagnosis in a smallpox outbreak is important. Specimens should be collected by someone who has recently been vaccinated (or is vaccinated that day) and who wears gloves and a mask. To obtain vesicular or pustular fluid, it is often necessary to open lesions with the blunt edge of a scalpel. The fluid can then be harvested on a cotton swab. Scabs can be picked off with forceps. Specimens should be deposited in a vacutainer tube that should be sealed with adhesive tape at the juncture of stopper and tube. This tube, in turn, should be enclosed in a second durable, watertight container. State or local health department laboratories should immediately be contacted regarding the shipping of specimens. Laboratory examination requires high-containment (BL-4) facilities and should be undertaken only in designated laboratories with the appropriate training and equipment. Once it is established that the epidemic is caused by smallpox virus, clinically typical cases would not require further laboratory confirmation.

Smallpox infection can be rapidly confirmed in the laboratory by electron microscopic examination of vesicular or pustular fluid or scabs. Although all orthopoxviruses exhibit identically appearing brick-shaped virions, history taking and clinical picture readily identify cowpox and vaccinia. Although smallpox and monkeypox virions may be indistinguishable, naturally occurring monkeypox is found only in tropical rain forest areas of Africa. Definitive laboratory identification and characterization of the virus involves growth of the virus in cell culture or on chorioallantoic egg membrane and characterization of strains by use of various biologic assays, including polymerase chain reaction techniques and restriction fragment-length polymorphisms.[27-29] The latter studies can be completed within a few hours.

PREEXPOSURE PREVENTIVE VACCINATION

Before 1972, smallpox vaccination was recommended for all US children at age 1 year. Most states required that each child be vaccinated before school en-

try. The only other requirement for vaccination was for military recruits and tourists visiting foreign countries. Most countries required that the individual be successfully vaccinated within a 3-year period prior to entering the country. Routine vaccination in the United States stopped in 1972 and since then, few persons younger than 27 years have been vaccinated. The US Census Bureau reported that in 1998, approximately 114 million persons, or 42% of the US population, were aged 29 years or younger.[30]

In addition, the immune status of those who were vaccinated more than 27 years ago is not clear. The duration of immunity, based on the experience of naturally exposed susceptible persons, has never been satisfactorily measured. Neutralizing antibodies are reported to reflect levels of protection, although this has not been validated in the field. These antibodies have been shown to decline substantially during a 5- to 10-year period.[24] Thus, even those who received the recommended single-dose vaccination as children do not have lifelong immunity. However, among a group who had been vaccinated at birth and at ages 8 and 18 years as part of a study, neutralizing antibody levels remained stable during a 30-year period.[31] Because comparatively few persons today have been successfully vaccinated on more than 1 occasion, it must be assumed that the population at large is highly susceptible to infection.

In the United States, a limited reserve supply of vaccine that was produced by Wyeth Laboratories, Lancaster, Pa, in the 1970s is in storage. This supply is believed to be sufficient to vaccinate between 6 and 7 million persons. This vaccine, now under the control of the CDC, consists of vaccine virus (New York Board of Health strain) grown on scarified calves. After purification, it was freeze-dried in rubber-stoppered vials that contain sufficient vaccine for at least 50 doses when a bifurcated needle is used. It is stored at −20°C (James LeDuc, PhD, oral communication, 1998). Although quantities of vaccine have also been retained

©1999 American Medical Association. All rights reserved.

Reprinted with permission from *JAMA*; June 9, 1999, Vol 281, No. 22

by a number of other countries, none have reserves large enough to meet more than their own potential emergency needs. WHO has 500 000 doses.[32]

There are no manufacturers now equipped to produce smallpox vaccine in large quantities. The development and licensure of a tissue cell culture vaccine and the establishment of a new vaccine production facility is estimated to require at least 36 months (Thomas Monath, MD, unpublished data, 1999).

Because of the small amounts of vaccine available, a preventive vaccination program to protect individuals such as emergency and health care personnel is not an option at this time. When additional supplies of vaccine are procured, a decision to undertake preventive vaccination of some portion of the population will have to weigh the relative risk of vaccination complications against the threat of contracting smallpox.

A further deterrent to extensive vaccination is the fact that presently available supplies of vaccinia immune globulin (VIG), also maintained by the CDC, are very limited in quantity. The working group recommends VIG for the treatment of severe cutaneous reactions occurring as a complication of vaccination.[33,34] Vaccinia immune globulin has also been given along with vaccination to protect those who needed vaccination but who were at risk of experiencing vaccine-related complications.[33] It has been estimated that if 1 million persons were vaccinated, as many as 250 persons would experience adverse reactions of a type that would require administration of VIG (James LeDuc, PhD, oral communication, 1998). How much VIG would be needed to administer with vaccine to those at risk is unknown.

POSTEXPOSURE THERAPY

At this time, the best that can be offered to the patient infected with smallpox is supportive therapy plus antibiotics as indicated for treatment of occasional secondary bacterial infections. No antiviral substances have yet proved effective for the treatment of smallpox, and the working group is not aware of any reports that suggest any an-

tiviral product is therapeutic. Encouraging initial reports in the 1960s describing the therapeutic benefits of the thiosemicarbazones, cytosine arabinoside, and adenine arabinoside proved questionable on further study.[21,35,36]

Recent studies on tissue culture, mice, and a small number of monkeys have suggested the possibility that cidofovir, a nucleoside analog DNA polymerase inhibitor, might prove useful in preventing smallpox infection if administered within 1 or 2 days after exposure (John Huggins, PhD, oral communication, 1998). At this time, there is no evidence that cidofovir is more effective than vaccination in this early period. Moreover, the potential utility of this drug is limited, given the fact that it must be administered intravenously and its use is often accompanied by serious renal toxicity.[37]

POSTEXPOSURE INFECTION CONTROL

A smallpox outbreak poses difficult public health problems because of the ability of the virus to continue to spread throughout the population unless checked by vaccination and/or isolation of patients and their close contacts.

A clandestine aerosol release of smallpox, even if it infected only 50 to 100 persons to produce the first generation of cases, would rapidly spread in a now highly susceptible population, expanding by a factor of 10 to 20 times or more with each generation of cases.[2,10,38] Between the time of an aerosol release of smallpox virus and diagnosis of the first cases, an interval as long as 2 weeks or more is apt to occur because of the average incubation period of 12 to 14 days and the lapse of several additional days before a rash was sufficiently distinct to suggest the diagnosis of smallpox. By that time, there would be no risk of further environmental exposure from the original aerosol release because the virus is fully inactivated within 2 days.

As soon as the diagnosis of smallpox is made, all individuals in whom smallpox is suspected should be iso-

lated immediately and all household and other face-to-face contacts should be vaccinated and placed under surveillance. Because the widespread dissemination of smallpox virus by aerosol poses a serious threat in hospitals, patients should be isolated in the home or other nonhospital facility whenever possible. Home care for most patients is a reasonable approach, given the fact that little can be done for a patient other than to offer supportive therapy.

In the event of an aerosol release of smallpox and a subsequent outbreak, the rationale for vaccinating patients suspected to have smallpox at this time is to ensure that some with a mistaken diagnosis are not placed at risk of acquiring smallpox. Vaccination administered within the first few days after exposure and perhaps as late as 4 days may prevent or significantly ameliorate subsequent illness.[39] An emergency vaccination program is also indicated that would include all health care workers at clinics or hospitals that might receive patients; all other essential disaster response personnel, such as police, firefighters, transit workers, public health staff, and emergency management staff; and mortuary staff who might have to handle bodies. The working group recommends that all such personnel for whom vaccination is not contraindicated should be vaccinated immediately irrespective of prior vaccination status.

Vaccination administered within 4 days of first exposure has been shown to offer some protection against acquiring infection and significant protection against a fatal outcome.[15] Those who have been vaccinated at some time in the past will normally exhibit an accelerated immune response. Thus, it would be prudent, when possible, to assign those who had been previously vaccinated to duties involving close patient contact.

It is important that discretion be used in identifying contacts of patients to ensure, to the extent that is possible, that vaccination and adequate surveillance measures are focused on those at great-

©1999 American Medical Association. All rights reserved.

Reprinted with permission from *JAMA*; June 9, 1999, Vol 281, No. 22

est risk. Specifically, it is recommended that *contacts* be defined as persons who have been in the same household as the infected individual or who have been in face-to-face contact with the patient after the onset of fever. Experience during the smallpox global eradication program showed that patients did not transmit infection until after the prodromal fever had given way to the rash stage of illness.[17,18]

Isolation of all contacts of exposed patients would be logistically difficult and, in practice, should not be necessary. Because contacts, even if infected, are not contagious until onset of rash, a practical strategy calls for all contacts to have temperatures checked at least once each day, preferably in the evening. Any increase in temperature higher than 38°C (101°F) during the 17-day period following last exposure to the case would suggest the possible development of smallpox[2] and be cause for isolating the patient immediately, preferably at home, until it could be determined clinically and/or by laboratory examination whether the contact had smallpox. All close contacts of the patients should be promptly vaccinated.

Although cooperation by most patients and contacts in observing isolation could be ensured through counseling and persuasion, there may be some for whom forcible quarantine will be required. Some states and cities in the United States, but not all, confer broad discretionary powers on health authorities to ensure the safety of the public's health and, at one time, this included powers to quarantine. Under epidemic circumstances, this could be an important power to have. Thus, each state and city should review its statutes as part of its preparedness activities.

During the smallpox epidemics in the 1960s and 1970s in Europe, there was considerable public alarm whenever outbreaks occurred and, often, a demand for mass vaccination throughout a very widespread area, even when the vaccination coverage of the population was high.[2] In the United States, where few people now have protective levels of immunity, such levels of con-

cern must be anticipated. However, the US vaccine supply is limited at present; thus, vaccine would have to be carefully conserved and used in conjunction with measures to implement rapid isolation of smallpox patients.

HOSPITAL EPIDEMIOLOGY AND INFECTION CONTROL

Smallpox transmission within hospitals has long been recognized as a serious problem. For this reason, separate hospitals for smallpox patients were used for more than 200 years. Throughout the 1970s, both England and Germany had fully equipped standby hospitals in case smallpox should be imported.[2] Infections acquired in hospitals may occur as the result of droplets spread from patients to staff and visitors in reasonably close contact or by a fine particle aerosol. In 1 such occurrence in Germany, a smallpox patient with a cough, although isolated in a single room, infected persons on 3 floors of a hospital.[10] Persons with the usually fatal hemorrhagic or malignant forms of the disease pose a special problem because they often remain undiagnosed until they are near death and extremely contagious. A number of outbreaks have occurred in laundry workers who handled linens and blankets used by patients.[15] The working group recommends that in an outbreak setting, all hospital employees as well as patients in the hospital be vaccinated. For individuals who are immunocompromised or for whom vaccination is otherwise contraindicated, VIG should be provided, if available. If it is not available, a judgment will have to be made regarding the relative risks of acquiring the disease in contrast with the risks associated with vaccination.

In the event of a limited outbreak with few cases, patients should be admitted to the hospital and confined to rooms that are under negative pressure and equipped with high-efficiency particulate air filtration. In larger outbreaks, home isolation and care should be the objective for most patients. However, not all will be able to be so accommodated and, to limit nosocomial infections, authorities should

consider the possibility of designating a specific hospital or hospitals for smallpox care. All persons isolated as such and those caring for them should be immediately vaccinated. Employees for whom vaccination is contraindicated should be furloughed.

Standard precautions using gloves, gowns, and masks should be observed. All laundry and waste should be placed in biohazard bags and autoclaved before being laundered or incinerated. A special protocol should be developed for decontaminating rooms after they are vacated by patients (see "Decontamination" section).

Laboratory examination requires high-containment (BL-4) facilities and should be undertaken only in designated laboratories with the appropriate trained personnel and equipment. Specific recommendations for safe specimen transport are described in the section on "Differential Diagnosis and Diagnostic Tests."

Protecting against the explosive spread of virus from the hemorrhagic or malignant case is difficult. Such cases occurring during the course of an outbreak may be detected if staff is alert to the possibility that any severe, acute, prostrating illness must be considered smallpox until proven otherwise.

Patients who die of smallpox should be cremated whenever possible and mortuary workers should be vaccinated.

VACCINE ADMINISTRATION AND COMPLICATIONS

Smallpox vaccine is currently approved by the US Food and Drug Administration (FDA) for use only in persons in special-risk categories, including laboratory workers directly involved with smallpox or closely related orthopoxviruses. Under epidemic circumstances, widespread vaccination would be indicated, as recommended by the working group.

Vaccination has been successfully and safely administered to persons of all ages, from birth onward.[40] However, there are certain groups for whom elective vaccination has not been recommended be-

©1999 American Medical Association. All rights reserved.

Reprinted with permission from *JAMA*; June 9, 1999, Vol 281, No. 22

cause of the risk of complications. Under epidemic circumstances, however, such contraindications will have to be weighed against the grave risks posed by smallpox. If available, VIG can be administered concomitantly with vaccination to minimize the risk of complications in these persons.

Figure 3. Vaccination With the Bifurcated Needle

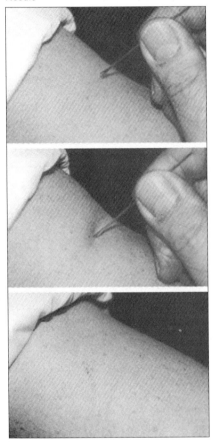

The requisite amount of reconstituted vaccine is held between the prongs of the needle and vaccination is done by multiple punctures; 15 strokes, at right angles to the skin over the deltoid muscle, are rapidly made within an area of about 5 mm in diameter.

Vaccination is normally performed using the bifurcated needle (FIGURE 3). A sterile needle is inserted into an ampoule of reconstituted vaccine and, on withdrawal, a droplet of vaccine sufficient for vaccination is held by capillarity between the 2 tines. The needle is held at right angles to the skin; the wrist of the vaccinator rests against the arm. Fifteen perpendicular strokes of the needle are rapidly made in an area of about 5 mm in diameter.[41,42] The strokes should be sufficiently vigorous so that a trace of blood appears at the vaccination site after 15 to 30 seconds. After vaccination, excess vaccine should be wiped from the site with gauze that should be discarded in a hazardous waste receptacle. The site should be covered with a loose, nonocclusive bandage to deter the individual from touching the site and perhaps transferring virus to other parts of the body.

After about 3 days, a red papule appears at the vaccination site and becomes vesicular on about the fifth day (FIGURE 4). By the seventh day, it becomes the typical Jennerian pustule—whitish, umbilicated, multilocular, containing turbid lymph and surrounded by an erythematous areola that may continue to expand for 3 more days. Regional lymphadenopathy and fever is not uncommon. As many as 70% of children have 1 or more days of temperature higher than 39°C (100°F) between days 4 and 14.[43] The pustule gradually dries, leaving a dark crust, which normally falls off after about 3 weeks.

A successful vaccination for those with partial immunity may manifest a gradient of responses. These range from what appears to be a primary take (as

described herein) to an accelerated reaction in which there may be little more than a papule surrounded by erythema that reaches a peak between 3 and 7 days. A response that reaches a peak in erythema within 48 hours represents a hypersensitivity reaction and does not signify that growth of the vaccinia virus has occurred.[2] Persons exhibiting such a reaction should be revaccinated.

Complications

The frequency of complications associated with use of the New York Board of Health strain (the strain used throughout the United States and Canada for vaccine) is the lowest for any established vaccinia virus strain, but the risks are not inconsequential.[44,45] Data on complications gathered by the CDC in 1968 are shown in TABLE 1. Complications occurred most frequently among primary vaccinees.

Postvaccinial Encephalitis. Postvaccinial encephalitis occurred at a rate of 1 case per 300 000 vaccinations and was observed only in primary vaccinees; one fourth of these cases were fatal and several had permanent neurological residua. Between 8 and 15 days after vaccination, encephalitic symptoms developed—fever, headache, vomiting, drowsiness, and, sometimes, spastic paralysis, meningitic signs, coma, and convulsions. Cerebrospinal fluid usually showed a pleocytosis. Recovery was either complete or associated with residual paralysis and other central nervous system symptoms and, sometimes, death. There was no treatment.

Progressive Vaccinia (Vaccinia Gangrenosa). Cases of progressive vaccinia occurred both among primary vaccinees and revaccinees. It was a frequently fatal complication among those with immune deficiency disorders. The vaccinial lesion failed to heal and progressed to involve adjacent skin with necrosis of tissue, spreading to other parts of the skin, to bones, and to viscera. Vaccinia immune globulin was used for this problem.[34,46] One case in a soldier with acquired immunodeficiency syndrome was successfully

Figure 4. Typical Appearance of an Evolving Primary Vaccination Take

Day 0	Day 3	Day 7	Day 10	Day 14

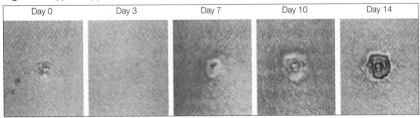

Reproduced with permission from the Centers for Disease Control and Prevention.[3]

©1999 American Medical Association. All rights reserved.

Reprinted with permission from *JAMA*; June 9, 1999, Vol 281, No. 22

treated with VIG and ribavirin. These treatment strategies were off-label and would be considered experimental.[26]

Eczema Vaccinatum. A sometimes serious complication, eczema vaccinatum occurred in some vaccinees and contacts with either active or healed eczema. Vaccinial skin lesions extended to cover all or most of the area once or currently afflicted with eczema. Vaccinia immune globulin was therapeutic.[46]

Generalized Vaccinia. A secondary eruption almost always following primary vaccination, generalized vaccinia resulted from blood-borne dissemination of virus. Lesions emerged between 6 and 9 days after vaccination and were either few in number or generalized. This complication was usually self-limited. In severe cases, VIG was indicated.[46]

Inadvertent Inoculation. Transmission to close contacts or autoinoculation to sites such as face, eyelid, mouth, and genitalia sometimes occurred. Most lesions healed without incident, although VIG was useful in some cases of periocular implantation.

Miscellaneous. Many different rashes have been associated with vaccination. Most common are erythema multiforme and variously distributed urticarial, maculopapular, and blotchy erythematous eruptions, which normally clear without therapy.

Groups at Special Risk for Complications

Consensus recommendations for special-risk groups as set forth herein reflect the best clinical and science-based judgment of the working group

and do not necessarily correspond to FDA-approved uses.

Five groups of persons are ordinarily considered at special risk of smallpox vaccine complications: (1) persons with eczema or other significant exfoliative skin conditions; (2) patients with leukemia, lymphoma, or generalized malignancy who are receiving therapy with alkylating agents, antimetabolites, radiation, or large doses of corticosteroids; (3) patients with HIV infection; (4) persons with hereditary immune deficiency disorders; and (5) pregnant women. If persons with contraindications have been in close contact with a smallpox patient or the individual is at risk for occupational reasons, VIG, if available, may be given simultaneously with vaccination in a dose of 0.3 mL/kg of body weight to prevent complications. This does not alter vaccine efficacy. If VIG is not available, vaccine administration may still be warranted, given the far higher risk of an adverse outcome from smallpox infection than from vaccination.

VIG Therapy for Complications

Vaccinia immune globulin is valuable in treating patients with progressive vaccinia, eczema vaccinatum, severe generalized vaccinia, and periocular infections resulting from inadvertent inoculation. It is administered intramuscularly in a dose of 0.6 mL/kg of body weight. Because the dose is large (eg, 42 mL for a person weighing 70 kg), the product is given intramuscularly in divided doses over a 24- to 36-hour period and may be repeated, if necessary, after 2 to 3 days if improvement is not occurring.[47] Because the availability of

VIG is so limited, its use should be reserved for the most serious cases. Vaccinia immune globulin, as well as vaccinia vaccine, is made available by the CDC through state health departments. Consultative assistance in the diagnosis and management of patients with complications can be obtained through state health departments.

DECONTAMINATION

Vaccinia virus, if released as an aerosol and not exposed to UV light, may persist for as long as 24 hours or somewhat longer under favorable conditions.[9] It is believed that variola virus would exhibit similar properties. However, by the time patients had become ill and it had been determined that an aerosol release of smallpox virus had occurred, there would be no viable smallpox virus in the environment. Vaccinia virus, if released as an aerosol, is almost completely destroyed within 6 hours in an atmosphere of high temperature (31°C-33°C) and humidity (80%) (TABLE 2).[9] In cooler temperatures (10°C-11°C) and lower humidity (20%), nearly two thirds of a vaccinia aerosol survives for as long as 24 hours.[9] It is believed that variola would behave similarly.

The occurrence of smallpox infection among personnel who handled laundry from infected patients is well documented[15] and it is believed that virus in such material remains viable for extended periods. Thus, special precautions need to be taken to ensure that all bedding and clothing of smallpox patients is autoclaved or laundered in hot water to which bleach has been added. Disinfectants that are used for standard hospital infection control, such as

Table 1. Complications of Smallpox Vaccination in the United States for 1968—Centers for Disease Control and Prevention National Survey[45]

Vaccination Status, Age, y	Estimated No. of Vaccinations	No. of Cases						
		Postvaccinial Encephalitis*	Progressive Vaccinia*	Eczema Vaccinatum*	Generalized Vaccinia	Accidental Infection	Other	Total
Primary vaccination†	5 594 000	16 (4)	5 (2)	58	131	142	66	418
Revaccination	8 574 000	0	6 (2)	8	10	7	9	40
Contacts	. . .‡	0	0	60 (1)	2	44	8	114
Total	14 168 000	16 (4)	11 (4)	126 (1)	143	193	83	572

*Data in parentheses indicate number of deaths attributable to vaccination.
†Data include 31 patients with unknown vaccination status.
‡Ellipses indicate contacts were not vaccinated.

©1999 American Medical Association. All rights reserved.

Reprinted with permission from *JAMA*; June 9, 1999, Vol 281, No. 22

hypochlorite and quaternary ammonia, are effective for cleaning surfaces possibly contaminated with virus.

Virus in scabs is more durable. At a temperature of 35°C and 65% relative humidity, the virus has persisted for 3 weeks.[48] At cooler temperatures (26°C), the virus has survived for 8 weeks at high relative humidity and 12 weeks at a relative humidity less than 10%.[48] Dutch investigators demonstrated that it was possible to isolate variola virus from scabs that had been sitting on a shelf for 13 years.[49] It is unlikely, however, that the smallpox virus, bound in the fibrin matrix of a scab, is infectious in humans. This is borne out by studies conducted during the eradication program and by surveillance for cases in newly smallpox-free areas.[2] It was reasoned that if the virus were able to persist in nature and infect humans, there would be cases occurring for which no source could be identified. Cases of this type were not observed. Rather, when cases were found, there were antecedent human cases with whom they had direct contact.

RESEARCH

Priority should be directed to 3 areas of smallpox research: vaccines, immunotherapy and drugs, and diagnostics.

The working group recommends that an emergency stockpile of at least 40 million doses of vaccine and a standby manufacturing capacity to produce more is a critical need. At a minimum, this quantity of vaccine would be needed in the control of an epidemic during the first 4 to 8 weeks after an attack. Smallpox vaccine, contained in glass-sealed ampoules and stored at –20°C, retains its potency almost indefinitely. However, several steps are necessary before manufacturing can begin. The traditional method for producing vaccine on the scarified flank of a calf is no longer acceptable because the product inevitably contains some microbial contaminants, however stringent the purification measures. Contemporary vaccines require the use of tissue cell cultures. Thus, as a first step, the traditional New York Board of Health strain needs to be grown in a suitable tissue cell culture and comparative studies performed of the reactogenicity and immunogenicity of calf-derived and tissue cell culture vaccines. This should be a comparatively straightforward exercise. The cost of such a stockpile should be comparatively modest because the vaccine would be packaged in 50-dose rather than costly single-dose containers. In the mid-1970s, 40 million doses would have cost less than $5 million (D.A.H., unpublished data, 1975).

The frequency of vaccine complications is sufficiently great to recommend development, if possible, of a more attenuated strain that, hopefully, would retain full efficacy. Development of an entirely new, genetically engineered strain would be both costly and time consuming. Moreover, it would be difficult at this time to justify its use in large numbers of human subjects to evaluate safety. There is, however, a candidate at-tenuated strain that was developed and field tested in Japan in the mid-1970s (a Lister strain–derived vaccine[50] that has been produced in volume in rabbit kidney cell culture and has been given to more than 100 000 persons in Japan). Research showed no severe complications among the first 30 000 vaccinees.[51] The cutaneous responses to vaccination were much less severe and far fewer vaccinees developed fever. More than 95% developed a Jennerian pustule; immunogenicity, as measured by neutralizing antibody, was slightly lower than for nonattenuated strains.

Vaccinia immune globulin has been used for the treatment of vaccine complications and for administration with vaccine to those for whom vaccine is otherwise contraindicated. Production of VIG should be a high priority for research. An alternative to VIG is also needed because VIG is difficult to produce and cumbersome to administer. Immunotherapy using humanized monoclonal antibodies is an alternative that should be explored. Studies of antiviral agents or drugs, already approved or near approval for marketing for use in other viral diseases, have suggested that 1 or more such products might prove useful.

Finally, a simple, rapid diagnostic test to identify variola virus in the oropharynx during the prodrome or early in the exanthematous phase of illness would be of considerable help in triage of suspected patients during the course of an outbreak.

SUMMARY

The specter of resurgent smallpox is ominous, especially given the enormous efforts that have been made to eradicate what has been characterized as the most devastating of all the pestilential diseases. Unfortunately, the threat of an aerosol release of smallpox is real and the potential for a catastrophic scenario is great unless effective control measures can quickly be brought to bear.

Early detection, isolation of infected individuals, surveillance of contacts, and a focused selective vaccina-

Table 2. Viability of Vaccinia Virus in Aerosols at Various Intervals After Spraying[9]

| Temperature, °C | Relative Humidity, % | Viable Vaccinia, %* | | | |
		1 h	4 h	6 h	23 h
10.5-11.5	20	82	79	81	66
	50	83	92	77	59
	82-84	79	59	60	27
21.0-23.0	18-19	66	46	45	15
	48-51	86	57	50	12
	82-84	66	24	18	Trace
31.5-33.5	17-19	61	51	33	13
	50	51	26	15	Trace
	80-83	36	5.9	1.2	Trace

*Initial titer of $10^{7.7}$ plaque-forming units per milliliter of McIlvaine buffer, containing 1% dialyzed horse serum.

©1999 American Medical Association. All rights reserved.

Reprinted with permission from JAMA; June 9, 1999, Vol 281, No. 22

tion program are the essential items of a control program. Educating health care professionals about the diagnostic features of smallpox should permit early detection; advance regionwide planning for isolation and care of infected individuals in their homes as appropriate and in hospitals when home care is not an option will be critical to deter spread. Ultimately, success in controlling a burgeoning epidemic will depend on the availability of adequate supplies of vaccine and VIG. An adequate stockpile of those commodities would offer a relatively inexpensive safeguard against tragedy.

Ex Officio Participants in the Working Group on Civilian Biodefense: George Curlin, MD, National Institutes of Health, Bethesda, Md; Margaret Hamburg, MD, and William Roub, PhD, Office of Assistant Secretary for Planning and Evaluation, DHHS, Washington, DC; Robert Knouss, MD, Office of Emergency Preparedness, DHHS, Rockville, Md; Marcelle Layton, MD, Office of Communicable Disease, New York City Health Department, New York, NY; and Brian Malkin and Stuart Nightingale, MD, FDA, Rockville, Md.
Funding/Support: Funding for this study primarily was provided by each participant's institution or agency. The Johns Hopkins Center for Civilian Biodefense Studies provided travel funds for 3 members of the group.
Disclaimers: In many cases, the indication and dosages and other information are not consistent with current FDA-approved labeling. The recommendations on the use of drugs and vaccine for uses not approved by the FDA do not represent the official views of the FDA or of any of the federal agencies whose scientists participated in these discussions. Unlabeled uses of the products recommended are noted in the sections of this article in which these products are discussed. Where unlabeled uses are indicated, information used as the basis for the recommendations is discussed.
The views, opinions, assertions, and findings contained herein are those of the authors and should not be construed as official US Department of Defense or US Department of Army positions, policies, or decisions unless so designated by other documentation.
Additional Articles: This article is second in a series entitled *Medical and Public Health Management Following the Use of a Biological Weapon: Consensus Statements of the Working Group on Civilian Biodefense.* See reference 1.
Acknowledgment: The working group wishes to thank Isao Arita, MD, Agency for Cooperation in International Health, Kumamoto, Japan; Joel Bremen, MD, DTPH, Fogarty International Center, Bethesda; Joseph Esposito, PhD, and Brian Mahy, PhD, ScD, CDC, Atlanta, Ga; Frank Fenner, MD, Australian National University, Canberra; and Ralph Henderson, MD, WHO, Geneva, Switzerland.

REFERENCES

1. Inglesby TV, Henderson DA, Bartlett JG, et al. Anthrax as a biological weapon: medical and public health management. *JAMA.* 1999;281:1735-1745.
2. Fenner F, Henderson DA, Arita I, Jezek Z, Ladnyi ID. *Smallpox and Its Eradication.* Geneva, Switzerland: World Health Organization; 1988:1460.
3. Stearn EW, Stearn AE. *The Effect of Smallpox on the Destiny of the Amerindian.* Boston, Mass: Bruce Humphries; 1945.
4. Hopkins DR. *Princes and Peasants.* Chicago, Ill: University of Chicago Press; 1983.
5. World Health Organization. *The Global Eradication of Smallpox: Final Report of the Global Commission for the Certification of Smallpox Eradication.* Geneva, Switzerland: World Health Organization; 1980.
6. Breman JG, Henderson DA. Poxvirus dilemmas: monkeypox, smallpox and biological terrorism. *N Engl J Med.* 1998;339:556-559.
7. Institute of Medicine. *Assessment of Future Scientific Need for Live Variola Virus.* Washington, DC: National Academy Press; 1999.
8. Alibek K. *Biohazard.* New York, NY: Random House Inc; 1999.
9. Harper GJ. Airborne micro-organisms: survival test with four viruses. *J Hyg.* 1961;59:479-486.
10. Wehrle PF, Posch J, Richter KH, Henderson DA. An airborne outbreak of smallpox in a German hospital and its significance with respect to other recent outbreaks in Europe. *Bull World Health Organ.* 1970; 43:669-679.
11. Chapin CV, Smith J. Permanency of the mild type of smallpox. *J Prev Med.* 1932;1:1-29.
12. Esposito JJ, Knight JC. Orthopox DNA: a comparison of restriction profiles and maps. *Virology.* 1985; 143:230-251.
13. Chapin CV. Variation in the type of infectious disease as shown by the history of smallpox in the United States, 1895-1912. *J Infect Dis.* 1913;13:171-196.
14. Anders W, Sosch J. Die Pockenausbruche 1961/61 in Nordrhein-Westfalen. *Bundesgesundheitsblatt.* 1962;17:265-269.
15. Dixon CW. *Smallpox.* London, England: J & A Churchill Ltd; 1962:1460.
16. Joarder AK, Tarantola D, Tulloch J. *The Eradication of Smallpox From Bangladesh, New Delhi.* Geneva, Switzerland: WHO Regional Publications; 1980.
17. Mack TM. Smallpox in Europe, 1950-71. *J Infect Dis.* 1972;125:161-169.
18. Mack TM, Thomas DB, Khan MM. Epidemiology of smallpox in West Pakistan, II: determinants of intravillage spread other than acquired immunity. *Am J Epidemiol.* 1972;95:157-168.
19. Rao AR. *Infected Inanimate Objects (Fomites) and Their Role in Transmission of Smallpox.* Geneva, Switzerland: World Health Organization; 1972. WHO/SE/72.40.
20. Fenner F, Wittek R, Dumbell KR. *The Orthopoxviruses.* San Diego, Calif: Academic Press; 1988:432.
21. Jezek Z, Fenner F. *Human Monkeypox.* Basel, Switzerland: S Karger; 1988.
22. Sarkar JK, Mitra AC, Mukherjee MK, De SK. Virus excretion in smallpox, 2: excretion in the throat of household contacts. *Bull World Health Organ.* 1973; 48:523-527.
23. Rao AR. *Smallpox.* Bombay, India: Kothari Book Depot; 1972.
24. Downie AW, McCarthy K. The antibody response in man following infection with viruses of the pox group, III: antibody response in smallpox. *J Hyg.* 1958;56:479-487.
25. Marsden JP. Variola minor: a personal analysis of 13,686 cases. *Bull Hyg.* 1948;23:735-746.
26. Redfield RR, Wright CD, James WD, Jones ST, Brown C, Burke D. Disseminated vaccinia in a military recruit with human immunodeficiency virus (HIV). *N Engl J Med.* 1987;316:673-676.
27. Esposito JJ, Massung RF. Poxvirus infections in humans. In: Murray PR, Tenover F, Baron EJ, eds. *Clinical Microbiology.* Washington, DC: American Society of Microbiology; 1995:1131-1138.
28. Knight JC, Massung RF, Esposito JJ. Polymerase chain reaction identification of smallpox virus. In: *PCR: Protocols for Diagnosis of Human and Animal Viral Disease.* Heidelberg, Germany: Springer-Verlag; 1995: 297-302.
29. Ropp SL, Knight JC, Massung RF, Esposito JJ. PCR strategy for identification and differentiation of small-pox and other orthopoxviruses. *J Clin Microbiol.* 1995; 33:2069-2076.
30. US Bureau of the Census. *Resident Population of the United States: Estimates, by Age and Sex.* Washington, DC: US Bureau of the Census; 1998.
31. El-Ad R, Roth Y, Winder A. The persistence of neutralizing antibodies after revaccination against small-pox. *J Infect Dis.* 1990;161:446-448.
32. World Health Organization. Smallpox vaccine and seed virus survey. Working document for the meeting of the WHO Ad Hoc Expert Committee on Orthopoxvirus Infections; January 14-15, 1999; Geneva, Switzerland.
33. Sharp JCM, Fletcher WB. Experience of antivaccinia immunoglobulin in the United Kingdom. *Lancet.* 1973;1:656-659.
34. Kempe CH. Studies on smallpox and complications of smallpox vaccination. *Pediatrics.* 1960;26: 176-189.
35. Koplan J, Monsur KA, Foster SO, et al. Treatment of variola major with adenine arabinoside. *J Infect Dis.* 1975;131:34-39.
36. Monsur KA, Hossain MS, Huq F, Rahaman MM, Haque MQ. Treatment of variola major with cytosine arabinoside. *J Infect Dis.* 1975;131:40-43.
37. Lalezari JP, Staagg RJ, Kuppermann BD, et al. Intravenous cidofovir for peripheral cytomegalovirus retinitis in patients with AIDS: a randomized, controlled trial. *Ann Intern Med.* 1997;126:257-263.
38. O'Toole T. Smallpox: a case history. *Emerg Infect Dis.* In press.
39. Dixon CW. Smallpox in Tripolitania, 1946: an epidemiological and clinical study of 500 cases, including trials of penicillin treatment. *J Hyg.* 1948;46:351-377.
40. Centers for Disease Control and Prevention. Vaccinia (smallpox) vaccine recommendations of the immunization practices advisory committee. *MMWR Morb Mortal Wkly Rep.* 1990;40(RR-14):445-448.
41. World Health Organization. *WHO Expert Committee on Smallpox Eradication.* Geneva, Switzerland: World Health Organization; 1972:493. WHO technical report series.
42. Henderson DA, Arita I, Shafa E. Studies of the bifurcated needle and recommendations for its use. Geneva, Switzerland: World Health Organization; 1972. WHO Smallpox Eradications Paper SE/72.5.
43. McIntosh K, Cherry JD, Benenson AS. Standard percutaneous (smallpox) revaccination of children who received primary percutaneous vaccination. *J Infect Dis.* 1990;161:445-448.
44. Wyeth Smallpox Vaccine [package insert]. Lancaster, Pa: Wyeth Laboratories Inc; 1988.
45. Lane JM, Ruben FL, Neff JM, Millar JD. Complications of smallpox vaccination, 1968: national surveillance in the United States. *N Engl J Med.* 1969;281:1201-1208.
46. Goldstein VA, Neff JM, Lande JM, Koplan J. Smallpox vaccination reactions, prophylaxis and therapy of complications. *Pediatrics.* 1975;55:342-347.
47. Centers for Disease Control and Prevention. Vaccinia (smallpox) vaccine: recommendations of the Immunization Practices Advisory Committee. *MMWR Morb Mortal Wkly Rep.* 1991;40:1-10.
48. Huq F. Effect of temperature and relative humidity on variola virus in crusts. *Bull World Health Organ.* 1976;54:710-712.
49. Wolff HL, Croon JJ. The survival of smallpox virus (variola minor) in natural circumstances. *Bull World Health Organ.* 1968;38:492-493.
50. Hashizume S, Yoshizawa H, Morita M, Suzuki K. Properties of attenuated mutant of vaccinia virus, LC16m8, derived from Lister strain. In: Quinnan GV, ed. *Vaccine Virus as Vectors for Vaccine Antigens.* Amsterdam, the Netherlands: Elsevier Science Publishing; 1985:87-99.
51. Hirayama M. Smallpox vaccination in Japan. In: Fukumi H, ed. *The Vaccination: Theory and Practice.* Tokyo: International Medical Foundation of Japan; 1975:113-124.

©1999 American Medical Association. All rights reserved.

Plague as a Biological Weapon
Medical and Public Health Management

Thomas V. Inglesby, MD

David T. Dennis, MD, MPH

Donald A. Henderson, MD, MPH

John G. Bartlett, MD

Michael S. Ascher, MD

Edward Eitzen, MD, MPH

Anne D. Fine, MD

Arthur M. Friedlander, MD

Jerome Hauer, MPH

John F. Koerner, MPH, CIH

Marcelle Layton, MD

Joseph McDade, PhD

Michael T. Osterholm, PhD, MPH

Tara O'Toole, MD, MPH

Gerald Parker, PhD, DVM

Trish M. Perl, MD, MSc

Philip K. Russell, MD

Monica Schoch-Spana, PhD

Kevin Tonat, DrPH, MPH

for the Working Group
on Civilian Biodefense

Objective The Working Group on Civilian Biodefense has developed consensus-based recommendations for measures to be taken by medical and public health professionals following the use of plague as a biological weapon against a civilian population.

Participants The working group included 25 representatives from major academic medical centers and research, government, military, public health, and emergency management institutions and agencies.

Evidence MEDLINE databases were searched from January 1966 to June 1998 for the Medical Subject Headings *plague*, *Yersinia pestis*, *biological weapon*, *biological terrorism*, *biological warfare*, and *biowarfare*. Review of the bibliographies of the references identified by this search led to subsequent identification of relevant references published prior to 1966. In addition, participants identified other unpublished references and sources. Additional MEDLINE searches were conducted through January 2000.

Consensus Process The first draft of the consensus statement was a synthesis of information obtained in the formal evidence-gathering process. The working group was convened to review drafts of the document in October 1998 and May 1999. The final statement incorporates all relevant evidence obtained by the literature search in conjunction with final consensus recommendations supported by all working group members.

Conclusions An aerosolized plague weapon could cause fever, cough, chest pain, and hemoptysis with signs consistent with severe pneumonia 1 to 6 days after exposure. Rapid evolution of disease would occur in the 2 to 4 days after symptom onset and would lead to septic shock with high mortality without early treatment. Early treatment and prophylaxis with streptomycin or gentamicin or the tetracycline or fluoroquinolone classes of antimicrobials would be advised.

JAMA. 2000;283:2281-2290   www.jama.com

THIS IS THE THIRD ARTICLE IN A series entitled *Medical and Public Health Management Following the Use of a Biological Weapon: Consensus Statements of the Working Group on Civilian Biodefense.*[1,2] The working group has identified a limited number of agents that, if used as weapons, could cause disease and death in sufficient numbers to cripple a city or region. These agents also comprise the top of the list of "Critical Biological Agents" recently developed by the Centers for Disease Control and Prevention (CDC).[3] *Yersinia pestis*, the causative agent of plague, is one of the most serious of these. Given the availability of *Y pestis* around the world, capacity for its mass production and aerosol dissemination, difficulty in preventing such activities, high fatality rate of pneumonic plague, and potential for secondary spread of cases during an epidemic, the potential use of plague as a biological weapon is of great concern.

CONSENSUS METHODS

The working group comprised 25 representatives from major academic medical centers and research, government, military, public health, and emergency management institutions and agencies.

MEDLINE databases were searched from January 1966 to June 1998 using the Medical Subject Headings (MeSH) *plague*, *Yersinia pestis*, *biological weapon*, *biological terrorism*, *biological warfare*, and *biowarfare*. Review of the bibliographies of the references identified by

Author Affiliations: Center for Civilian Biodefense Studies, Johns Hopkins University Schools of Medicine (Drs Inglesby, Bartlett, and Perl) and Public Health (Drs Henderson, O'Toole, Russell, and Schoch-Spana and Mr Koerner), Baltimore, Md; National Center for Infectious Diseases, Centers for Disease Control and Prevention, Fort Collins, Colo (Dr Dennis), and Atlanta, Ga (Dr McDade); Viral and Rickettsial Diseases Laboratory, California Department of Health Services, Berkeley (Dr Ascher); United States Army Medical Research Institute of Infectious Diseases, Frederick, Md (Drs Eitzen, Friedlander, and Parker); Science Application International Corporation, McLean, Va (Mr Hauer); Office of Communicable Disease, New York City Health Department, New York, NY (Drs Fine and Layton); Office of Emergency Preparedness, Department of Health and Human Services, Rockville, Md (Dr Tonat); and Infection Control Advisory Network Inc, Eden Prairie, Minn (Dr Osterholm).
Corresponding Author and Reprints: Thomas V. Inglesby, MD, Johns Hopkins Center for Civilian Biodefense Studies, Johns Hopkins University, Candler Bldg, Suite 850, 111 Market Place, Baltimore, MD 21202 (e-mail: tvi@jhsph.edu).

©2000 American Medical Association. All rights reserved.

Reprinted with permission from *JAMA*; May 3, 2000, Vol 283, No. 17

this search led to subsequent identification of relevant references published prior to 1966. In addition, participants identified other unpublished references and sources in their fields of expertise. Additional MEDLINE searches were conducted through January 2000 during the review and revisions of the statement.

The first draft of the consensus statement was a synthesis of information obtained in the initial formal evidence-gathering process. Members of the working group were asked to make formal written comments on this first draft of the document in September 1998. The document was revised incorporating changes suggested by members of the working group, which was convened to review the second draft of the document on October 30, 1998. Following this meeting and a second meeting of the working group on May 24, 1999, a third draft of the document was completed, reviewed, and revised. Working group members had a final opportunity to review the document and suggest revisions. The final document incorporates all relevant evidence obtained by the literature search in conjunction with consensus recommendations supported by all working group members.

The assessment and recommendations provided herein represent the best professional judgment of the working group based on data and expertise currently available. The conclusions and recommendations need to be regularly reassessed as new information becomes available.

HISTORY AND POTENTIAL AS A BIOTERRORIST AGENT

In AD 541, the first recorded plague pandemic began in Egypt and swept across Europe with attributable population losses of between 50% and 60% in North Africa, Europe, and central and southern Asia.[4] The second plague pandemic, also known as the *black death* or *great pestilence*, began in 1346 and eventually killed 20 to 30 million people in Europe, one third of the European population.[5] Plague spread slowly and inexorably from village to village by infected

rats and humans or more quickly from country to country by ships. The pandemic lasted more than 130 years and had major political, cultural, and religious ramifications. The third pandemic began in China in 1855, spread to all inhabited continents, and ultimately killed more than 12 million people in India and China alone.[4] Small outbreaks of plague continue to occur throughout the world.[4,5]

Advances in living conditions, public health, and antibiotic therapy make future pandemics improbable. However, plague outbreaks following use of a biological weapon are a plausible threat. In World War II, a secret branch of the Japanese army, Unit 731, is reported to have dropped plague-infected fleas over populated areas of China, thereby causing outbreaks of plague.[6] In the ensuing years, the biological weapons programs of the United States and the Soviet Union developed techniques to aerosolize plague directly, eliminating dependence on the unpredictable flea vector. In 1970, the World Health Organization (WHO) reported that, in a worst-case scenario, if 50 kg of *Y pestis* were released as an aerosol over a city of 5 million, pneumonic plague could occur in as many as 150 000 persons, 36 000 of whom would be expected to die.[7] The plague bacilli would remain viable as an aerosol for 1 hour for a distance of up to 10 km. Significant numbers of city inhabitants might attempt to flee, further spreading the disease.[7]

While US scientists had not succeeded in making quantities of plague organisms sufficient to use as an effective weapon by the time the US offensive program was terminated in 1970, Soviet scientists were able to manufacture large quantities of the agent suitable for placing into weapons.[8] More than 10 institutes and thousands of scientists were reported to have worked with plague in the former Soviet Union.[8] In contrast, few scientists in the United States study this disease.[9]

There is little published information indicating actions of autonomous groups or individuals seeking to develop plague as a weapon. However, in 1995 in Ohio,

a microbiologist with suspect motives was arrested after fraudulently acquiring *Y pestis* by mail.[10] New antiterrorism legislation was introduced in reaction.

EPIDEMIOLOGY
Naturally Occurring Plague

Human plague most commonly occurs when plague-infected fleas bite humans who then develop bubonic plague. As a prelude to human epidemics, rats frequently die in large numbers, precipitating the movement of the flea population from its natural rat reservoir to humans. Although most persons infected by this route develop bubonic plague, a small minority will develop sepsis with no bubo, a form of plague termed *primary septicemic plague*. Neither bubonic nor septicemic plague spreads directly from person to person. A small percentage of patients with bubonic or septicemic plague develop secondary pneumonic plague and can then spread the disease by respiratory droplet. Persons contracting the disease by this route develop primary pneumonic plague.[11]

Plague remains an enzootic infection of rats, ground squirrels, prairie dogs, and other rodents on every populated continent except Australia.[4] Worldwide, on average in the last 50 years, 1700 cases have been reported annually.[4] In the United States, 390 cases of plague were reported from 1947 to 1996, 84% of which were bubonic, 13% septicemic, and 2% pneumonic. Concomitant case fatality rates were 14%, 22%, and 57%, respectively.[12] Most US cases were in New Mexico, Arizona, Colorado, and California. Of the 15 cases following exposure to domestic cats with plague, 4 were primary pneumonic plague.[13] In the United States, the last case of human-to-human transmission of plague occurred in Los Angeles in 1924.[14,15]

Although pneumonic plague has rarely been the dominant manifestation of the disease, large outbreaks of pneumonic plague have occurred.[16] In an outbreak in Manchuria in 1910-1911, as many as 60 000 persons developed pneumonic plague; a second large Manchurian pneumonic plague outbreak occurred in 1920-1921.[16,17] As

©2000 American Medical Association. All rights reserved.

Reprinted with permission from *JAMA*; May 3, 2000, Vol 283, No. 17

would be anticipated in the preantibiotic era, nearly 100% of these cases were reported to be fatal.[16,17] Reports from the Manchurian outbreaks suggested that indoor contacts of affected patients were at higher risk than outdoor contacts and that cold temperature, increased humidity, and crowding contributed to increased spread.[14,15] In northern India, there was an epidemic of pneumonic plague with 1400 deaths reported at about the same time.[15] While epidemics of pneumonic plague of this scale have not occurred since, smaller epidemics of pneumonic plague have occurred recently. In 1997 in Madagascar, 1 patient with bubonic plague and secondary pneumonic infection transmitted pneumonic plague to 18 persons, 8 of whom died.[18]

Plague Following Use of a Biological Weapon

The epidemiology of plague following its use as a biological weapon would differ substantially from that of naturally occurring infection. Intentional dissemination of plague would most probably occur via an aerosol of *Y pestis*, a mechanism that has been shown to produce disease in nonhuman primates.[19] A pneumonic plague outbreak would result with symptoms initially resembling those of other severe respiratory illnesses. The size of the outbreak would depend on factors including the quantity of biological agent used, characteristics of the strain, environmental conditions, and methods of aerosolization. Symptoms would begin to occur 1 to 6 days following exposure, and people would die quickly following onset of symptoms.[16] Indications that plague had been artificially disseminated would be the occurrence of cases in locations not known to have enzootic infection, in persons without known risk factors, and in the absence of prior rodent deaths.

MICROBIOLOGY AND VIRULENCE FACTORS

Y pestis is a nonmotile, gram-negative bacillus, sometimes coccobacillus, that shows bipolar (also termed *safety pin*) staining with Wright, Giemsa, or Way-

son stain (**FIGURE 1**).[20] *Y pestis* is a lactose nonfermenter, urease and indole negative, and a member of the Enterobacteriaceae family.[21] It grows optimally at 28°C on blood agar or MacConkey agar, typically requiring 48 hours for observable growth, but colonies are initially much smaller than other Enterobacteriaceae and may be overlooked. *Y pestis* has a number of virulence factors that enable it to survive in humans by facilitating use of host nutrients, causing damage to host cells, and subverting phagocytosis and other host defense mechanisms.[4,11,21,22]

PATHOGENESIS AND CLINICAL MANIFESTATIONS
Naturally Occurring Plague

In most cases of naturally occurring plague, the bite by a plague-infected flea leads to the inoculation of up to thousands of organisms into a patient's skin. The bacteria migrate through cutaneous lymphatics to regional lymph nodes where they are phagocytosed but resist destruction. They rapidly multiply, causing destruction and necrosis of lymph node architecture with subsequent bacteremia, septicemia, and endotoxemia that can lead quickly to shock, disseminated intravascular coagulation, and coma.[21]

Patients typically develop symptoms of bubonic plague 2 to 8 days after being bitten by an infected flea. There is sudden onset of fever, chills, and weakness and the development of an acutely swollen tender lymph node, or bubo, up to 1 day later.[23] The bubo most typically develops in the groin, axilla, or cervical region (**FIGURE 2**, A) and is often so painful that it prevents patients from moving the affected area of the body. Buboes are 1 to 10 cm in diameter, and the overlying skin is erythematous.[21] They are extremely tender, nonfluctuant, and warm and are often associated with considerable surrounding edema, but seldom lymphangitis. Rarely, buboes become fluctuant and suppurate. In addition, pustules or skin ulcerations may occur at the site of the flea bite in a minority of patients. A small minority of patients infected by fleas develop *Y pes-*

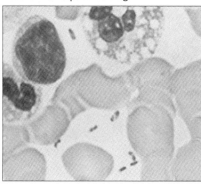

Figure 1. Peripheral Blood Smear From Patient With Septicemic Plague

Smear shows characteristic bipolar staining of *Yersinia pestis* bacilli (Wright-Giemsa stain; magnification, ×1000). Figure from Centers for Disease Control and Prevention, Division of Vector-Borne Infectious Diseases, Fort Collins, Colo.

tis septicemia without a discernable bubo, the form of disease termed *primary septicemic plague.*[23] Septicemia can also arise secondary to bubonic plague.[21] Septicemic plague may lead to disseminated intravascular coagulation, necrosis of small vessels, and purpuric skin lesions (Figure 2, B). Gangrene of acral regions such as the digits and nose may also occur in advanced disease, a process believed responsible for the name *black death* in the second plague pandemic (Figure 2, C).[21] However, the finding of gangrene would not be expected to be helpful in diagnosing the disease in the early stages of illness when early antibiotic treatment could be lifesaving.

Secondary pneumonic plague develops in a minority of patients with bubonic or primary septicemic plague—approximately 12% of total cases in the United States over the last 50 years.[4] This process, termed *secondary pneumonic plague*, develops via hematogenous spread of plague bacilli to the lungs. Patients commonly have symptoms of severe bronchopneumonia, chest pain, dyspnea, cough, and hemoptysis.[16,21]

Primary pneumonic plague resulting from the inhalation of plague bacilli occurs rarely in the United States.[12] Reports of 2 recent cases of primary pneumonic plague, contracted after handling cats with pneumonic plague, reveal that both patients had pneumonic symptoms as well as prominent gastro-

©2000 American Medical Association. All rights reserved.

Reprinted with permission from *JAMA*; May 3, 2000, Vol 283, No. 17

Figure 2. Patients With Naturally Occurring Plague

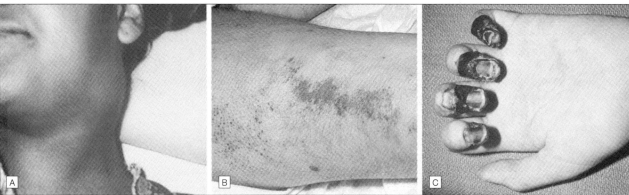

A, Cervical bubo in patient with bubonic plague; B, petechial and ecchymotic bleeding into the skin in patient with septicemic plague; and C, gangrene of the digits during the recovery phase of illness of patient shown in B. In plague following the use of a biological weapon, presence of cervical bubo is rare; purpuric skin lesions and necrotic digits occur only in advanced disease and would not be helpful in diagnosing the disease in the early stages of illness when antibiotic treatment can be life-saving. Figures from Centers for Disease Control and Prevention, Division of Vector-Borne Infectious Diseases, Fort Collins, Colo.

Figure 3. Chest Radiograph of Patient With Primary Pneumonic Plague

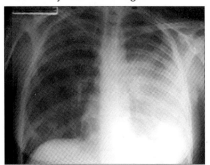

Radiograph shows extensive lobar consolidation in left lower and left middle lung fields. Figure from Centers for Disease Control and Prevention, Division of Vector-Borne Infectious Diseases, Fort Collins, Colo.

intestinal symptoms including nausea, vomiting, abdominal pain, and diarrhea. Diagnosis and treatment were delayed more than 24 hours after symptom onset in both patients, both of whom died.[24,25]

Less common plague syndromes include plague meningitis and plague pharyngitis. Plague meningitis follows the hematogenous seeding of bacilli into the meninges and is associated with fever and meningismus. Plague pharyngitis follows inhalation or ingestion of plague bacilli and is associated with cervical lymphadenopathy.[21]

Plague Following Use of a Biological Weapon

The pathogenesis and clinical manifestations of plague following a biologi-

cal attack would be notably different than naturally occurring plague. Inhaled aerosolized *Y pestis* bacilli would cause primary pneumonic plague. The time from exposure to aerosolized plague bacilli until development of first symptoms in humans and nonhuman primates has been found to be 1 to 6 days and most often, 2 to 4 days.[12,16,19,26] The first sign of illness would be expected to be fever with cough and dyspnea, sometimes with the production of bloody, watery, or less commonly, purulent sputum.[16,19,27] Prominent gastrointestinal symptoms, including nausea, vomiting, abdominal pain, and diarrhea, might be present.[24,25]

The ensuing clinical findings of primary pneumonic plague are similar to those of any severe rapidly progressive pneumonia and are quite similar to those of secondary pneumonic plague. Clinicopathological features may help distinguish primary from secondary pneumonic plague.[11] In contrast to secondary pneumonic plague, features of primary pneumonic plague would include absence of buboes (except, rarely, cervical buboes) and, on pathologic examination, pulmonary disease with areas of profound lobular exudation and bacillary aggregation.[11] Chest radiographic findings are variable but bilateral infiltrates or consolidation are common (**FIGURE 3**).[22]

Laboratory studies may reveal leukocytosis with toxic granulations, co-

agulation abnormalities, aminotransferase elevations, azotemia, and other evidence of multiorgan failure. All are nonspecific findings associated with sepsis and systemic inflammatory response syndrome.[11,21]

The time from respiratory exposure to death in humans is reported to have been between 2 to 6 days in epidemics during the preantibiotic era, with a mean of 2 to 4 days in most epidemics.[16]

DIAGNOSIS

Given the rarity of plague infection and the possibility that early cases are a harbinger of a larger epidemic, the first clinical or laboratory suspicion of plague must lead to immediate notification of the hospital epidemiologist or infection control practitioner, health department, and the local or state health laboratory. Definitive tests can thereby be arranged rapidly through a state reference laboratory or, as necessary, the Diagnostic and Reference Laboratory of the CDC and early interventions instituted.

The early diagnosis of plague requires a high index of suspicion in naturally occurring cases and even more so following the use of a biological weapon. There are no effective environmental warning systems to detect an aerosol of plague bacilli.[28]

The first indication of a clandestine terrorist attack with plague would most likely be a sudden outbreak of illness presenting as severe pneumonia and

©2000 American Medical Association. All rights reserved.

Reprinted with permission from *JAMA*; May 3, 2000, Vol 283, No. 17

sepsis. If there are only small numbers of cases, the possibility of them being plague may be at first overlooked given the clinical similarity to other bacterial or viral pneumonias and that few Western physicians have ever seen a case of pneumonic plague. However, the sudden appearance of a large number of previously healthy patients with fever, cough, shortness of breath, chest pain, and a fulminant course leading to death should immediately suggest the possibility of pneumonic plague or inhalational anthrax.[1] The presence of hemoptysis in this setting would strongly suggest plague (TABLE 1).[22]

There are no widely available rapid diagnostic tests for plague.[28] Tests that would be used to confirm a suspected diagnosis—antigen detection, IgM enzyme immunoassay, immunostaining, and polymerase chain reaction—are available only at some state health departments, the CDC, and military laboratories.[21] The routinely used passive hemagglutination antibody detection assay is typically only of retrospective value since several days to weeks usually pass after disease onset before antibodies develop.

Microbiologic studies are important in the diagnosis of pneumonic plague. A Gram stain of sputum or blood may reveal gram-negative bacilli or coccobacilli.[4,21,29] A Wright, Giemsa, or Wayson stain will often show bipolar staining (Figure 1), and direct fluorescent antibody testing, if available, may be positive. In the unlikely event that a cervical bubo is present in pneumonic plague, an aspirate (obtained with a 20-gauge needle and a 10-mL syringe containing 1-2 mL of sterile saline for infusing the node) may be cultured and similarly stained (Table 1).[22]

Cultures of sputum, blood, or lymph node aspirate should demonstrate growth approximately 24 to 48 hours after inoculation. Most microbiology laboratories use either automated or semiautomated bacterial identification systems. Some of these systems may misidentify Y pestis.[12,30] In laboratories without automated bacterial identification, as many as 6 days may be required for

Table 1. Diagnosis of Pneumonic Plague Infection Following Use of a Biological Weapon

Epidemiology and symptoms	Sudden appearance of many persons with fever, cough, shortness of breath, hemoptysis, and chest pain
	Gastrointestinal symptoms common (eg, nausea, vomiting, abdominal pain, and diarrhea)
	Patients have fulminant course and high mortality
Clinical signs	Tachypnea, dyspnea, and cyanosis
	Pneumonic consolidation on chest examination
	Sepsis, shock, and organ failure
	Infrequent presence of cervical bubo
	(Purpuric skin lesions and necrotic digits only in advanced disease)
Laboratory studies	Sputum, blood, or lymph node aspirate
	Gram-negative bacilli with bipolar (safety pin) staining on Wright, Giemsa, or Wayson stain
	Rapid diagnostic tests available only at some health departments, the Centers for Disease Control and Prevention, and military laboratories
	Pulmonary infiltrates or consolidation on chest radiograph
Pathology	Lobular exudation, bacillary aggregation, and areas of necrosis in pulmonary parenchyma

identification, and there is some chance that the diagnosis may be missed entirely. Approaches for biochemical characterization of Y pestis are described in detail elsewhere.[20]

If a laboratory using automated or nonautomated techniques is notified that plague is suspected, it should split the culture: 1 culture incubated at 28°C for rapid growth and the second culture incubated at 37°C for identification of the diagnostic capsular (F_1) antigen. Using these methods, up to 72 hours may be required following specimen procurement to make the identification (May Chu, PhD, CDC, Fort Collins, Colo, written communication, April 9, 1999). Antibiotic susceptibility testing should be performed at a reference laboratory because of the lack of standardized susceptibility testing procedures for Y pestis. A process establishing criteria and training measures for laboratory diagnosis of this disease is being undertaken jointly by the Association of Public Health Laboratories and the CDC.

VACCINATION

The US-licensed formaldehyde-killed whole bacilli vaccine was discontinued by its manufacturers in 1999 and is no longer available. Plans for future licensure and production are unclear. This killed vaccine demonstrated efficacy in preventing or ameliorating bubonic disease, but it does not prevent or amelio-

rate the development of primary pneumonic plague.[19,31] It was used in special circumstances for individuals deemed to be at high risk of developing plague, such as military personnel working in plague endemic areas, microbiologists working with Y pestis in the laboratory, or researchers working with plague-infected rats or fleas. Research is ongoing in the pursuit of a vaccine that protects against primary pneumonic plague.[22,32]

THERAPY

Recommendations for the use of antibiotics following a plague biological weapon exposure are conditioned by the lack of published trials in treating plague in humans, limited number of studies in animals, and possible requirement to treat large numbers of persons. A number of possible therapeutic regimens for treating plague have yet to be adequately studied or submitted for approval to the Food and Drug Administration (FDA). For these reasons, the working group offers consensus recommendations based on the best available evidence. The recommendations do not necessarily represent uses currently approved by the FDA or an official position on the part of any of the federal agencies whose scientists participated in these discussions. Recommendations will need to be revised as further relevant information becomes available.

©2000 American Medical Association. All rights reserved.

Reprinted with permission from *JAMA*; May 3, 2000, Vol 283, No. 17

In the United States during the last 50 years, 4 of the 7 reported primary pneumonic plague patients died.[12] Fatality rates depend on various factors including time to initiation of antibiotics, access to advanced supportive care, and the dose of inhaled bacilli. The fatality rate of patients with pneumonic plague when treatment is delayed more than 24 hours after symptom onset is extremely high.[14,24,25,33]

Historically, the preferred treatment for plague infection has been streptomycin, an FDA-approved treatment for plague.[21,34,35] Administered early during the disease, streptomycin has reduced overall plague mortality to the 5% to 14% range.[12,21,34] However, streptomycin is infrequently used in the United States and only modest supplies are available.[35] Gentamicin is not FDA approved for the treatment of plague but has been used successfully[36-39] and is recommended as an acceptable alternative by experts.[23,40] In 1 case series, 8 patients with plague were treated with gentamicin with morbidity or mortality equivalent to that of patients treated with streptomycin (Lucy Boulanger, MD, Indian Health Services, Crown Point, NM, written communication, July 20, 1999). In vitro studies and an in vivo study in mice show equal or improved activity of gentamicin against many strains of Y pestis when compared with streptomycin.[41,42] In addition, gentamicin is widely available, inexpensive, and can be given once daily.[35]

Tetracycline and doxycycline also have been used in the treatment and prophylaxis of plague; both are FDA approved for these purposes. In vitro studies have shown that Y pestis susceptibility to tetracycline[43] and doxycycline[41,44] is equivalent to that of the aminoglycosides. In another investigation, 13% of Y pestis strains in Madagascar were found to have some in vitro resistance to tetracycline.[45] Experimental murine models of Y pestis infection have yielded data that are difficult to extrapolate to humans. Some mouse studies have shown doxycycline to be a highly efficacious treatment of infection[44,46] or prophylaxis[47] against na-turally occurring plague strains. Experimental murine infection with F_1-deficient variants of Y pestis have shown decreased efficacy of doxycycline,[47,48] but only 1 human case of F_1-deficient plague infection has been reported.[49] Russell and colleagues[50] reported poor efficacy of doxycycline against plague-infected mice, but the dosing schedules used in this experiment would have failed to maintain drug levels above the minimum inhibitory concentration due to the short half-life of doxycycline in mice. In another study, doxycycline failed to prevent death in mice intraperitoneally infected with 29 to 290000 times the median lethal inocula of Y pestis.[51]

There are no controlled clinical trials comparing either tetracycline or doxycycline to aminoglycoside in the treatment of plague, but anecdotal case series and a number of medical authorities support use of this class of antimicrobials for prophylaxis and for therapy in the event that streptomycin or gentamicin cannot be administered.[23,27,38-40,52-54] Based on evidence from in vitro studies, animal studies, and uncontrolled human data, the working group recommends that the tetracycline class of antibiotics be used to treat pneumonic plague if aminoglycoside therapy cannot be administered. This might be the case in a mass casualty scenario when parenteral therapy was either unavailable or impractical. Doxycycline would be considered pharmacologically superior to other antibiotics in the tetracycline class for this indication, because it is well absorbed without food interactions, is well distributed with good tissue penetration, and has a long half-life.[35]

The fluoroquinolone family of antimicrobials has demonstrated efficacy in animal studies. Ciprofloxacin has been demonstrated to be at least as efficacious as aminoglycosides and tetracyclines in studies of mice with experimentally induced pneumonic plague.[44,50,51] In vitro studies also suggest equivalent or greater activity of ciprofloxacin, levofloxacin, and ofloxacin against Y pestis when compared with aminoglycosides or tetracyclines.[41,55] However, there have been no trials of fluoroquinolones in human plague, and they are not FDA approved for this indication.

Chloramphenicol has been used to treat plague infection and has been recommended for treatment of plague meningitis because of its ability to cross the blood-brain barrier.[21,34] However, human clinical trials demonstrating the superiority of chloramphenicol in the therapy of classic plague infection or plague meningitis have not been performed. It has been associated with dose dependent hematologic abnormalities and with rare idiosyncratic fatal aplastic anemia.[35]

A number of different sulfonamides have been used successfully in the treatment of human plague infection: sulfathiazole,[56] sulfadiazine, sulfamerazine, and trimethoprim-sulfamethoxazole.[57,58] The 1970 WHO analysis reported that sulfadiazine reduced mortality for bubonic plague but was ineffective against pneumonic plague and was less effective than tetracycline overall.[59] In a study comparing trimethoprim-sulfamethoxazole with streptomycin, patients treated with trimethoprim-sulfamethoxazole had a longer median duration of fever and a higher incidence of complications.[58] Authorities have generally considered trimethoprim-sulfamethoxazole a second-tier choice.[21,23,34] Some have recommended sulfonamides only in the setting of pediatric prophylaxis.[22] No sulfonamides have been FDA approved for the treatment of plague.

Antimicrobials that have been shown to have poor or only modest efficacy in animal studies have included rifampin, aztreonam, ceftazidime, cefotetan, and cefazolin; these antibiotics should not be used.[42]

Antibiotic resistance patterns must also be considered in making treatment recommendations. Naturally occurring antibiotic resistance to the tetracycline class of drugs has occurred rarely.[4] Recently, a plasmid-mediated multidrug-resistant strain was isolated in Madagascar.[60] A report published by Russian scientists cited quinolone-resistant Y pestis.[61] There have been assertions that Russian scientists have en-

©2000 American Medical Association. All rights reserved.

gineered multidrug-resistant strains of *Y pestis*,[8] although there is as yet no scientific publication confirming this.

Recommendations for Antibiotic Therapy

The working group treatment recommendations are based on literature reports on treatment of human disease, reports of studies in animal models, reports on in vitro susceptibility testing, and antibiotic safety. Should antibiotic susceptibility testing reveal resistance, proper antibiotic substitution would need to be made.

In a contained casualty setting, a situation in which a modest number of patients require treatment, the working group recommends parenteral antibiotic therapy (TABLE 2). Preferred parenteral forms of the antimicrobials streptomycin or gentamicin are recommended. However, in a mass casualty setting, intravenous or intramuscular therapy may not be possible for reasons of patient care logistics and/or exhaustion of equipment and antibiotic supplies, and parenteral therapy will need to be supplanted by oral therapy. In a mass casualty setting, the working group recommends oral therapy, preferably with doxycycline (or tetracycline) or ciprofloxacin (Table 2).

Patients with pneumonic plague will require substantial advanced medical supportive care in addition to antimicrobial therapy. Complications of gramnegative sepsis would be expected, including adult respiratory distress syndrome, disseminated intravascular coagulation, shock, and multiorgan failure.[23]

Once it was known or strongly suspected that pneumonic plague cases were occurring, anyone with fever or cough in the presumed area of exposure should be immediately treated with antimicrobials for presumptive pneumonic plague. Delaying therapy until confirmatory testing is performed would greatly decrease survival.[59] Clinical deterioration of patients despite early initiation of empiric therapy could signal antimicrobial resistance and should be promptly evaluated.

Table 2. Working Group Recommendations for Treatment of Patients With Pneumonic Plague in the Contained and Mass Casualty Settings and for Postexposure Prophylaxis*

Patient Category	Recommended Therapy
Contained Casualty Setting	
Adults	Preferred choices Streptomycin, 1 g IM twice daily
	Gentamicin, 5 mg/kg IM or IV once daily or 2 mg/kg loading dose followed by 1.7 mg/kg IM or IV 3 times daily†
	Alternative choices Doxycycline, 100 mg IV twice daily or 200 mg IV once daily
	Ciprofloxacin, 400 mg IV twice daily‡
	Chloramphenicol, 25 mg/kg IV 4 times daily§
Children‖	Preferred choices Streptomycin, 15 mg/kg IM twice daily (maximum daily dose, 2 g)
	Gentamicin, 2.5 mg/kg IM or IV 3 times daily†
	Alternative choices Doxycycline, If ≥45 kg, give adult dosage
	If <45 kg, give 2.2 mg/kg IV twice daily (maximum, 200 mg/d)
	Ciprofloxacin, 15 mg/kg IV twice daily‡
	Chloramphenicol, 25 mg/kg IV 4 times daily§
Pregnant women¶	Preferred choice Gentamicin, 5 mg/kg IM or IV once daily or 2 mg/kg loading dose followed by 1.7 mg/kg IM or IV 3 times daily†
	Alternative choices Doxycycline, 100 mg IV twice daily or 200 mg IV once daily
	Ciprofloxacin, 400 mg IV twice daily‡
Mass Casualty Setting and Postexposure Prophylaxis#	
Adults	Preferred choices Doxycycline, 100 mg orally twice daily††
	Ciprofloxacin, 500 mg orally twice daily‡
	Alternative choice Chloramphenicol, 25 mg/kg orally 4 times daily§**
Children‖	Preferred choice Doxycycline,†† If ≥45 kg, give adult dosage
	If <45 kg, then give 2.2 mg/kg orally twice daily
	Ciprofloxacin, 20 mg/kg orally twice daily
	Alternative choices Chloramphenicol, 25 mg/kg orally 4 times daily§**
Pregnant women¶	Preferred choices Doxycycline, 100 mg orally twice daily††
	Ciprofloxacin, 500 mg orally twice daily
	Alternative choices Chloramphenicol, 25 mg/kg orally 4 times daily§**

*These are consensus recommendations of the Working Group on Civilian Biodefense and are not necessarily approved by the Food and Drug Administration. See "Therapy" section for explanations. One antimicrobial agent should be selected. Therapy should be continued for 10 days. Oral therapy should be substituted when patient's condition improves. IM indicates intramuscularly; IV, intravenously.
†Aminoglycosides must be adjusted according to renal function. Evidence suggests that gentamicin, 5 mg/kg IM or IV once daily, would be efficacious in children, although this is not yet widely accepted in clinical practice. Neonates up to 1 week of age and premature infants should receive gentamicin, 2.5 mg/kg IV twice daily.
‡Other fluoroquinolones can be substituted at doses appropriate for age. Ciprofloxacin dosage should not exceed 1 g/d in children.
§Concentration should be maintained between 5 and 20 µg/mL. Concentrations greater than 25 µg/mL can cause reversible bone marrow suppression.[35,62]
‖Refer to "Management of Special Groups" for details. In children, ciprofloxacin dose should not exceed 1 g/d, chloramphenicol should not exceed 4 g/d. Children younger than 2 years should not receive chloramphenicol.
¶Refer to "Management of Special Groups" for details and for discussion of breastfeeding women. In neonates, gentamicin loading dose of 4 mg/kg should be given initially.[63]
#Duration of treatment of plague in mass casualty setting is 10 days. Duration of postexposure prophylaxis to prevent plague infection is 7 days.
**Children younger than 2 years should not receive chloramphenicol. Oral formulation available only outside the United States.
††Tetracycline could be substituted for doxycycline.

©2000 American Medical Association. All rights reserved.

Reprinted with permission from *JAMA*; May 3, 2000, Vol 283, No. 17

Management of Special Groups

Consensus recommendations for special groups as set forth in the following reflect the clinical and evidence-based judgments of the working group and do not necessarily correspond to FDA approved use, indications, or labeling.

Children. The treatment of choice for plague in children has been streptomycin or gentamicin.[21,40] If aminoglycosides are not available or cannot be used, recommendations for alternative antimicrobial treatment with efficacy against plague are conditioned by balancing risks associated with treatment against those posed by pneumonic plague. Children aged 8 years and older can be treated with tetracycline antibiotics safely.[35,40] However, in children younger than 8 years, tetracycline antibiotics may cause discolored teeth, and rare instances of retarded skeletal growth have been reported in infants.[35] Chloramphenicol is considered safe in children except for children younger than 2 years who are at risk of "gray baby syndrome."[35,40] Some concern exists that fluoroquinolone use in children may cause arthropathy,[35] although fluoroquinolones have been used to treat serious infections in children.[64] No comparative studies assessing efficacy or safety of alternative treatment strategies for plague in children has or can be performed.

Given these considerations, the working group recommends that children in the contained casualty setting receive streptomycin or gentamicin. In a mass casualty setting or for postexposure prophylaxis, we recommend that doxycycline be used. Alternatives are listed for both settings (Table 2). The working group assessment is that the potential benefits of these antimicrobials in the treating of pneumonic plague infection substantially outweigh the risks.

Pregnant Women. It has been recommended that aminoglycosides be avoided in pregnancy unless severe illness warrants,[35,65] but there is no more efficacious treatment for pneumonic plague. Therefore, the working group recommends that pregnant women in

the contained casualty setting receive gentamicin (Table 2). Since streptomycin has been associated with rare reports of irreversible deafness in children following fetal exposure, this medication should be avoided if possible.[35] The tetracycline class of antibiotics has been associated with fetal toxicity including retarded skeletal growth,[35] although a large case-control study of doxycycline use in pregnancy showed no significant increase in teratogenic risk to the fetus.[66] Liver toxicity has been reported in pregnant women following large doses of intravenous tetracycline (no longer sold in the United States), but it has also been reported following oral administration of tetracycline to nonpregnant individuals.[35] Balancing the risks of pneumonic plague infection with those associated with doxycycline use in pregnancy, the working group recommends that doxycycline be used to treat pregnant women with pneumonic plague if gentamicin is not available.

Of the oral antibiotics historically used to treat plague, only trimethoprim-sulfamethoxazole has a category C pregnancy classification[65]; however, many experts do not recommend trimethoprim-sulfamethoxazole for treatment of pneumonic plague. Therefore, the working group recommends that pregnant women receive oral doxycycline for mass casualty treatment or postexposure prophylaxis. If the patient is unable to take doxycycline or the medication is unavailable, ciprofloxacin or other fluoroquinolones would be recommended in the mass casualty setting (Table 2).

The working group recommendation for treatment of breastfeeding women is to provide the mother and infant with the same antibiotic based on what is most safe and effective for the infant: gentamicin in the contained casualty setting and doxycycline in the mass casualty setting. Fluoroquinolones would be the recommended alternative (Table 2).

Immunosuppressed Persons. The antibiotic treatment or postexposure prophylaxis for pneumonic plague among those who are immunosuppressed has

not been studied in human or animal models of pneumonic plague infection. Therefore, the consensus recommendation is to administer antibiotics according to the guidelines developed for immunocompetent adults and children.

POSTEXPOSURE PROPHYLAXIS RECOMMENDATIONS

The working group recommends that in a community experiencing a pneumonic plague epidemic, all persons developing a temperature of 38.5°C or higher or new cough should promptly begin parenteral antibiotic treatment. If the resources required to administer parenteral antibiotics are unavailable, oral antibiotics should be used according to the mass casualty recommendations (Table 2). For infants in this setting, tachypnea would also be an additional indication for immediate treatment.[29] Special measures would need to be initiated for treatment or prophylaxis of those who are either unaware of the outbreak or require special assistance, such as the homeless or mentally handicapped persons. Continuing surveillance of patients would be needed to identify individuals and communities at risk requiring postexposure prophylaxis.

Asymptomatic persons having household, hospital, or other close contact with persons with untreated pneumonic plague should receive postexposure antibiotic prophylaxis for 7 days[29] and watch for fever and cough. Close contact is defined as contact with a patient at less than 2 meters.[16,31] Tetracycline, doxycycline, sulfonamides, and chloramphenicol have each been used or recommended as postexposure prophylaxis in this setting.[16,22,29,31,59] Fluoroquinolones could also be used based on studies in mice.[51]

The working group recommends the use of doxycycline as the first choice antibiotic for postexposure prophylaxis; other recommended antibiotics are noted (Table 2). Contacts who develop fever or cough while receiving prophylaxis should seek prompt medical attention and begin antibiotic treatment as described in Table 2.

©2000 American Medical Association. All rights reserved.

Reprinted with permission from *JAMA*; May 3, 2000, Vol 283, No. 17

INFECTION CONTROL

Previous public health guidelines have advised strict isolation for all close contacts of patients with pneumonic plague who refuse prophylaxis.[29] In the modern setting, however, pneumonic plague has not spread widely or rapidly in a community,[4,14,24] and therefore isolation of close contacts refusing antibiotic prophylaxis is not recommended by the working group. Instead, persons refusing prophylaxis should be carefully watched for the development of fever or cough during the first 7 days after exposure and treated immediately should either occur.

Modern experience with person-to-person spread of pneumonic plague is limited; few data are available to make specific recommendations regarding appropriate infection control measures. The available evidence indicates that person-to-person transmission of pneumonic plague occurs via respiratory droplets; transmission by droplet nuclei has not been demonstrated.[14-17] In large pneumonic plague epidemics earlier this century, pneumonic plague transmission was prevented in close contacts by wearing masks.[14,16,17] Commensurate with this, existing national infection control guidelines recommend the use of disposable surgical masks to prevent the transmission of pneumonic plague.[29,67]

Given the available evidence, the working group recommends that, in addition to beginning antibiotic prophylaxis, persons living or working in close contact with patients with confirmed or suspect pneumonic plague that have had less than 48 hours of antimicrobial treatment should follow respiratory droplet precautions and wear a surgical mask. Further, the working group recommends avoidance of unnecessary close contact with patients with pneumonic plague until at least 48 hours of antibiotic therapy and clinical improvement has taken place. Other standard respiratory droplet precautions (gown, gloves, and eye protection) should be used as well.[29,31]

The patient should remain isolated during the first 48 hours of antibiotic therapy and until clinical improvement occurs.[29,31,59] If large numbers of patients make individual isolation impossible, patients with pneumonic plague may be cohorted while undergoing antibiotic therapy. Patients being transported should also wear surgical masks. Hospital rooms of patients with pneumonic plague should receive terminal cleaning in a manner consistent with standard precautions, and clothing or linens contaminated with body fluids of patients infected with plague should be disinfected as per hospital protocol.[29]

Microbiology laboratory personnel should be alerted when Y pestis is suspected. Four laboratory-acquired cases of plague have been reported in the United States.[68] Simple clinical materials and cultures should be processed in biosafety level 2 conditions.[31,69] Only during activities involving high potential for aerosol or droplet production (eg, centrifuging, grinding, vigorous shaking, and animal studies) are biosafety level 3 conditions necessary.[69]

Bodies of patients who have died following infection with plague should be handled with routine strict precautions.[29] Contact with the remains should be limited to trained personnel, and the safety precautions for transporting corpses for burial should be the same as those when transporting ill patients.[70] Aerosol-generating procedures, such as bone-sawing associated with surgery or postmortem examinations, would be associated with special risks of transmission and are not recommended. If such aerosol-generating procedures are necessary, then high-efficiency particulate air filtered masks and negative-pressure rooms should be used as would be customary in cases in which contagious biological aerosols, such as *Mycobacterium tuberculosis*, are deemed a possible risk.[71]

ENVIRONMENTAL DECONTAMINATION

There is no evidence to suggest that residual plague bacilli pose an environmental threat to the population following the dissolution of the primary aerosol. There is no spore form in the Y pestis life cycle, so it is far more susceptible to environmental conditions than sporulating bacteria such as *Bacillus anthracis*. Moreover, Y pestis is very sensitive to the action of sunlight and heating and does not survive long outside the host.[72] Although some reports suggest that the bacterium may survive in the soil for some time,[72] there is no evidence to suggest environmental risk to humans in this setting and thus no need for environmental decontamination of an area exposed to an aerosol of plague. In the WHO analysis, in a worst case scenario, a plague aerosol was estimated to be effective and infectious for as long as 1 hour.[7] In the setting of a clandestine release of plague bacilli, the aerosol would have dissipated long before the first case of pneumonic plague occurred.

ADDITIONAL RESEARCH

Improving the medical and public health response to an outbreak of plague following the use of a biological weapon will require additional knowledge of the organism, its genetics, and pathogenesis. In addition, improved rapid diagnostic and standard laboratory microbiology techniques are necessary. An improved understanding of prophylactic and therapeutic antibiotic regimens would be of benefit in defining optimal antibiotic strategy.

Ex officio participants in the Working Group on Civilian Biodefense: George Counts, MD, National Institutes of Health, Margaret Hamburg, MD, Assistant Secretary for Planning and Evaluation, Robert Knouss, MD, Office of Emergency Preparedness, Brian Malkin, Food and Drug Administration, Stuart Nightingale, MD, Food and Drug Administration, and William Raub, PhD, Office of Assistant Secretary for Planning and Evaluation, Department of Health and Human Services.
Funding/Support: Funding for the development of this working group document was primarily provided by each representative's individual institution or agency; the Johns Hopkins Center for Civilian Biodefense Studies provided travel funds for 5 members of the group (Drs Ascher, Fine, Layton, and Osterholm and Mr Hauer).
Acknowledgment: We thank Christopher Davis, OBE, MD, PhD, ORAQ Consultancy, Marlborough, England; Edward B. Hayes, MD, Centers for Disease Control and Prevention (CDC), Atlanta, Ga; May Chu, PhD, CDC, Fort Collins, Colo; Timothy Townsend, MD, Johns Hopkins University, Baltimore, Md; Jane Wong, MS, California Department of Health, Berkeley; and Paul A. Pham, PharmD, Johns Hopkins University, for their review of the manuscript and Molly D'Esopo for administrative support.

REFERENCES

1. Inglesby TV, Henderson DA, Bartlett JG, et al. Anthrax as a biological weapon: medical and public health management. *JAMA.* 1999;281:1735-1745.
2. Henderson DA, Inglesby TV, Bartlett JG, et al. Small-

©2000 American Medical Association. All rights reserved.

pox as a biological weapon: medical and public health management. *JAMA*. 1999;281:2127-2137.

3. Centers for Disease Control and Prevention. *Critical Biological Agents for Public Health Preparedness: Summary of Selection Process and Recommendations*. October 16, 1999. Unpublished report.

4. Perry RD, Fetherston JD. *Yersinia pestis*—etiologic agent of plague. *Clin Microbiol Rev*. 1997; 10:35-66.

5. Slack P. The black death past and present. *Trans R Soci Trop Med Hyg*. 1989;83:461-463.

6. Harris SH. *Factories of Death*. New York, NY: Routledge; 1994:78, 96.

7. *Health Aspects of Chemical and Biological Weapons*. Geneva, Switzerland: World Health Organization; 1970:98-109

8. Alibek K, Handelman S. *Biohazard*. New York, NY: Random House; 1999.

9. Hughes J. *Nation's Public Health Infrastructure Regarding Epidemics and Bioterrorism* [congressional testimony]. Washington, DC: Appropriations Committee, US Senate; June 2, 1998.

10. Carus WS. *Bioterrorism and Biocrimes: The Illicit Use of Biological Agents in the 20th Century*. Washington, DC: Center for Counterproliferation Research, National Defense University; 1998.

11. Dennis D, Meier F. Plague. In: Horsburgh CR, Nelson AM, eds. *Pathology of Emerging Infections*. Washington, DC: ASM Press; 1997:21-47.

12. Centers for Disease Control and Prevention. Fatal human plague. *MMWR Morb Mortal Wkly Rep*. 1997;278:380-382.

13. Centers for Disease Control and Prevention. Human plague—United States, 1993-1994. *MMWR Morb Mortal Wkly Rep*. 1994;43:242-246.

14. Meyer K. Pneumonic plague. *Bacteriol Rev*. 1961; 25:249-261.

15. Kellogg WH. An epidemic of pneumonic plague. *Am J Public Health*. 1920;10:599-605.

16. Wu L-T. *A Treatise on Pneumonic Plague*. Geneva, Switzerland: League of Nations Health Organization; 1926.

17. Chernin E. Richard Pearson Strong and the Manchurian epidemic of pneumonic plague, 1910-1911. *J Hist Med Allied Sci*. 1989;44:296-319.

18. Ratsitorahina M, Chanteau S, Rahalison L, Ratsifasoamanana L, Boisier P. Epidemiological and diagnostic aspects of the outbreak of pneumonic plague in Madagascar. *Lancet*. 2000;355:111-113.

19. Speck RS, Wolochow H. Studies on the experimental epidemiology of respiratory infections: experimental pneumonic plague in *Macaccus rhesus*. *J Infect Dis*. 1957;100:58-69.

20. Aleksic S, Bockemuhl J. *Yersinia* and other enterobacteriaceae. In: Murray P, ed. *Manual of Clinical Microbiology*. Washington, DC: American Society for Microbiology; 1999:483-496.

21. Butler T. *Yersinia* species (including plague). In: Mandell GL, Bennett JE, Dolin R, eds. *Principles and Practice of Infectious Diseases*. New York, NY: Churchill Livingstone; 1995:2070-2078.

22. McGovern TW, Friedlander A. Plague. In: Zajtchuk R, Bellamy RF, eds. *Medical Aspects of Chemical and Biological Warfare*. Bethesda, Md: Office of the Surgeon General; 1997:479-502.

23. Campbell GL, Dennis DT. Plague and other *Yersinia* infections. In: Fauci AS, Braunwald E, Isselbacher KJ, et al, eds. *Harrison's Principles of Internal Medicine*. New York, NY: McGraw-Hill; 1998: 975-983.

24. Centers for Disease Control and Prevention. Pneumonic plague—Arizona. *MMWR Morb Mortal Wkly Rep*. 1992;41:737-739.

25. Werner SB, Weidmer CE, Nelson BC, Nygaard GS, Goethals RM, Poland JD. Primary plague pneumonia contracted from a domestic cat in South Lake Tahoe, California. *JAMA*. 1984;251:929-931.

26. Finegold MJ, Petery JJ, Berendt RF, Adams HR. Studies on the pathogenesis of plague. *J Infect Dis*. 1968;53:99-114.

27. Poland JD, Dennis DT. Plague. In: Evans AS, Brachman PS, eds. *Bacterial Infections of Humans: Epidemiology and Control*. New York, NY: Plenum Medical Book Co; 1998:545-558.

28. Institute of Medicine National Research Council. Detection and measurement of biological agents. In: *Chemical and Biological Terrorism: Research and Development to Improve Civilian Medical Response*. Washington, DC: National Academy Press; 1999:95.

29. American Public Health Association. Plague. In: Benenson AS, ed. *Control of Communicable Diseases Manual*. Washington, DC: American Public Health Association; 1995:353-358.

30. Wilmoth BA, Chu MC, Quan TC. Identification of *Yersinia pestis* by BBL crystal enteric/nonfermenter identification system. *J Clin Microbiol*. 1996;34:2829-2830.

31. Centers for Disease Control and Prevention. Prevention of plague: recommendations of the Advisory Committee on Immunization Practice (ACIP). *MMWR Morb Mortal Wkly Rep*. 1996;45(RR-14):1-15.

32. Titball RW, Eley S, Williamson ED, Dennis DT. Plague. In: Plotkin S, Mortimer EA, eds. *Vaccines*. Philadelphia, Pa: WB Saunders; 1999:734-742.

33. McCrumb FR, Mercier S, Robic J, et al. Chloramphenicol and terramycin in the treatment of pneumonic plague. *Am J Med*. 1953;14:284-293.

34. Barnes AM, Quan TJ. Plague. In: Gorbach SL, Bartlett JG, Blacklow NR, eds. *Infectious Diseases*. Philadelphia, Pa: WB Saunders Co; 1992:1285-1291.

35. American Hospital Formulary Service. *AHFS Drug Information*. Bethesda, Md: American Society of Health System Pharmacists; 2000.

36. Wong TW. Plague in a pregnant patient. *Trop Doct*. 1986;16:187-188.

37. Lewiecki EM. Primary plague septicemia. *Rocky Mt Med J*. 1978;75:201-202.

38. Welty TK, Grabman J, Kompare E, et al. Nineteen cases of plague in Arizona. *West J Med*. 1985; 142:641-646.

39. Crook LD, Tempest B. Plague: a clinical review of 27 cases. *Arch Intern Med*. 1992;152:1253-1256.

40. Committee on Infectious Diseases. Plague. In: Peter G, ed. *1997 Redbook*. Elk Grove Village, Ill: American Academy of Pediatrics; 1997:408-410.

41. Smith MD, Vinh SX, Hoa NT, Wain J, Thung D, White NJ. In vitro antimicrobial susceptibilities of strains of *Yersinia pestis*. *Antimicrob Agents Chemother*. 1995;39:2153-2154.

42. Byrne WR, Welkos SL, Pitt ML, et al. Antibiotic treatment of experimental pneumonic plague in mice. *Antimicrob Agents Chemother*. 1998;42:675-681.

43. Lyamuya EF, Nyanda P, Mohammedali H, Mhalu FS. Laboratory studies on *Yersinia pestis* during the 1991 outbreak of plague in Lushoto, Tanzania. *J Trop Med Hyg*. 1992;95:335-338.

44. Bonacorsi SP, Scavizzi MR, Guiyoule A, Amouroux JH, Carniel E. Assessment of a fluoroquinolone, three β-lactams, two aminoglycosides, and a cycline in the treatment of murine *Yersinia pestis* infection. *Antimicrob Agents Chemother*. 1994;38:481-486.

45. Rasoamanana B, Coulanges P, Michel P, Rasolofonirina N. Sensitivity of *Yersinia pestis* to antibiotics: 277 strains isolated in Madagascar between 1926 and 1989. *Arch Inst Pasteur Madagascar*. 1989;56: 37-53.

46. Makarovskaia LN, Shcherbaniuk AI, Ryzhkova VV, Sorokina TB. Effectiveness of doxycycline in experimental plague. *Antibiot Khimioter*. 1993;38:48-50.

47. Samokhodkina ED, Ryzhko IV, Shcherbaniuk AI, Kasatkina IV, Tsuraeva RI, Zhigalova TA. Doxycycline in the prevention of experimental plague induced by plague microbe variants. *Antibiot Khimioter*. 1992;37:26-28.

48. Ryzhko IV, Samokhodkina ED, Tsuraeva RI, Shcherbaniuk AI, Tsetskhladze NS. Characteristics of etiotropic therapy of plague infection induced by atypical strains of F_1-phenotype plague microbe. *Antibiot Khimioter*. 1998;43:24-28.

49. Davis KJ, Fritz DL, Pitt ML, Welkos SL, Worsham

PL, Friedlander A. Pathology of experimental pneumonic plague produced by fraction-1 positive and fraction-1 negative *Yersinia pestis* in African Green Monkeys. *Arch Pathol Lab Med*. 1996;120:156-163.

50. Russell P, Eley SM, Green M, et al. Efficacy of doxycycline and ciprofloxacin against experimental *Yersinia pestis* infection. *J Antimicrob Chemother*. 1998;41: 301-305.

51. Russell P, Eley SM, Bell DL, Manchee RJ, Titball RW. Doxycycline or ciprofloxacin prophylaxis and therapy against experimental *Y. pestis* infection in mice. *J Antimicrob Chemother*. 1996;37:769-774.

52. Butler T. Plague. In: Strickland GT, ed. *Tropical Medicine*. Philadelphia, Pa: WB Saunders Co; 1991: 408-416.

53. *Expert Committee on Plague*. Geneva, Switzerland: World Health Organization; 1959. Technical Report Series 165.

54. Burkle FM. Plague as seen in South Vietnamese children. *Clin Pediatr*. 1973;12:291-298.

55. Frean JA, Arntzen L, Capper T, Bryskier A, Klugman KP. In vitro activities of 14 antibiotics against 100 human isolates of *Yersinia pestis* from a Southern African plague focus. *Antimicrob Agents Chemother*. 1996;40:2646-2647.

56. Brygoo ER, Gonon M. Une epidemie de peste pulmonaire dans le Nor-Est de Madagascar. *Bull Soc Pathol Exot*. 1958;51:47-66.

57. Nguyen VI, Nguyen DH, Pham VD, Nguyen VL. Peste bubonique et septicemique traitée avec succes par du trimethoprime-sulfamethoxazole. *Bull Soc Pathol Exot*. 1972;769-779.

58. Butler TJ, Levin J, Linh NN, Chau DM, Adickman M, Arnold K. *Yersinia pestis* infection in Vietnam. *J Infect Dis*. 1976;133:493-499.

59. *WHO Expert Committee on Plague: Third Report*. Geneva, Switzerland: World Health Organization; 1970:1-25. Technical Report Series 447.

60. Galimand M, Guiyoule A, Gerbaud G, et al. Multidrug resistance in *Yersinia pestis* mediated by a transferable plasmid. *N Engl J Med*. 1997;337:677-680.

61. Ryzhko IV, Shcherbaniuk AI, Samokhodkina ED, et al. Virulence of rifampicin and quinolone resistant mutants of strains of plague microbe with Fra+ and Fra– phenotypes. *Antibiot Khimioter*. 1994;39: 32-36.

62. Scott JL, Finegold SM, Belkin GA, et al. A controlled double blind study of the hematologic toxicity of chloramphenicol. *N Engl J Med*. 1965;272: 113-142.

63. Watterberg KL, Kelly HW, Angelus P, Backstrom C. The need for a loading dose of gentamicin in neonates. *Ther Drug Monit*. 1989;11:16-20.

64. Consensus Report of the International Society of Chemotherapy Commission: use of fluoroquinolones in pediatrics. *Pediatr Infect Dis J*. 1995;14:1-9.

65. Sakala E. *Obstetrics and Gynecology*. Baltimore, Md: Williams & Wilkins; 1997:945.

66. Cziel A, Rockenbauer M. Teratogenic study of doxycycline. *Obstet Gynecol*. 1997;89:524-528.

67. Garner JS. Guidelines for isolation precautions in hospitals: Hospital Infection Control Practices Advisory Committee. *Infect Control Hosp Epidemiol*. 1996; 17:53-80.

68. Burmeister RW, Tigertt WD, Overholt EL. Laboratory-acquired pneumonic plague. *Ann Intern Med*. 1962;56:789-800.

69. Morse S, McDade J. Recommendations for working with pathogenic bacteria. *Methods Enzymol*. 1994; 235:1-26.

70. *Safety Measures for Use in Outbreaks in Communicable Disease Outbreaks*. Geneva, Switzerland: World Health Organization; 1986.

71. Gershon RR, Vlahov D, Cejudo JA, et al. Tuberculosis risk in funeral home employees. *J Occup Environ Med*. 1998;40:497-503.

72. Freeman BA. *Yersinia; Pasturella; Francisella; Actinobacillus*. In: *Textbook of Microbiology*. Philadelphia, Pa: WB Saunders Co; 1985:513-530.

©2000 American Medical Association. All rights reserved.

Tularemia as a Biological Weapon
Medical and Public Health Management

David T. Dennis, MD, MPH

Thomas V. Inglesby, MD

Donald A. Henderson, MD, MPH

John G. Bartlett, MD

Michael S. Ascher, MD

Edward Eitzen, MD, MPH

Anne D. Fine, MD

Arthur M. Friedlander, MD

Jerome Hauer, MHS

Marcelle Layton, MD

Scott R. Lillibridge, MD

Joseph E. McDade, PhD

Michael T. Osterholm, PhD, MPH

Tara O'Toole, MD, MPH

Gerald Parker, PhD, DVM

Trish M. Perl, MD, MSc

Philip K. Russell, MD

Kevin Tonat, DrPH, MPH

for the Working Group on
Civilian Biodefense

Objective The Working Group on Civilian Biodefense has developed consensus-based recommendations for measures to be taken by medical and public health professionals if tularemia is used as a biological weapon against a civilian population.

Participants The working group included 25 representatives from academic medical centers, civilian and military governmental agencies, and other public health and emergency management institutions and agencies.

Evidence MEDLINE databases were searched from January 1966 to October 2000, using the Medical Subject Headings *Francisella tularensis*, *Pasteurella tularensis*, *biological weapon*, *biological terrorism*, *bioterrorism*, *biological warfare*, and *biowarfare*. Review of these references led to identification of relevant materials published prior to 1966. In addition, participants identified other references and sources.

Consensus Process Three formal drafts of the statement that synthesized information obtained in the formal evidence-gathering process were reviewed by members of the working group. Consensus was achieved on the final draft.

Conclusions A weapon using airborne tularemia would likely result 3 to 5 days later in an outbreak of acute, undifferentiated febrile illness with incipient pneumonia, pleuritis, and hilar lymphadenopathy. Specific epidemiological, clinical, and microbiological findings should lead to early suspicion of intentional tularemia in an alert health system; laboratory confirmation of agent could be delayed. Without treatment, the clinical course could progress to respiratory failure, shock, and death. Prompt treatment with streptomycin, gentamicin, doxycycline, or ciprofloxacin is recommended. Prophylactic use of doxycycline or ciprofloxacin may be useful in the early postexposure period.

JAMA. 2001;285:2763-2773   www.jama.com

I know of no other infection of animals communicable to man that can be acquired from sources so numerous and so diverse. In short, one can but feel that the status of tularemia, both as a disease in nature and of man, is one of potentiality.

R. R. Parker[1]

TULAREMIA, A BACTERIAL ZOONO-sis, is the subject of this fifth article in a series providing recommendations for medical and public health management following use of various agents as biological weapons of terrorism.[2-5] The causative agent of tularemia, *Francisella tularensis*, is one of the most infectious pathogenic bacteria known, requiring inoculation or inhalation of as few as 10 organisms to cause disease.[6,7] Humans become incidentally infected through diverse environmental exposures and can develop severe and sometimes fatal illness but do not transmit infection to others. The Working Group on Civilian Biodefense considers *F tularensis* to be a dangerous potential biological weapon because of its extreme infectivity, ease of dissemination, and substantial capacity to cause illness and death.[8-11]

CONSENSUS METHODS

The working group comprised 25 representatives from academic medical centers, civilian and military governmental agencies, and other public health and emergency management institutions. This group followed a specified process in developing a consensus statement. MEDLINE databases from January 1966 to October 2000 were searched

Author Affiliations: National Center for Infectious Diseases, Centers for Disease Control and Prevention, Atlanta, Ga (Drs Dennis, Lillibridge, and McDade); Center for Civilian Biodefense Studies, Johns Hopkins University Schools of Medicine (Drs Inglesby, Bartlett, and Perl) and Public Health (Drs Henderson, O'Toole, and Russell), Baltimore, Md; Viral and Rickettsial Diseases Laboratory, California Department of Health Services, Berkeley (Dr Ascher); US Army Medical Research Institute of Infectious Diseases, Ft Detrick, Md (Drs Eitzen, Friedlander, and Parker); Bureau of Communicable Disease, New York City Health Department

(Drs Fine and Layton), and Kroll Associates (Mr Hauer), New York, NY; ican Inc, Eden Prairie, Minn (Dr Osterholm); and Office of Emergency Preparedness, Department of Health and Human Services, Rockville, Md (Dr Tonat).
Ex Officio Participants in the Working Group on Civilian Biodefense are listed at the end of this article. **Corresponding Author and Reprints:** David T. Dennis, MD, MPH, Division of Vector-Borne Infectious Diseases, National Center for Infectious Diseases, Centers for Disease Control and Prevention, PO Box 2087, Fort Collins, CO 80522 (e-mail: dtd1@cdc.gov).

©2001 American Medical Association. All rights reserved.

Reprinted with permission from *JAMA*; June 6, 2001, Vol 285, No. 21

using the Medical Subject Headings *Francisella tularensis*, *Pasteurella tularensis*, *biological weapon*, *biological terrorism*, *bioterrorism*, *biological warfare*, and *biowarfare*. Review of the bibliographies of these references led to identification of relevant materials published prior to 1966. In addition, participants identified other published and unpublished references and sources for review.

The first draft of the consensus statement was a synthesis of information obtained in the formal evidence-gathering process. Members of the working group were asked to make written comments on this first draft in May 1999. Subsequent revised drafts were reviewed and edited until full consensus of the working group was achieved.

HISTORY AND POTENTIAL AS A BIOLOGICAL WEAPON

Tularemia was first described as a plague-like disease of rodents in 1911 and, shortly thereafter, was recognized as a potentially severe and fatal illness in humans.[12] Tularemia's epidemic potential became apparent in the 1930s and 1940s, when large waterborne outbreaks occurred in Europe and the Soviet Union[13-15] and epizootic-associated cases occurred in the United States.[16,17] As well, *F tularensis* quickly gained notoriety as a virulent laboratory hazard.[18,19] Public health concerns impelled substantial early investigations into tularemia's ecology, microbiology, pathogenicity, and prevention.[19-22]

Francisella tularensis has long been considered a potential biological weapon. It was one of a number of agents studied at Japanese germ warfare research units operating in Manchuria between 1932 and 1945[23]; it was also examined for military purposes in the West. A former Soviet Union biological weapons scientist, Ken Alibeck, has suggested that tularemia outbreaks affecting tens of thousands of Soviet and German soldiers on the eastern European front during World War II may have been the result of intentional use.[24] Following the war, there were continuing military studies of tularemia. In the

1950s and 1960s, the US military developed weapons that would disseminate *F tularensis* aerosols[10]; concurrently, it conducted research to better understand the pathophysiology of tularemia and to develop vaccines and antibiotic prophylaxis and treatment regimens. In some studies, volunteers were infected with *F tularensis* by direct aerosol delivery systems and by exposures in an aerosol chamber.[10] A live attenuated vaccine was developed that partially protected against respiratory and intracutaneous challenges with the virulent SCHU S-4 strain of *F tularensis*,[6,7] and various regimens of streptomycin, tetracyclines, and chloramphenicol were found to be effective in prophylaxis and treatment.[25-27] By the late 1960s, *F tularensis* was one of several biological weapons stockpiled by the US military.[10] According to Alibeck, a large parallel effort by the Soviet Union continued into the early 1990s and resulted in weapons production of *F tularensis* strains engineered to be resistant to antibiotics and vaccines.[24]

In 1969, a World Health Organization expert committee estimated that an aerosol dispersal of 50 kg of virulent *F tularensis* over a metropolitan area with 5 million inhabitants would result in 250 000 incapacitating casualties, including 19 000 deaths.[28] Illness would be expected to persist for several weeks and disease relapses to occur during the ensuing weeks or months. It was assumed that vaccinated individuals would be only partially protected against an aerosol exposure. Referring to this model, the Centers for Disease Control and Prevention (CDC) recently examined the expected economic impact of bioterrorist attacks and estimated the total base costs to society of an *F tularensis* aerosol attack to be $5.4 billion for every 100 000 persons exposed.[9]

The United States terminated its biological weapons development program by executive order in 1970 and, by 1973, had destroyed its entire biological arsenal.[10] Since then, the US Army Medical Research Institute of Infectious Diseases has been responsible for defensive medical research on *F tu-*

larensis and other potential biological warfare agents to better protect the US military, including protocols on decontamination, prophylaxis, clinical recognition, laboratory diagnosis, and medical management.[29] The CDC operates a national program for bioterrorism preparedness and response that incorporates a broad range of public health partnerships.[30,31]

EPIDEMIOLOGY
Geographic Distribution and Human Exposures

Tularemia occurs throughout much of North America and Eurasia.[15,21,22,32] In the United States, human cases have been reported from every state except Hawaii; however, most cases occur in south-central and western states (especially Missouri, Arkansas, Oklahoma, South Dakota, and Montana).[33-35] In Eurasia, the disease is also widely endemic, although the greatest numbers of human cases are reported from northern and central Europe, especially Scandinavian countries and those of the former Soviet Union.[36,37] Tularemia is almost entirely a rural disease, although urban and suburban exposures occasionally do occur.[38-41]

Throughout its range, *F tularensis* is found in widely diverse animal hosts and habitats and can be recovered from contaminated water, soil, and vegetation.[15,20-22,32] A variety of small mammals, including voles, mice, water rats, squirrels, rabbits, and hares, are natural reservoirs of infection. They acquire infection through bites by ticks, flies, and mosquitoes, and by contact with contaminated environments. Although enzootic cycles of *F tularensis* typically occur without notice, epizootics with sometimes extensive die-offs of animal hosts may herald outbreaks of tularemia in humans.[16,22,42,43] Humans become infected with *F tularensis* by various modes, including bites by infective arthropods,[42,44-47] handling infectious animal tissues or fluids,[17,48,49] direct contact with or ingestion of contaminated water, food, or soil,[13,20,40,50,51] and inhalation of infective aerosols.[43,52-56] Persons of all ages

©2001 American Medical Association. All rights reserved.

Reprinted with permission from *JAMA*; June 6, 2001, Vol 285, No. 21

and both sexes appear to be equally susceptible to tularemia. Certain activities, such as hunting, trapping, butchering, and farming, are most likely to expose adult men. Laboratory workers are especially vulnerable to infection, either by accidentally inoculating themselves or by inhaling aerosolized organisms.[18,22,56-58] Ordinary exposures during examination of an open culture plate can cause infection. Although *F tularensis* is highly infectious and pathogenic, its transmission from person to person has not been documented.

Incidence

The worldwide incidence of tularemia is not known, and the disease is probably greatly underrecognized and underreported. In the United States, reported cases have dropped sharply from several thousand per year prior to 1950 to less than 200 per year in the 1990s.[33-35] Between 1985 and 1992, 1409 cases and 20 deaths were reported in the United States, for a mean of 171 cases per year and a case-fatality rate of 1.4%.[34] Persons in all age groups were affected, but most were children younger than 10 years and adults aged 50 years or older. Of 1298 cases for which information on sex was available, 942 (72.6%) occurred in males, and males outnumbered females in all age groups. Most cases occur in June through September, when arthropod-borne transmission is most common.[17,35,59] Cases in winter usually occur among hunters and trappers who handle infected animal carcasses.[17,35,48] In the United States, cases are mostly sporadic or occur in small clusters[34,35,49]; in Eurasia, waterborne, arthropod-borne, and airborne outbreaks involving hundreds of persons have been reported.[40,43,44,51,53-55]

Natural Occurrences of Inhalational Tularemia

The largest recorded airborne tularemia outbreak occurred in 1966-1967 in an extensive farming area of Sweden.[43] This outbreak involved more than 600 patients infected with strains of the milder European biovar of *F tularensis*

(*F tularensis* biovar palaearctica) [type B]), most of whom acquired infection while doing farm work that created contaminated aerosols. Case exposures and disease onsets occurred during a period of months but peaked during the winter, when rodent-infested hay was being sorted and moved from field storage sites to barns. Among 140 serologically confirmed cases thought to have been infected by inhalation, most had typical acute symptoms of fever, fatigue, chills, headache, and malaise; only 14 (10%) of confirmed patients had symptoms of pneumonia, such as dyspnea and chest pains. Patients generally responded well to tetracycline, and no deaths were reported. Inhalational tularemia in the United States has involved only single cases or small clusters of cases, variously resulting from laboratory exposures,[18,56,57] disturbance of contaminated animal carcasses,[38,39,41] and suspected infective environmental aerosols.[41,52] Cases of inhalational tularemia in the United States are thought to be due mostly to the more virulent *F tularensis* biovar tularensis (type A) and usually follow an acute and severe course, with prominent pneumonitis. Some cases, however, have radiographic evidence of pleuropneumonia with minimal or absent respiratory signs on physical examination.[39,41,52]

Although airborne *F tularensis* would be expected to principally cause primary pleuropneumonic infection, some exposures might contaminate the eye, resulting in ocular tularemia; penetrate broken skin, resulting in ulceroglandular or glandular disease; or cause oropharyngeal disease with cervical lymphadenitis. In the aforementioned Swedish outbreak, conjunctivitis was reported in 26% of 140 confirmed cases and an infected ulcer of the skin was reported in nearly 12%; pharyngitis was reported in 31% and oral ulcers in about 9% of the cases; and 32% of these patients had various exanthemas, such as erythema multiforme and erythema nodosum.[43] Tularemia outbreaks arising from similar agricultural exposures have been reported from Finland,[53] mostly presenting with general constitutional

symptoms rather than specific manifestations of pneumonia; enlargement of hilar nodes was the principal radiographic finding in these cases.[54]

Inhalational Tularemia Following Use as a Biological Weapon

Although *F tularensis* could be used as a weapon in a number of ways, the working group believes that an aerosol release would have the greatest adverse medical and public health consequences. Release in a densely populated area would be expected to result in an abrupt onset of large numbers of cases of acute, nonspecific febrile illness beginning 3 to 5 days later (incubation range, 1-14 days), with pleuropneumonitis developing in a significant proportion of cases during the ensuing days and weeks. Public health authorities would most likely become aware of an outbreak of unusual respiratory disease in its early stages, but this could be difficult to distinguish from a natural outbreak of community-acquired infection, especially influenza or various atypical pneumonias. The abrupt onset of large numbers of acutely ill persons, the rapid progression in a relatively high proportion of cases from upper respiratory symptoms and bronchitis to life-threatening pleuropneumonitis and systemic infection affecting, among others, young, previously healthy adults and children should, however, quickly alert medical professionals and public health authorities to a critical and unexpected public health event and to bioterrorism as a possible cause (TABLE 1). Until the etiology became clear, clinicians would need to work closely with epidemiologists and diagnostic laboratories to differentiate the illness from various community-acquired pneumonias and to determine if it could have resulted from use of one of several potential bioterrorism weapons agents, such as those causing tularemia, plague, anthrax, or Q fever.[2,4,29]

In general, tularemia would be expected to have a slower progression of illness and a lower case-fatality rate than either inhalational plague or anthrax. Plague would most likely progress very

©2001 American Medical Association. All rights reserved.

Reprinted with permission from *JAMA*; June 6, 2001, Vol 285, No. 21

Table 1. Diagnosis of Inhalational Tularemia Following Use of a Biological Weapon

Clinical Findings

Sudden onset of acute febrile illness, progressing in some patients to pharyngitis, bronchiolitis, pneumonitis, pleuritis, hilar lymphadenitis. Complications of overwhelming untreated infection may lead to sepsis and inflammatory response syndrome.

Epidemiology

Point-source outbreak pattern; likely urban, nonagricultural setting. Unexpected severe respiratory illness in otherwise healthy persons. Risk related to degree of exposure with no differences in susceptibility by age or sex.

Microbiology

Small, gram-negative coccobacilli in direct stain of respiratory secretions. Sputum, tracheobronchial secretions, and blood should be cultured using cysteine-enriched medium. Antimicrobial susceptibility of isolates should be determined. Direct fluorescent antibody stain is first-line, rapid identification procedure at reference laboratories. Polymerase chain reaction and antigen detection procedures may also provide rapid identification. Microagglutination assay can detect serum antibodies beginning 10 days after illness onset. Virulence testing and molecular genetic characterizations are performed at specialized laboratories.

Pathology

Histological findings of acute suppurative necrosis followed by granulomatous reactions. Target organs include lungs, lymph nodes, spleen, liver, and kidney.

Radiology

Peribronchial infiltrates leading to bronchopneumonia in 1 or more lobes, often accompanied by pleural effusion and enlarged hilar nodes. Signs may be absent or minimal, with only 1 or several small, discrete pulmonary infiltrates, or scattered granulomatous lesions of lung parenchyma or pleura.

rapidly to severe pneumonia, with copious watery or purulent sputum production, hemoptysis, respiratory insufficiency, sepsis, and shock.[4] Inhalational anthrax would be differentiated by its characteristic radiological findings of prominent symmetric mediastinal widening and absence of bronchopneumonia.[2] As well, anthrax patients would be expected to develop fulminating, toxic, and fatal illness despite antibiotic treatment.[29] Milder forms of inhalational tularemia could be clinically indistinguishable from Q fever; establishing a diagnosis of either would be problematic without reference laboratory testing. Presumptive laboratory diagnoses of plague or anthrax would be expected to be made relatively quickly, although microbiological confirmation could take days. Isolation and identification of F tularensis using routine laboratory procedures could take several weeks.

Once a substantial cluster of cases of inhalational tularemia had been identified, epidemiological findings should suggest a bioterrorist event. The abrupt onset and single peak of cases would implicate a point-source exposure without secondary transmission. Among exposed persons, attack rates would likely be similar across sex and age groups, and risk would be related to degree of exposure to the point source (Table 1). An outbreak of inhalational tularemia in an urban setting should trigger a high level of suspicion of an intentional event, since all reported inhalational tularemia outbreaks have occurred in rural areas.

MICROBIOLOGY AND VIRULENCE FACTORS

Francisella tularensis is a small, nonmotile, aerobic, gram-negative coccobacillus. It has a thin lipopolysaccharide-containing envelope and is a hardy non–spore-forming organism that survives for weeks at low temperatures in water, moist soil, hay, straw, and decaying animal carcasses.[21,22,60,61] *Francisella tularensis* has been divided into 2 major subspecies (biovars) by virulence testing, biochemical reactions, and epidemiological features.[62] *Francisella tularensis* biovar tularensis (type A) may be highly virulent in humans and animals, produces acid from glycerol, demonstrates citrulline ureidase activity, and is the most common biovar isolated in North America.[22,60] *Francisella tularensis* biovar palaearctica (type B) is relatively avirulent, does not produce acid from glycerol, and does not demonstrate citrulline ureidase activity. In Europe and Asia, all human tularemia is thought to be caused by the milder type B strains, although recent studies there have identified naturally occurring *F tularensis* related to *F tularensis* biovar tularensis.[63,64] A few rapidly growing strains of *F tularensis* have been recovered from the blood of immunocompromised patients not showing seroreactivity to *F tularensis*.[65]

Transformed plasmids have been engineered to express chloramphenicol and tetracycline resistance in *F tularensis*.[66] Virulent, streptomycin-resistant *F tularensis* strains have been examined in biowarfare agent studies both in the United States and the Soviet Union.[24,27,56] Although *F tularensis* virulence factors are poorly understood and characterized,[67,68] it is possible that strain virulence could be enhanced through laboratory manipulation.

PATHOGENESIS AND CLINICAL MANIFESTATIONS
Pathogenesis

Francisella tularensis can infect humans through the skin, mucous membranes, gastrointestinal tract, and lungs. It is a facultative intracellular bacterium that multiplies within macrophages.[68,69] The major target organs are the lymph nodes, lungs and pleura, spleen, liver, and kidney.[19,20,49,70-72] Untreated, bacilli inoculated into skin or mucous membranes multiply, spread to the regional lymph nodes and further multiply, and may then disseminate to organs throughout the body. Bacteremia may be common in the early phase of infection. The initial tissue reaction to infection is a focal, intensely suppurative necrosis consisting largely of accumulations of polymorphonuclear leukocytes, followed by invasion of macrophages, epithelioid cells, and lymphocytes. Suppurative lesions become granulomatous, and histopathological examination of the granulomas shows a central necrotic, sometimes caseating zone surrounded by a layer of epithelioid cells, multinucleated giant cells, and fibroblasts in a radial arrange-

©2001 American Medical Association. All rights reserved.

Reprinted with permission from *JAMA*; June 6, 2001, Vol 285, No. 21

ment, typical of other granulomatous conditions, such as tuberculosis and sarcoidosis.[20,70,71]

Monkeys that inhaled the virulent SCHU S-4 strain of *F tularensis* (type A) developed acute bronchiolitis within 24 hours of exposure to 1-μm particles and within 48 hours of exposure to 8-μm particles.[73] By 72 hours following challenge, inflammation was present in peribronchial tissues and alveolar septa. Bronchopneumonia was most pronounced in animals exposed to the smaller particles and was characterized by tracheobronchial lymph node enlargement and reddish, firm, 0.2- to 0.5-cm-diameter discrete inflammatory lesions scattered throughout the lungs. In the absence of treatment, the disease progressed to pneumonic consolidation and organization, granuloma formation, and eventual chronic interstitial fibrosis.

Humans with inhalational exposures also develop hemorrhagic inflammation of the airways early in the course of illness, which may progress to bronchopneumonia.[54] Histopathological examination of affected lungs shows alveolar spaces filled with an exudate of mononuclear cells. Pleuritis with adhesions and effusion and hilar lymphadenopathy are common radiological and pathological findings.[70,72]

Clinical Manifestations

The primary clinical forms of tularemia vary in severity and presentation according to virulence of the infecting organism, dose, and site of inoculum. Primary disease presentations include ulceroglandular, glandular, oculoglandular, oropharyngeal, pneumonic, typhoidal, and septic forms.[19,20,49,70,72,74,75] The term *typhoidal tularemia* has been used to describe illness in tularemia patients with systemic infections manifesting as fever and other constitutional signs without cutaneous or mucosal membrane lesions or regional lymphadenitis. Sometimes, these patients present with prominent gastrointestinal manifestations, such as diarrhea and pain. Confusion is created when *typhoidal tularemia* is used to describe the illness in patients infected by

inhalation, especially when there are signs of pleuropneumonic disease; this usage can be misleading and has been discouraged.[54,75]

The onset of tularemia is usually abrupt, with fever (38°C-40°C), headache, chills and rigors, generalized body aches (often prominent in the low back), coryza, and sore throat. A pulse-temperature dissociation has been noted in as many as 42% of patients.[49] A dry or slightly productive cough and substernal pain or tightness frequently occur with or without objective signs of pneumonia, such as purulent sputum, dyspnea, tachypnea, pleuritic pain, or hemoptysis.[7,19,26,70,74] Nausea, vomiting, and diarrhea sometimes occur. Sweats, fever and chills, progressive weakness, malaise, anorexia, and weight loss characterize the continuing illness. Studies of volunteers have shown that *F tularensis* aerosol exposures can incapacitate some persons in the first 1 or 2 days of illness, and significant impairment in performing tasks can continue for days after antibiotic treatment is begun.[76] In untreated tularemia, symptoms often persist for several weeks and, sometimes, for months, usually with progressive debility. Any form of tularemia may be complicated by hematogenous spread, resulting in secondary pleuropneumonia, sepsis, and, rarely, meningitis.[74,77]

Prior to the advent of antibiotics, the overall mortality from infections with the more severe type A strains was in the range of 5% to 15%, and fatality rates as high as 30% to 60% were reported for untreated pneumonic and severe systemic forms of disease.[72,78] Currently, the overall case-fatality rate of reported cases in the United States is less than 2%.[34,49] Type B infections are rarely fatal.

In ulceroglandular tularemia, the form that typically arises from handling a contaminated carcass or following an infective arthropod bite, a local cutaneous papule appears at the inoculation site at about the time of onset of generalized symptoms, becomes pustular, and ulcerates within a few days of its first appearance. The ulcer is ten-

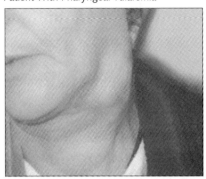

Figure 1. Cervical Lymphadenitis in a Patient With Pharyngeal Tularemia

Patient has marked swelling and fluctuant suppuration of several anterior cervical nodes. Infection was acquired by ingestion of contaminated food or water. Source: World Health Organization.

der, generally has an indolent character, and may be covered by an eschar. Typically, one or more regional afferent lymph nodes may become enlarged and tender within several days of the appearance of the papule. Even with antibiotic treatment, the affected nodes may become fluctuant and rupture. In oculoglandular tularemia, which follows direct contamination of the eye, ulceration occurs on the conjunctiva, accompanied by pronounced chemosis, vasculitis, and regional lymphadenitis. Glandular tularemia is characterized by lymphadenopathy without an ulcer.

Oropharyngeal tularemia is acquired by drinking contaminated water, ingesting contaminated food, and, sometimes, by inhaling contaminated droplets or aerosols.[14,20,36,43,50,51,79] Affected persons may develop stomatitis but more commonly develop exudative pharyngitis or tonsillitis, sometimes with ulceration. Pronounced cervical or retropharyngeal lymphadenopathy may occur (FIGURE 1).[74,79]

Tularemia pneumonia can be the direct result of inhaling contaminated aerosols or be secondary to hematogenous spread from a distal site. An aerosol release of *F tularensis* would be expected to result in acute illness with signs and symptoms of 1 or more of pharyngitis, bronchiolitis, pleuropneumonitis, and hilar lymphadenitis, accompanied by various manifesta-

©2001 American Medical Association. All rights reserved.

Reprinted with permission from *JAMA*; June 6, 2001, Vol 285, No. 21

Figure 2. Chest Radiograph of a Patient With Pulmonary Tularemia

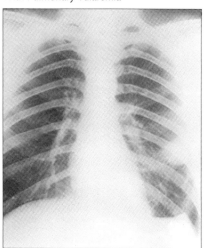

Infiltrates in left lower lung, tenting of diaphragm, probably caused by pleural effusion, and enlargement of left hilum. Source: Armed Forces Institute of Pathology.

Box. Clinicians Caring for Patients With Suspected Tularemia Should Immediately Contact Their:

(1) Hospital epidemiologist or infection control practitioner and

(2) Local or state health departments

Consult your local telephone operator, the telephone directory under "governmental listings," or the Internet at http://www.cdc.gov/other .htm#states or http://www.astho.org /state.html

If the local and state health departments are unavailable, contact the Centers for Disease Control and Prevention at (970) 221-6400 or http://www.cdc.gov/ncidod/dvbid /dvbid.htm

tions of systemic illness. Inhalational exposures, however, commonly result in an initial clinical picture of systemic illness without prominent signs of respiratory disease.[7,43,53,56] The earliest pulmonary radiographic findings of inhalational tularemia may be peribronchial infiltrates, typically advancing to bronchopneumonia in 1 or more lobes, and often accompanied by pleural effusions and hilar lymphadenopathy (FIGURE 2).[72,75] Signs may, however, be minimal or absent, and some patients will show only 1 or several small, discrete pulmonary infiltrates or scattered granulomatous lesions of lung parenchyma or pleura. Although volunteers challenged with aerosols of virulent *F tularensis* (type A) regularly developed systemic symptoms of acute illness 3 to 5 days following exposure, only 25% to 50% of participants had radiological evidence of pneumonia in the early stages of infection.[7,26] On the other hand, pulmonary infection can sometimes rapidly progress to severe pneumonia, respiratory failure, and death.[72,80] Lung abscesses occur infrequently.[75]

Typhoidal tularemia is used to describe systemic illness in the absence of signs indicating either site of inoculation or anatomic localization of infection. This should be differentiated from inhalational tularemia with pleuropneumonic disease.[54,75]

Tularemia sepsis is potentially severe and fatal. As in typhoidal tularemia, nonspecific findings of fever, abdominal pain, diarrhea, and vomiting may be prominent early in the course of illness. The patient typically appears toxic and may develop confusion and coma. Unless treated promptly, septic shock and other complications of systemic inflammatory response syndrome may ensue, including disseminated intravascular coagulation and bleeding, acute respiratory distress syndrome, and organ failure.[80]

DIAGNOSIS

Tularemia in humans occurs infrequently, resulting in a low index of diagnostic suspicion among clinicians and laboratorians. Since rapid diagnostic testing for tularemia is not widely available, the first indication of intentional tularemia might follow recognition by public health authorities of a clustering of acute, severe respiratory illness with unusual epidemiological features (Table 1). Suspicion of tularemia might be triggered in alert clini-cians encountering patients with findings of atypical pneumonia, pleuritis, and hilar lymphadenopathy. Identification of *F tularensis* in clinical specimens may be missed or delayed for days or weeks when procedures for routine microbiological screening of bacterial pathogens are followed, and it is unlikely that a serendipitous laboratory identification would be the sentinel event that alerted authorities to a major bioterrorism action.

Physicians who suspect inhalational tularemia should promptly collect specimens of respiratory secretions and blood and alert the laboratory to the need for special diagnostic and safety procedures. *Francisella tularensis* may be identified by direct examination of secretions, exudates, or biopsy specimens using direct fluorescent antibody or immunohistochemical stains.[81-83] By light microscopy, the organism is characterized by its small size ($0.2 \mu m \times 0.2$-$0.7 \mu m$), pleomorphism, and faint staining. It does not show the bipolar staining characteristics of *Yersinia pestis*,[4] the agent of plague, and is easily distinguished from the large gram-positive rods characteristic of vegetative forms of *Bacillus anthracis* (FIGURE 3).[2] Microscopic demonstration of *F tularensis* using fluorescent-labeled antibodies is a rapid diagnostic procedure performed in designated reference laboratories in the National Public Health Laboratory Network; test results can be made available within several hours of receiving the appropriate specimens if the laboratory is alerted and prepared. Suspicion of inhalational tularemia must be promptly reported to local or state public health authorities so timely epidemiological and environmental investigations can be made (BOX).

Growth of *F tularensis* in culture is the definitive means of confirming the diagnosis of tularemia.[60,81] *Francisella tularensis* can be grown from pharyngeal washings, sputum specimens, and even fasting gastric aspirates in a high proportion of patients with inhalational tularemia.[56] It is only occasionally isolated from the blood. *Fran-*

©2001 American Medical Association. All rights reserved.

Reprinted with permission from *JAMA*; June 6, 2001, Vol 285, No. 21

Figure 3. Gram Stain Smears of the Agents of Anthrax (*Bacillus anthracis*), Plague (*Yersinia pestis*), and Tularemia (*Francisella tularensis*), Demonstrating Comparative Morphology, Size, and Staining Characteristics

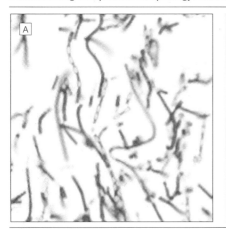

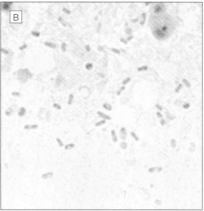

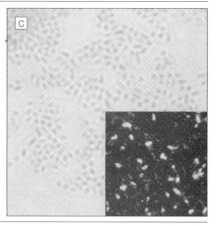

A, *B anthracis* is a large (0.5-1.2 µm × 2.5-10.0 µm), chain-forming, gram-positive rod that sporulates under certain conditions (Gram stain of organism from culture; original magnification ×250); B, *Y pestis* is a gram-negative, plump, non–spore-forming, bipolar-staining bacillus that is approximately 0.5-0.8 µm × 1-3 µm (Gram stain of smear from infected tissue; original magnification ×250); C, *F tularensis* is a small (0.2 µm × 0.2-0.7 µm), pleomorphic, poorly staining, gram-negative coccobacillus (Gram stain of organism from culture; original magnification ×500) (inset, direct immunofluorescence of smear of *F tularensis*; original magnification ×400. Sources: A and B, Sherif Zaki, Centers for Disease Control and Prevention; C, Armed Forces Institute of Pathology.

cisella tularensis grows best in cysteine-enriched broth and thioglycollate broth and on cysteine heart blood agar, buffered charcoal-yeast agar, and chocolate agar. Selective agar (such as chocolate agar selective for *Neisseria gonorrhea* isolation) may be useful when culturing materials from non-sterile sites, such as sputum. Inoculated media should be incubated at 37°C. Although growth may be visible as early as 24 to 48 hours after inoculation, growth may be delayed and cultures should be held for at least 10 days before discarding. Under ideal conditions, bacterial colonies on cysteine-enriched agar are typically 1 mm in diameter after 24 to 48 hours of incubation and 3 to 5 mm in diameter by 96 hours.[60,81] On cysteine heart agar, *F tularensis* colonies are characteristically opalescent and do not discolor the medium (FIGURE 4).

Antigen detection assays, polymerase chain reaction, enzyme-linked immunoassays, immunoblotting, pulsed-field gel electrophoresis, and other specialized techniques may be used to identify *F tularensis* and to characterize strains.[84-87] These procedures are usually performed only in research and reference laboratories, however. In laboratories where advanced methods are

established, results of antigen detection and polymerase chain reaction analyses can be obtained within several hours of receipt of isolates. Typically, serum antibody titers do not attain diagnostic levels until 10 or more days after onset of illness, and serology would provide minimal useful information for managing an outbreak. Serological confirmation of cases, however, may be of value for forensic or epidemiological purposes. Most laboratories use tube agglutination or microagglutination tests that detect combined immunoglobulin M and immunoglobulin G.[84,85] A 4-fold change in titer between acute and convalescent serum specimens, a single titer of at least 1:160 for tube agglutination or 1:128 for microagglutination is diagnostic for *F tularensis* infection. Information on reference diagnostic testing and shipping/handling of specimens can be obtained from state public health laboratories and from the Division of Vector-Borne Infectious Diseases, CDC, Fort Collins, Colo (telephone: [970] 221-6400; e-mail: dvbid@cdc.gov).

VACCINATION

Beginning in the 1930s, the Soviet Union used a live attenuated vaccine to immunize tens of millions of persons living in tularemia-endemic areas.[88] In

Figure 4. *Francisella tularensis* Growth at 72 Hours After Inoculation

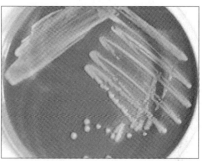

These *Francisella tularensis* colonies show characteristic opalescence on cysteine heart agar with sheep blood (cultured at 37°C for 72 hours). Source: Centers for Disease Control and Prevention.

the United States, a live attenuated vaccine derived from the avirulent live vaccine strain has been used to protect laboratorians routinely working with *F tularensis*; until recently, this vaccine was available as an investigational new drug.[89] It is currently under review by the US Food and Drug Administration (FDA), and its future availability is undetermined.

In a retrospective study of civilians working with *F tularensis* at a US Army research facility, the incidence of accidental acute inhalational tularemia among laboratorians declined from 5.70 cases per 1000 person-years of risk at

©2001 American Medical Association. All rights reserved.

Reprinted with permission from *JAMA*; June 6, 2001, Vol 285, No. 21

Table 2. Working Group Consensus Recommendations for Treatment of Patients With Tularemia in a Contained Casualty Setting*

Contained Casualty Recommended Therapy

Adults

Preferred choices
   Streptomycin, 1 g IM twice daily
   Gentamicin, 5 mg/kg IM or IV once daily†
Alternative choices
   Doxycycline, 100 mg IV twice daily
   Chloramphenicol, 15 mg/kg IV 4 times daily†
   Ciprofloxacin, 400 mg IV twice daily†

Children

Preferred choices
   Streptomycin, 15 mg/kg IM twice daily (should not exceed 2 g)
   Gentamicin, 2.5 mg/kg IM or IV 3 times daily†
Alternative choices
   Doxycycline; if weight ≥45 kg, 100 mg IV twice daily; if weight <45 kg, give 2.2 mg/kg IV twice daily
   Chloramphenicol, 15 mg/kg IV 4 times daily†
   Ciprofloxacin, 15 mg/kg IV twice daily†‡

Pregnant Women

Preferred choices
   Gentamicin, 5 mg/kg IM or IV once daily†
   Streptomycin, 1 g IM twice daily
Alternative choices
   Doxycycline, 100 mg IV twice daily
   Ciprofloxacin, 400 mg IV twice daily†

*Treatment with streptomycin, gentamicin, or ciprofloxacin should be continued for 10 days; treatment with doxycycline or chloramphenicol should be continued for 14-21 days. Persons beginning treatment with intramuscular (IM) or intravenous (IV) doxycycline, ciprofloxacin, or chloramphenicol can switch to oral antibiotic administration when clinically indicated.
†Not a US Food and Drug Administration–approved use.
‡Ciprofloxacin dosage should not exceed 1 g/d in children.

Table 3. Working Group Consensus Recommendations for Treatment of Patients With Tularemia in a Mass Casualty Setting and for Postexposure Prophylaxis*

Mass Casualty Recommended Therapy

Adults

Preferred choices
   Doxycycline, 100 mg orally twice daily
   Ciprofloxacin, 500 mg orally twice daily†

Children

Preferred choices
   Doxycycline; if ≥45 kg, give 100 mg orally twice daily; if <45 kg, give 2.2 mg/kg orally twice daily
   Ciprofloxacin, 15 mg/kg orally twice daily†‡

Pregnant Women

Preferred choices
   Ciprofloxacin, 500 mg orally twice daily†
   Doxycycline, 100 mg orally twice daily

*One antibiotic, appropriate for patient age, should be chosen from among alternatives. The duration of all recommended therapies in Table 3 is 14 days.
†Not a US Food and Drug Administration–approved use.
‡Ciprofloxacin dosage should not exceed 1 g/d in children.

a time when a killed vaccine was in use to 0.27 cases per 1000 person-years of risk after introduction of the live vaccine.[58] Although the incidence of ulceroglandular disease remained unchanged in the 2 periods, signs and symptoms were considered milder among those who received the live vaccine. In volunteer studies, the live attenuated vaccine did not protect all recipients against aerosol challenges with virulent *F tularensis*.[7,26]

Correlates of protective immunity appear about 2 weeks following natural infection or vaccination. Given the short incubation period of tularemia and incomplete protection of current vaccines against inhalational tularemia, vaccination is not recommended for postexposure prophylaxis. The working group recommends use of the live vaccine strain only for laboratory personnel routinely working with *F tularensis*.

TREATMENT
Contained Casualty Situation

Adults. In a contained casualty situation, in which logistics permit individual medical management, the working group recommends parenteral antimicrobial therapy for tularemia (**TABLE 2**). Streptomycin is the drug of choice.[49,74,90,91] Gentamicin, which is more widely available and may be used intravenously, is an acceptable alternative.[49,74,90-93] Treatment with aminoglycosides should be continued for 10 days. Tetracyclines and chloramphenicol are also used to treat tularemia[49,74,90]; however, relapses and primary treatment failures occur at a higher rate with these bacteriostatic agents than with aminoglycosides, and they should be given for at least 14 days to reduce chance of relapse.[27,74,90] Fluoroquinolones, which have intracellular activity, are promising candidates for treating tularemia. Ciprofloxacin, which is not labeled for use in tularemia, has been shown to be active against *F tularensis* in vitro[94] and in animals[95] and has been used to successfully treat tularemia in both adults and chil-

dren.[90,94,96,97] Treatment with ciprofloxacin should be continued for 10 days. In persons beginning treatment with parenteral doxycycline, ciprofloxacin, or chloramphenicol, therapy can be switched to oral antibiotic administration when clinically indicated. Very limited experiences in treating tularemia patients with β-lactam and macrolide antibiotics have been reported, and treatment failures have occurred.[98] Use of β-lactam and macrolide antibiotics in treating tularemia is neither FDA-approved nor recommended by the working group.

Children. In children, streptomycin or gentamicin is recommended by the working group as first-line treatment in a contained casualty situation (Table 2). Doxycycline, ciprofloxacin (≤1 g/d), and chloramphenicol can be used as alternatives to aminoglycosides. Fluoroquinolones have been reported to cause cartilage damage in immature animals and are not FDA-approved for use in children. However, short courses of these agents have not been associated with arthropathy in pediatric patients, and the potential risks of their use must be weighed against their benefits in treating serious infections.[96,99,100]

Mass Casualty Situation

Doxycycline and ciprofloxacin, administered orally, are the preferred choices for treatment in the mass casualty setting, for both adults and children (**TABLE 3**). The ciprofloxacin dosage for children should not exceed 1 g/d. In a mass casualty situation, the working group believes the benefits to children from short courses of doxycycline or fluoroquinolones (Table 3) outweigh the risks of their use.

Since it is unknown whether drug-resistant organisms might be used in a bioterrorist event, antimicrobial susceptibility testing of isolates should be conducted quickly and treatments altered according to test results and clinical responses.

Antibiotics for treating patients infected with tularemia in a bioterrorism scenario are included in a national pharmaceutical stockpile

©2001 American Medical Association. All rights reserved.

Reprinted with permission from *JAMA*; June 6, 2001, Vol 285, No. 21

maintained by the CDC, as are ventilators and other emergency equipment needed to respond to situations of large numbers of critically ill persons that strip local and state resources.[30]

Management of Special Groups

Pregnant Women. In a contained casualty situation, short courses of gentamicin are likely to pose a low risk to fetuses when used to treat tularemia in pregnant women (Table 2). Rare cases of fetal nerve deafness and renal damage have been reported with other aminoglycosides but have not been reported with gentamicin. The benefits of gentamicin in treating pregnant women with tularemia are expected to outweigh any potential risk to fetuses. In a mass casualty situation, oral ciprofloxacin is considered the best alternative to gentamicin for pregnant women (Table 3).

Immunosuppressed Persons. There is scant experience in treating tularemia in immunocompromised patients. However, considering the greater occurrence in immunocompetent patients of tularemia relapses and treatment failures following use of bacteriostatic antimicrobial agents compared with aminoglycosides, streptomycin or gentamicin should be used when possible to treat patients with known immune dysfunction in either contained casualty or mass casualty situations (Table 2).

POSTEXPOSURE ANTIBIOTIC RECOMMENDATIONS

Persons beginning treatment with streptomycin, gentamicin, doxycycline, or ciprofloxacin in the incubation period of tularemia and continuing treatment daily for 14 days might be protected against symptomatic infection. In studies of aerosol challenge with infective doses of the virulent SCHU S-4 strain of *F tularensis*, each of 8 volunteers given oral dosages of tetracycline, 1 g/d for 28 days, and each of 8 volunteers given tetracycline, 2 g/d for 14 days, were fully protected when treatment was begun 24 hours following challenge.[27] Two of 10 volunteers given tetracycline, 1 g/d for only 5 days,

developed symptomatic tularemia after antibiotic treatment was stopped.

In the unlikely event that authorities quickly become aware that an *F tularensis* biological weapon has been used and are able to identify and reach exposed persons during the early incubation period, the working group recommends that exposed persons be prophylactically treated with 14 days of oral doxycycline or ciprofloxacin (Table 3). In a circumstance in which the weapon attack has been covert and the event is discovered only after persons start to become ill, persons potentially exposed should be instructed to begin a fever watch. Persons who develop an otherwise unexplained fever or flulike illness within 14 days of presumed exposure should begin treatment as outlined in Tables 2 and 3.

In the laboratory, persons who have had potentially infective exposures to *F tularensis* should be administered oral postexposure antibiotic prophylaxis if the risk of infection is high (eg, spill, centrifuge accident, or needlestick). If the risk is low, exposed persons can be placed on a fever watch and treated if they develop symptoms.

Postexposure prophylactic antibiotic treatment of close contacts of tularemia patients is not recommended since human-to-human transmission of *F tularensis* is not known to occur.

INFECTION CONTROL

Isolation is not recommended for tularemia patients, given the lack of human-to-human transmission. In hospitals, standard precautions[101] are recommended by the working group for treatment of patients with tularemia.

Microbiology laboratory personnel should be alerted when tularemia is clinically suspected. Routine diagnostic procedures can be performed in biological safety level 2 (BSL-2) conditions. Examination of cultures in which *F tularensis* is suspected should be carried out in a biological safety cabinet. Manipulation of cultures and other activities involving infectious materials with a potential for aerosol or droplet production (centrifuging, grinding, vig-

orous shaking, growing cultures in volume, animal studies) require BSL-3 conditions.[102] When *F tularensis* is presumptively identified in a routine BSL-2 clinical laboratory (level A), specimens should be forwarded to a BSL-3 laboratory (level B) (eg, a state public health laboratory) for confirmation of agent and other studies, such as antimicrobial susceptibility testing.[11] Bodies of patients who die of tularemia should be handled using standard precautions. Autopsy procedures likely to cause aerosols, such as bone sawing, should be avoided. Clothing or linens contaminated with body fluids of patients infected with *F tularensis* should be disinfected per standard precautions protocols.[101]

ENVIRONMENTAL DECONTAMINATION AND PROTECTION

Under natural conditions, *F tularensis* may survive for extended periods in a cold, moist environment. The working group lacks information on survival of intentionally dispersed particles but would expect a short half-life due to desiccation, solar radiation, oxidation and other environmental factors, and a very limited risk from secondary dispersal. In circumstances of a laboratory spill or intentional use in which authorities are concerned about an environmental risk (eg, inanimate surfaces wet with material thought to contain *F tularensis*), decontamination can be achieved by spraying the suspected contaminant with a 10% bleach solution (1 part household bleach and 9 parts water). After 10 minutes, a 70% solution of alcohol can be used to further clean the area and reduce the corrosive action of the bleach. Soap water can be used to flush away less hazardous contaminations. Persons with direct exposure to powder or liquid aerosols containing *F tularensis* should wash body surfaces and clothing with soap water. Standard levels of chlorine in municipal water sources should protect against waterborne infection.[60] Following an urban release, the risk to humans of acquiring tula-

©2001 American Medical Association. All rights reserved.

Reprinted with permission from *JAMA*; June 6, 2001, Vol 285, No. 21

remia from infected animals or arthropod bites is considered minimal and could be reduced by educating the public on simple avoidance of sick or dead animals and on personal protective measures against biting arthropods.

ADDITIONAL RESEARCH

Simple, rapid, and reliable diagnostic tests that could be used to identify persons infected with *F tularensis* in the mass exposure setting need to be developed. Further methods should be designed to rapidly define the molecular genetic characteristics of organisms, especially as they may relate to engineered attributes, such as enhanced virulence and resistance to antimicrobial agents or normally lethal environmental conditions. Complete sequencing and analysis of the genome of natural strains of *F tularensis* would provide an archival base for understanding genetic variants, functions of genes, and mechanisms of action useful in developing means to protect against *F tularensis*. Research is also needed to develop accurate and reliable procedures to rapidly detect *F tularensis* in environmental samples.

New technologies should be explored for developing active (eg, DNA-based) or passive (eg, monoclonal antibody–based) vaccines for rapid preexposure or postexposure protection.

Ex Officio Participants in the Working Group on Civilian Biodefense: George Counts, MD, CDC; Margaret Hamburg, MD, former assistant secretary for planning and evaluation, Department of Health and Human Services (DHHS); Robert Knouss, MD, Office of Emergency Preparedness, DHHS; Brian Malkin, Esq, formerly with the FDA; and Stuart Nightingale, MD, Office of the Assistant Secretary for Planning and Evaluation, DHHS.

Funding/Support: Funding for this study primarily was provided by each participant's institution or agency. The Johns Hopkins Center for Civilian Biodefense Studies provided travel funds for 5 of the group.

Disclaimers: In some instances, the indications, dosages, and other information in this article are not consistent with current approved labeling by the US Food and Drug Administration (FDA). The recommendations on use of drugs and vaccine for uses not approved by the FDA do not represent the official views of the FDA nor of any of the federal agencies whose scientists participated in these discussions. Unlabeled uses of the products recommended are noted in the sections of this article in which these products are discussed. Where unlabeled uses are indicated, information used as the basis for the recommendation is discussed.

The views, opinions, assertions, and findings contained herein are those of the authors and should not be construed as official US Department of Defense or US Department of Army positions, policies, or decisions unless so designated by other documentation.

Additional Articles: This article is the fifth in a series entitled *Medical and Public Health Management Following the Use of a Biological Weapon: Consensus Statements of the Working Group on Civilian Biodefense.* See references 2 through 5.

Acknowledgment: We thank May C. Chu, PhD, CDC, for assistance with laboratory diagnostic aspects of tularemia, and Edward B. Hayes, MD, CDC, for assistance with clinical and epidemiological aspects of tularemia.

REFERENCES

1. Parker RR. Recent studies of tick-borne diseases made at the United States Public Health Service Laboratory at Hamilton, Montana. In: Proceedings of the Fifth Pacific Congress; 1934:3367-3374.
2. Inglesby TV, Henderson DA, Bartlett JG, et al, for the Working Group on Civilian Biodefense. Anthrax as a biological weapon: medical and public health management. *JAMA.* 1999;281:1735-1745.
3. Henderson DA, Inglesby TV, Bartlett JG, et al, for the Working Group on Civilain Biodefense. Smallpox as a biological weapon: medical and public health management. *JAMA.* 1999;281:2127-2137.
4. Inglesby TV, Dennis DT, Henderson DA, et al, for the Working Group on Civilian Biodefense. Plague as a biological weapon: medical and public health management. *JAMA.* 2000;283:2281-2290.
5. Arnon SA, Schecter R, Inglesby TV, et al, for the Working Group on Civilain Biodefense. Botulinum toxin as a biological weapon: medical and public health management. *JAMA.* 2001;285:1059-1070.
6. Saslaw S, Eigelsbach HT, Wilson HE, Prior JA, Carhart S. Tularemia vaccine study, I: intracutaneous challenge. *Arch Intern Med.* 1961;107:121-133.
7. Saslaw S, Eigelsbach HT, Prior JA, Wilson HE, Carhart S. Tularemia vaccine study, II: respiratory challenge. *Arch Intern Med.* 1961;107:134-146.
8. World Health Organization. *Health Aspects of Chemical and Biological Weapons.* Geneva, Switzerland: World Health Organization; 1970:75-76.
9. Kaufmann AF, Meltzer MI, Schmid GP. The economic impact of a bioterrorist attack: are prevention and post-attack intervention programs justifiable? *Emerg Infect Dis.* 1997;2:83-94.
10. Christopher GW, Cieslak TJ, Pavlin JA, Eitzen EM. Biological warfare: a historical perspective. *JAMA.* 1997;278:412-417.
11. Centers for Disease Control and Prevention. Biological and chemical terrorism: strategic plan for preparedness and response: recommendations of the CDC Strategic Planning Workgroup. *MMWR Morb Mortal Wkly Rep.* 2000;49(RR-4):1-14.
12. Francis E. Tularemia. *JAMA.* 1925;84:1243-1250.
13. Karpoff SP, Antononoff NI. The spread of tularemia through water as a new factor in its epidemiology. *J Bacteriol.* 1936;32:243-258.
14. Silchenko VS. Epidemiological and clinical features of tularemia caused by waterborne infection. *Zh Mikrobiol Epidemiol Immunobiol.* 1957;28:788-795.
15. Gelman AC. The ecology of tularemia. In: May JM, ed. *Studies in Disease Ecology.* New York, NY: Hafner Publishing Co; 1961:89-108.
16. Jellison WL, Kohls GM. *Tularemia in Sheep and Sheep Industry Workers in Western United States.* Washington, DC: US Public Health Service; 1955:1-17. Public health monograph 28.
17. Francis E. Sources of infection and seasonal incidence of tularemia in man. *Public Health Rep.* 1937; 52:103-113.
18. Lake GC, Francis E. Six cases of tularemia occur-

ring in laboratory workers. *Public Health Rep.* 1922; 37:392-413.
19. Simpson WM. Tularemia (Francis' disease). *Ann Intern Med.* 1928;1:1007-1059.
20. Francis E. A summary of present knowledge of tularemia. *Medicine.* 1928;7:411-432.
21. Hopla CE. The ecology of tularemia. *Adv Vet Sci Comp Med.* 1974;18:25-53.
22. Jellison WL. *Tularemia in North America.* Missoula: University of Montana; 1974:1-276.
23. Harris S. Japanese biological warfare research on humans: a case study of microbiology and ethics. *Ann N Y Acad Sci.* 1992;666:21-52.
24. Alibek K. *Biohazard.* New York, NY: Random House; 1999:29-38.
25. McCrumb FR Jr, Snyder MJ, Woodward TE. Studies on human infection with *Pasteurella tularensis:* comparison of streptomycin and chloramphenicol in the prophylaxis of clinical disease. *Trans Assoc Am Physicians.* 1957;70:74-80.
26. McCrumb FR Jr. Aerosol infection in man with *Pasteurella tularensis. Bacteriol Rev.* 1961;25:262-267.
27. Sawyer WD, Dangerfield HG, Hogge AL, Crozier D. Antibiotic prophylaxis and therapy of airborne tularemia. *Bacteriol Rev.* 1966;30:542-548.
28. *Health Aspects of Chemical and Biological Weapons.* Geneva, Switzerland: World Health Organization; 1970:105-107.
29. Franz DR, Jahrling PB, Friedlander AM, et al. Clinical recognition and management of patients exposed to biological warfare agents. *JAMA.* 1997;278: 399-411.
30. Khan AS, Morse S, Lillibridge S. Public health preparedness for biological terrorism in the USA. *Lancet.* 2000;356:1179-1182.
31. Tucker JB. National health and medical services response to incidents of chemical and biological terrorism. *JAMA.* 1997;278:362-368.
32. Hopla CE, Hopla AK. Tularemia. In: Beran GW, Steele JH, eds. *Handbook of Zoonoses.* 2nd ed. Boca Raton, Fla: CRC Press; 1994:113-126.
33. Centers for Disease Control and Prevention. Summary of notifiable diseases, United States, 1997. *MMWR Morb Mortal Wkly Rep.* 1998;46:71-80.
34. Dennis DT. Tularemia. In: Wallace RB, ed. *Maxcy-Rosenau-Last Public Health and Preventive Medicine.* 14th ed. Stamford, Conn: Appleton & Lange; 1998:354-357.
35. Boyce JM. Recent trends in the epidemiology of tularemia in the United States. *J Infect Dis.* 1975;131: 197-199.
36. Tärnvik A, Sandström G, Sjöstedt A. Epidemiological analysis of tularemia in Sweden 1931-1993. *FEMS Immunol Med Microbiol.* 1996;13:201-204.
37. Pollitzer R. *History and Incidence of Tularemia in the Soviet Union: A Review.* Bronx, NY: Institute for Contemporary Russian Studies, Fordham University; 1967:1-103.
38. Halsted CC, Klasinghe HP. Tularemia pneumonia in urban children. *Pediatrics.* 1978;4:660-662.
39. Martone WJ, Marshall LW, Kaufmann AF, Hobbs JH, Levy ME. Tularemia pneumonia in Washington, DC. A report of three cases with possible common-source exposures. *JAMA.* 1979;23:2315-2317.
40. Rogutsky SV, Khramtsov MM, Avchinikov AV, et al. Epidemiological investigation of an outbreak of tularemia in the Smolensk region. *Zh Mikrobiol (Moscow).* 1997;2:33-37.
41. McCarthy VP, Murphy MD. Lawnmower tularemia. *Pediatr Infect Dis J.* 1990;9:298-299.
42. Klock LE, Olsen PF, Fukushima T. Tularemia epidemic associated with the deerfly. *JAMA.* 1973;226: 149-152.
43. Dahlstrand S, Ringertz O, Zetterberg B. Airborne tularemia in Sweden. *Scand J Infect Dis.* 1971;3:7-16.
44. Christenson B. An outbreak of tularemia in the northern part of central Sweden. *Scand J Infect Dis.* 1984;16:285-290.

©2001 American Medical Association. All rights reserved.

45. Warring WB, Ruffin JS. A tick-borne epidemic of tularemia. *N Engl J Med.* 1946;234:137-140.

46. Ohara Y, Sato T, Homma M. Arthropod-borne tularemia in Japan: clinical analysis of 1,374 cases observed between 1924 and 1996. *J Med Entomol.* 1998; 35:471-473.

47. Markowitz LE, Hynes NA, de la Cruz P, et al. Tick-borne tularemia: an outbreak of lymphadenopathy in children. *JAMA.* 1985;254:2922-2925.

48. Young LS, Bicknell DS, Archer BG, et al. Tularemia epidemic, Vermont, 1968: forty-seven cases linked to contact with muskrats. *N Engl J Med.* 1969;280: 1253-1260.

49. Evans ME, Gregory DW, Schaffner W, McGee ZA. Tularemia: a 30-year experience with 88 cases. *Medicine.* 1985;64:251-269.

50. Jellison WL, Epler DC, Kuhns E, Kohls GM. Tularemia in man from a domestic rural water supply. *Public Health Rep.* 1950;65:1219-1226.

51. Mignani E, Palmieri F, Fontana M, Marigo S. Italian epidemic of waterborne tularaemia. *Lancet.* 1988; 2:1423.

52. Teutsch SM, Martone WJ, Brink EW, et al. Pneumonic tularemia on Martha's Vineyard. *N Engl J Med.* 1979;301:826-828.

53. Syrjälä H, Kujala P, Myllylä V, Salminen A. Airborne transmission of tularemia in farmers. *Scand J Infect Dis.* 1985;17:371-375.

54. Syrjälä H, Sutinen S, Jokinen K, Nieminen P, Tuuponen T, Salminen A. Bronchial changes in airborne tularemia. *J Laryngol Otol.* 1986;100:1169-1176.

55. Puntigam F. Erkrankungen an torakalen formen der tularämia bei arbeitnehmern in Zuckerfabriken. *Z Hyg.* 1960;147:162-168.

56. Overholt EL, Tigertt WD, Kadull PJ, et al. An analysis of forty-two cases of laboratory-acquired tularemia. *Am J Med.* 1961;30:785-806.

57. Pike RM. Laboratory-associated infections: summary and analysis of 3921 cases. *Health Lab Sci.* 1976; 13:105-114.

58. Burke DS. Immunization against tularemia: analysis of the effectiveness of live *Francisella tularensis* vaccine in prevention of laboratory-acquired tularemia. *J Infect Dis.* 1977;135:55-60.

59. Centers for Disease Control and Prevention. Summary of notifiable diseases, United States, 1994. *MMWR Morb Mortal Wkly Rep.* 1995;43:3.

60. Bell JF. Tularemia. In: Steele JH, ed. *CRC Handbook Series in Zoonoses.* Vol 2. Boca Raton, Fla: CRC Press; 1980:161-193.

61. Pomanskaia LA. The survival times of the organisms of tularaemia on grain and straw. *J Microbiol Epidemiol Immunobiol.* 1957;28:597-603.

62. Wong JD, Shapiro DS. *Francisella.* In : Murray PR, ed. *Manual of Clinical Microbiology.* 7th ed. Washington, DC: ASM Press; 1999:647-651.

63. Johansson A, Ibrahim A, Goransson I, et al. Evaluation of PCR-based methods for discrimination of *Francisella* species and subspecies and development of a specific PCR that distinguishes the two major subspecies of *Francisella tularensis. J Clin Microbiol.* 2000; 38:4180-4185.

64. Gurycova D. First isolation of *Francisella tularensis* subspecies tularensis in Europe. *Eur J Epidemiol.* 1998;14:797-802.

65. Clarridge JE III, Raich TJ, Sjösted A, et al. Characterization of two unusual clinically significant *Francisella strains. J Clin Microbiol.* 1996;34:1995-2000.

66. Pavlov VM, Mokrievich, Volkovoy K. Cryptic plasmid pFNL10 from *Francisella novicida*-like F6168: the base of plasmid vectors for *Francisella tularensis. FEMS Immunol Med Microbiol.* 1996;13:253-256.

67. Sandström G, Sjöstedt A, Johansson T, Kuoppa K, Williams JC. Immunogenicity and toxicity of lipopolysaccharide from *Francisella tularensis* LVS. *FEMS Microbiol Immunol.* 1992;105:201-210.

68. Tärnvik A. Nature of protective immunity to *Francisella tularensis. Rev Infect Dis.* 1989;11:440-451.

69. Fortier AH, Green SJ, Polsinelli T, et al. Life and death of an intracellular pathogen: *Francisella tularensis* and the macrophage. *Immunol Ser.* 1994;60: 349-361.

70. Pullen RL, Stuart BM. Tularemia: analysis of 225 cases. *JAMA.* 1945;129:495-500.

71. Lillie RD, Francis EI. The pathology of tularaemia in man (*Homo sapiens*). In: *The Pathology of Tularaemia.* Washington, DC: US Government Printing Office; 1937:1-81. National Institute of Health Bulletin No. 167.

72. Stuart BM, Pullen RL. Tularemic pneumonia: Review of American literature and report of 15 additional cases. *Am J Med Sci.* 1945;210:223-236.

73. White JD, Rooney JR, Prickett PA, Derrenbacher EH, Beard CW, Griffith WR. Pathogenesis of experimental respiratory tularemia in monkeys. *J Infect Dis.* 1964;114:277-283.

74. Cross JT, Penn RL. *Francisella tularensis* (tularemia). In: Mandell GL, et al. eds. *Principles and Practice of Infectious Diseases.* Philadelphia, Pa: Churchill Livingstone; 2000:2393-2402.

75. Avery FW, Barnett TB. Pulmonary tularemia: a report of five cases and consideration of pathogenesis and terminology. *Am Rev Respir Dis.* 1967;95:584-591.

76. Alluisi EA, Beisel WR, Bartonelli PJ, Coates GD. Behavioral effects of tularaemia and sandfly fever in man. *J Infect Dis.* 1973;128:710-717.

77. Stuart BM, Pullen RL. Tularemic meningitis: review of the literature and report of a case with postmortem observations. *Arch Intern Med.* 1945;76:163-166.

78. American Public Health Association. Tularemia. In: Chin J, ed. *Control of Communicable Diseases Manual.* Washington, DC: American Public Health Association; 2000:532-535.

79. Amoss HL, Sprunt DH. Tularemia: review of literature of cases contracted by ingestion of rabbit and the report of additional cases with a necropsy. *JAMA.* 1936;106:1078-1080.

80. Sunderrajan EV, Hutton J, Marienfeld D. Adult respiratory distress syndrome secondary to tularemia pneumonia. *Arch Intern Med.* 1985;145:1435-1437.

81. Centers for Disease Control and Prevention. Basic laboratory protocols for the presumptive identification of *Francisella tularensis.* Available at: http://www.bt.cdc.gov/Agent/Tularemia/tularemia20010417.pdf. Accessed April 20, 2001.

82. White JD, McGavran MH. Identification of *Pasteurella tularensis* by immunofluorescence. *JAMA.* 1965;194:180-182.

83. Guarner J, Greer PW, Bartlett J, Chu MC, Shieh WJ, Zaki SR. Immunohistochemical detection of *Francisella tularensis* in formalin-fixed paraffin-embedded tissue. *Appl Immunohistochem Mol Morphol.* 1999;7:122-126.

84. Syrjälä H, Koskela P, Ripatti T, Salminen A, Herva E. Agglutination and ELISA methods in the diagnosis

of tularemia in different clinical forms and severities of the disease. *J Infect Dis.* 1986;153:142-145.

85. Bevanger L, Macland JA, Naess AI. Agglutinins and antibodies to *Francisella tularensis* outer membrane antigens in the early diagnosis of disease during an outbreak of tularemia. *J Clin Microbiol.* 1988; 26:433-437.

86. Grunow R, Splettstoesser W, McDonald S, et al. Detection of *Francisella tularensis* in biological specimens using a capture enzyme-linked immunosorbent assay, an immunochromatographic handheld assay, and a PCR. *Clin Diagn Lab Immunol.* 2000:7: 86-90.

87. Higgins JA, Hubalek Z, Halouzka J, et al. Detection of *Francisella tularensis* in infected mammals and vectors using a proble-based polymerase chain reaction. *Am J Trop Med Hyg.* 2000;62:310-318.

88. Sjöstedt A, Tärnvik A, Sandström G. *Francisella tularensis*: host-parasite interaction. *FEMS Immunol Med Microbiol.* 1996;13:181-184.

89. French GR, Plotkin SA. Miscellaneous limited-use vaccines. In: Plotkin S, Mortimer EA, eds. *Vaccine.* Philadelphia, Pa: WB Saunders; 1999:728-733.

90. Enderlin, G, Morales L, Jacobs RF, Cross TJ. Streptomycin and alternative agents for the treatment of tularemia: review of the literature. *Clin Infect Dis.* 1994; 19:42-47.

91. Jacobs RF, Narain JP. Tularemia in children. *Pediatr Infect Dis.* 1983;2:487-491.

92. Mason WL, Eigelsbach HT, Little SF, et al. Treatment of tularemia, including pulmonary tularemia, with gentamicin. *Am Rev Respir Dis.* 1980;121:39-45.

93. Cross JT, Schutze GE, Jacobs RF. Treatment of tularemia with gentamicin in pediatric patients. *Pediatr Infect Dis J.* 1995;14:151-152.

94. Syrjälä H, Schildt R, Räisäinen S. In vitro susceptibility of *Francisella tularensis* to fluoroquinolones and treatment of tularemia with norfloxacin and ciprofloxacin. *Eur J Clin Microbiol Infect Dis.* 1991;10: 68-70.

95. Russell P, Eley SM, Fulop MJ, Bell DL, Titball RW. The efficacy of ciprofloxacin and doxycycline against tularemia. *J Antimicrob Chemother.* 1998;41:461-465.

96. Limaye AP, Hooper CJ. Treatment of tularemia with fluoroquinolones: two cases and review. *Clin Infect Dis.* 1999;29:922-924.

97. Johansson A, Berglund L, Gothefors L, et al. Ciprofloxacin for treatment of tularemia in children. *Pediatr Infect Dis J.* 2000;19:449-453.

98. Cross JT, Jacobs RF. Tularemia: treatment failures with outpatient use of ceftriaxone. *Clin Infect Dis.* 1993;17:976-980.

99. Quinolones. In: *AHFS Drug Information 1999.* Bethesda, Md: American Society of Health-System Pharmacists; 1999:670-684.

100. American Academy of Pediatrics. Antimicrobials and related therapy. In: Peter G, ed. *Red Book 2000: Report of the Committee on Infectious Diseases.* 25th ed. Elk Grove Village, Ill: American Academy of Pediatrics; 2000:645-646.

101. Garner JS. Guideline for isolation precautions in hospitals. *Infect Control Hosp Epidemiol.* 1996;17: 51-80.

102. US Department of Health and Human Services. Laboratory biosafety level criteria. In: Richmond JY, McKinney RW, eds. *Biosafety in Microbiological and Biomedical Laboratories.* 4th ed. Washington, DC: Dept of Health and Human Services; 1999:17-52.

©2001 American Medical Association. All rights reserved.

Botulinum Toxin as a Biological Weapon
Medical and Public Health Management

Stephen S. Arnon, MD

Robert Schechter, MD

Thomas V. Inglesby, MD

Donald A. Henderson, MD, MPH

John G. Bartlett, MD

Michael S. Ascher, MD

Edward Eitzen, MD, MPH

Anne D. Fine, MD

Jerome Hauer, MPH

Marcelle Layton, MD

Scott Lillibridge, MD

Michael T. Osterholm, PhD, MPH

Tara O'Toole, MD, MPH

Gerald Parker, PhD, DVM

Trish M. Perl, MD, MSc

Philip K. Russell, MD

David L. Swerdlow, MD

Kevin Tonat, PhD, MPH

for the Working Group on Civilian Biodefense

Objective The Working Group on Civilian Biodefense has developed consensus-based recommendations for measures to be taken by medical and public health professionals if botulinum toxin is used as a biological weapon against a civilian population.

Participants The working group included 23 representatives from academic, government, and private institutions with expertise in public health, emergency management, and clinical medicine.

Evidence The primary authors (S.S.A. and R.S.) searched OLDMEDLINE and MEDLINE (1960–March 1999) and their professional collections for literature concerning use of botulinum toxin as a bioweapon. The literature was reviewed, and opinions were sought from the working group and other experts on diagnosis and management of botulism. Additional MEDLINE searches were conducted through April 2000 during the review and revisions of the consensus statement.

Consensus Process The first draft of the working group's consensus statement was a synthesis of information obtained in the formal evidence-gathering process. The working group convened to review the first draft in May 1999. Working group members reviewed subsequent drafts and suggested additional revisions. The final statement incorporates all relevant evidence obtained in the literature search in conjunction with final consensus recommendations supported by all working group members.

Conclusions An aerosolized or foodborne botulinum toxin weapon would cause acute symmetric, descending flaccid paralysis with prominent bulbar palsies such as diplopia, dysarthria, dysphonia, and dysphagia that would typically present 12 to 72 hours after exposure. Effective response to a deliberate release of botulinum toxin will depend on timely clinical diagnosis, case reporting, and epidemiological investigation. Persons potentially exposed to botulinum toxin should be closely observed, and those with signs of botulism require prompt treatment with antitoxin and supportive care that may include assisted ventilation for weeks or months. Treatment with antitoxin should not be delayed for microbiological testing.

JAMA. 2001;285:1059-1070   www.jama.com

THIS IS THE FOURTH ARTICLE IN A series entitled *Medical and Public Health Management Following the Use of a Biological Weapon: Consensus Statements of The Working Group on Civilian Biodefense*.[1-3] This article is the only one in the series to feature a biological toxin rather than a replicating agent. Botulinum toxin poses a major bioweapon threat because of its extreme potency and lethality; its ease of production, transport, and misuse; and the need for prolonged intensive care among affected persons.[4,5] An outbreak of botulism constitutes a medical emergency that requires prompt provision of botulinum antitoxin and, often, mechanical ventilation, and it constitutes a public health emergency that requires immediate intervention to prevent additional cases. Timely recognition of a botulism outbreak begins with an astute clinician who quickly notifies public health officials.

Botulinum toxin is the most poisonous substance known.[6,7] A single gram of crystalline toxin, evenly dispersed and inhaled, would kill more than 1 million people, although technical factors would make such dissemination difficult. The basis of the phenomenal potency of botulinum toxin is enzymatic; the toxin is a zinc proteinase that cleaves 1 or more of the fusion proteins by which neuronal vesicles release acetylcholine into the neuromuscular junction.[8]

It is regrettable that botulinum toxin still needs to be considered as a bioweapon at the historic moment when it has become the first biological toxin to become licensed for treatment of human disease. In the United States, botulinum toxin is currently licensed for treatment of cervical torticollis, strabismus, and blepharospasm associ-

Author Affiliations are listed at the end of this article.
Corresponding Author and Reprints: Stephen S. Arnon, MD, Infant Botulism Treatment and Prevention Program, California Department of Health Services, 2151 Berkeley Way, Room 506, Berkeley, CA 94704 (e-mail: sarnon@dhs.ca.gov).

©2001 American Medical Association. All rights reserved.

Reprinted with permission from *JAMA*; February 28, 2001, Vol 285, No. 8

ated with dystonia. It is also used "off label" for a variety of more prevalent conditions that include migraine headache, chronic low back pain, stroke, traumatic brain injury, cerebral palsy, achalasia, and various dystonias.[9-13]

CONSENSUS METHODS

The working group included 23 representatives from academic, government, and private institutions with expertise in public health, emergency management, and clinical medicine. The 2 primary authors (S.S.A. and R.S.) conducted a literature search on use of botulinum toxin as a bioweapon. The OLDMEDLINE and MEDLINE databases were queried for all articles published between January 1960 and March 1999 that contained words referring to biological warfare (*bioterrorism*, *biowarfare*, *terrorism*, *war*, *warfare*, and *weapon*) in combination with terms related to *Clostridium botulinum* (*bacillus*, *botulin*, *botulinal*, *botulinum*, *botulinus*, *botulism*, *clostridia*, *clostridial*, and *Clostridium*). The articles identified in the databases were fully reviewed. In addition, published and unpublished articles, books, monographs, and special reports in the primary authors' collections were reviewed. Additional MEDLINE searches were conducted through April 2000 during the review and revisions of the consensus statement.

The first draft of the consensus statement was a synthesis of information obtained in the formal evidence-gathering process. Members of the working group provided written and oral comments about the first draft at their meeting in May 1999. Working group members then reviewed subsequent drafts and suggested additional revisions. The final statement incorporates all relevant evidence obtained in the literature search in conjunction with final consensus recommendations supported by all working group members.

The assessment and recommendations provided herein represent the best professional judgment of the working group based on currently available data and expertise. These conclusions and recommendations should be regularly reassessed as new information becomes available.

HISTORY OF CURRENT THREAT

Terrorists have already attempted to use botulinum toxin as a bioweapon. Aerosols were dispersed at multiple sites in downtown Tokyo, Japan, and at US military installations in Japan on at least 3 occasions between 1990 and 1995 by the Japanese cult Aum Shinrikyō. These attacks failed, apparently because of faulty microbiological technique, deficient aerosol-generating equipment, or internal sabotage. The perpetrators obtained their *C botulinum* from soil that they had collected in northern Japan.[14,15]

Development and use of botulinum toxin as a possible bioweapon began at least 60 years ago.[16,17] The head of the Japanese biological warfare group (Unit 731) admitted to feeding cultures of *C botulinum* to prisoners with lethal effect during that country's occupation of Manchuria, which began in the 1930s.[18] The US biological weapons program first produced botulinum toxin during World War II. Because of concerns that Germany had weaponized botulinum toxin, more than 1 million doses of botulinum toxoid vaccine were made for Allied troops preparing to invade Normandy on D-Day.[19,20] The US biological weapons program was ended in 1969-1970 by executive orders of Richard M. Nixon, then president. Research pertaining to biowarfare use of botulinum toxin took place in other countries as well.[21]

Although the 1972 Biological and Toxin Weapons Convention prohibited offensive research and production of biological weapons, signatories Iraq and the Soviet Union subsequently produced botulinum toxin for use as a weapon.[22,23] Botulinum toxin was 1 of several agents tested at the Soviet site Aralsk-7 on Vozrozhdeniye Island in the Aral Sea.[23,24] A former senior scientist of the Russian civilian bioweapons program reported that the Soviets had attempted splicing the botulinum toxin gene from *C botulinum* into other bacteria.[25] With the economic difficulties in Russia after the demise of the Soviet

Union, some of the thousands of scientists formerly employed by its bioweapons program have been recruited by nations attempting to develop biological weapons.[25,26] Four of the countries listed by the US government as "state sponsors of terrorism" (Iran, Iraq, North Korea, and Syria)[27] have developed, or are believed to be developing, botulinum toxin as a weapon.[28,29]

After the 1991 Persian Gulf War, Iraq admitted to the United Nations inspection team to having produced 19 000 L of concentrated botulinum toxin, of which approximately 10 000 L were loaded into military weapons.[22,30] These 19 000 L of concentrated toxin are not fully accounted for and constitute approximately 3 times the amount needed to kill the entire current human population by inhalation. In 1990, Iraq deployed specially designed missiles with a 600-km range; 13 of these were filled with botulinum toxin, 10 with aflatoxin, and 2 with anthrax spores. Iraq also deployed special 400-lb (180-kg) bombs for immediate use; 100 bombs contained botulinum toxin, 50 contained anthrax spores, and 7 contained aflatoxin.[22,30] It is noteworthy that Iraq chose to weaponize more botulinum toxin than any other of its known biological agents.

Some contemporary analyses discount the potential of botulinum toxin as a bioweapon because of constraints in concentrating and stabilizing the toxin for aerosol dissemination. However, these analyses pertain to military uses of botulinum toxin to immobilize an opponent (William C. Patrick, unpublished data, 1998). In contrast, deliberate release of botulinum toxin in a civilian population would be able to cause substantial disruption and distress. For example, it is estimated that a point-source aerosol release of botulinum toxin could incapacitate or kill 10% of persons within 0.5 km downwind (William C. Patrick, unpublished data, 1998). In addition, terrorist use of botulinum toxin might be manifested as deliberate contamination of food. Misuse of toxin in this manner could produce either a large

©2001 American Medical Association. All rights reserved.

Reprinted with permission from *JAMA*; February 28, 2001, Vol 285, No. 8

botulism outbreak from a single meal or episodic, widely separated outbreaks.[31] In the United States, the Centers for Disease Control and Prevention (CDC) maintains a well-established surveillance system for human botulism based on clinician reporting that would promptly detect such events.[32]

MICROBIOLOGY AND VIRULENCE FACTORS

Clostridium botulinum is a spore-forming, obligate anaerobe whose natural habitat is soil, from which it can be isolated without undue difficulty. The species *C botulinum* consists of 4 genetically diverse groups that would not otherwise be designated as a single species except for their common characteristic of producing botulinum toxin.[33,34] Botulinum toxin exists in 7 distinct antigenic types that have been assigned the letters A through G. The toxin types are defined by their absence of cross-neutralization (eg, anti-A antitoxin does not neutralize toxin types B-G). The toxin types also serve as convenient epidemiological markers. In addition to *C botulinum*, unique strains of *Clostridium baratii* and *Clostridium butyricum* have the capacity to produce botulinum toxin.[35-37] Botulinum toxin is a simple dichain polypeptide that consists of a 100-kd "heavy" chain joined by a single disulfide bond to a 50-kd "light" chain; its 3-dimensional structure was recently resolved to 3.3 A.[38] The toxin's light chain is a Zn++-containing endopeptidase that blocks acetylcholine-containing vesicles from fusing with the terminal membrane of the motor neuron, resulting in flaccid muscle paralysis (FIGURE 1).[8]

The lethal dose of botulinum toxin for humans is not known but can be estimated from primate studies. By extrapolation, the lethal amounts of crystalline type A toxin for a 70-kg human would be approximately 0.09-0.15 µg intravenously or intramuscularly, 0.70-0.90 µg inhalationally, and 70 µg orally.[10,39-41] Therapeutic botulinum toxin represents an impractical bioterrorist weapon because a vial of the type A preparation currently licensed in the United States contains only about 0.3% of the estimated

human lethal inhalational dose and 0.005% of the estimated lethal oral dose.

PATHOGENESIS AND CLINICAL MANIFESTATIONS

Three forms of naturally occurring human botulism exist: foodborne, wound, and intestinal (infant and adult). Fewer than 200 cases of all forms of botulism are reported annually in the United States.[42] All forms of botulism result from absorption of botulinum toxin into the circulation from either a mucosal surface (gut, lung) or a wound. Botulinum toxin does not penetrate intact skin. Wound botulism and intestinal

Figure 1. Mechanism of Action of Botulinum Toxin

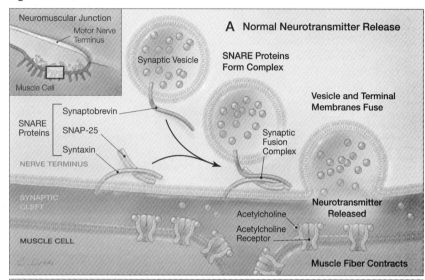

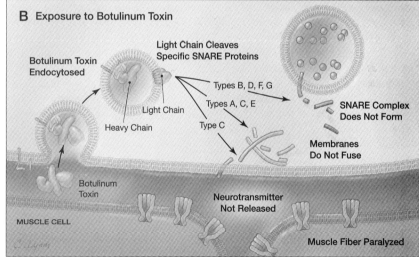

A, Release of acetylcholine at the neuromuscular junction is mediated by the assembly of a synaptic fusion complex that allows the membrane of the synaptic vesicle containing acetylcholine to fuse with the neuronal cell membrane. The synaptic fusion complex is a set of SNARE proteins, which include synaptobrevin, SNAP-25, and syntaxin. After membrane fusion, acetylcholine is released into the synaptic cleft and then bound by receptors on the muscle cell.
B, Botulinum toxin binds to the neuronal cell membrane at the nerve terminus and enters the neuron by endocytosis. The light chain of botulinum toxin cleaves specific sites on the SNARE proteins, preventing complete assembly of the synaptic fusion complex and thereby blocking acetylcholine release. Botulinum toxins types B, D, F, and G cleave synaptobrevin; types A, C, and E cleave SNAP-25; and type C cleaves syntaxin. Without acetylcholine release, the muscle is unable to contract.
SNARE indicates soluble NSF-attachment protein receptor; NSF, N-ethylmaleimide-sensitive fusion protein; and SNAP-25, synaptosomal-associated protein of 25 kd.

©2001 American Medical Association. All rights reserved.

Reprinted with permission from *JAMA*; February 28, 2001, Vol 285, No. 8

Figure 2. Seventeen-Year-Old Patient With Mild Botulism

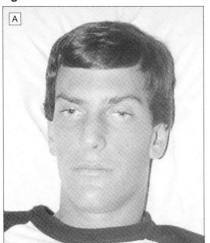
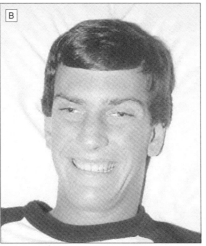

A, Patient at rest. Note bilateral mild ptosis, dilated pupils, disconjugate gaze, and symmetric facial muscles. B, Patient was requested to perform his maximum smile. Note absent periorbital smile creases, ptosis, disconjugate gaze, dilated pupils, and minimally asymmetric smile. As an indication of the extreme potency of botulinum toxin, the patient had 40×10^{-12} g/mL of type A botulinum toxin in his serum (ie, 1.25 mouse units/mL) when these photographs were taken.

Table 1. Symptoms and Signs of Foodborne Botulism, Types A and B*

	Cases, %
Symptoms	
Fatigue	77
Dizziness	51
Double vision	91
Blurred vision	65
Dysphagia	96
Dry mouth	93
Dysarthria	84
Sore throat	54
Dyspnea	60
Constipation	73
Nausea	64
Vomiting	59
Abdominal cramps	42
Diarrhea	19
Arm weakness	73
Leg weakness	69
Paresthesia	14
Signs	
Alert mental status	90
Ptosis	73
Gaze paralysis	65
Pupils dilated or fixed	44
Nystagmus	22
Facial palsy	63
Diminished gag reflex	65
Tongue weakness	58
Arm weakness	75
Leg weakness	69
Hyporeflexia or areflexia	40
Ataxia	17

*Data are from outbreaks of botulism reported in the United States in 1973-1974. The number of patients with available data varied from 35 to 55. Adapted from Hughes et al[44] with permission.

botulism are infectious diseases that result from production of botulinum toxin by *C botulinum* either in devitalized (ie, anaerobic) tissue[43] or in the intestinal lumen,[37] respectively. Neither would result from bioterrorist use of botulinum toxin.

A fourth, man-made form that results from aerosolized botulinum toxin is inhalational botulism. This mode of transmission has been demonstrated experimentally in primates,[39] has been attempted by bioterrorists,[14,15] and has been the intended outcome of at least 1 country's specially designed missiles and artillery shells.[22,30] Inhalational botulism has occurred accidentally in humans. A brief report from West Germany in 1962 described 3 veterinary personnel who were exposed to reaerosolized botulinum toxin while disposing of rabbits and guinea pigs whose fur was coated with aerosolized type A botulinum toxin. Type A botulinum toxin was detected in serum samples from all 3 affected individuals.[21]

Once botulinum toxin is absorbed, the bloodstream carries it to peripheral cholinergic synapses, principally, the neuromuscular junction, where it binds irreversibly. The toxin is then internalized and enzymatically blocks acetylcholine release (Figure 1). Accordingly, all forms of human botulism display virtually identical neurologic signs. However, the neurologic signs in naturally occurring foodborne botulism may be preceded by abdominal cramps, nausea, vomiting, or diarrhea.[44] These gastrointestinal symptoms are thought to be caused by other bacterial metabolites also present in the food[33] and may not occur if purified botulinum toxin is intentionally placed in foods or aerosols.

Botulism is an acute, afebrile, symmetric, descending flaccid paralysis that always begins in bulbar musculature. It is not possible to have botulism without having multiple cranial nerve palsies. Disease manifestations are similar regardless of botulinum toxin type. However, the extent and pace of paralysis may vary considerably among patients. Some patients may be mildly affected (**Figure 2**), while others may be so paralyzed that they appear comatose and require months of ventilatory support. The rapidity of onset and the severity of paralysis depend on the amount of toxin absorbed into the circulation. Recovery results from new motor axon twigs that sprout to reinnervate paralyzed muscle fibers, a process that, in adults, may take weeks or months to complete.[45,46]

Patients with botulism typically present with difficulty seeing, speaking, and/or swallowing (**TABLE 1** and **TABLE 2**). Prominent neurologic findings in all forms of botulism include ptosis, diplopia, blurred vision, often enlarged or sluggishly reactive pupils, dysarthria, dysphonia, and dysphagia.[5,44,47,48] The mouth may appear dry and the pharynx injected because of peripheral parasympathetic cholinergic blockade. Sensory changes are not observed except for infrequent circumoral and peripheral paresthesias from hyperventilation as a patient becomes frightened by onset of paralysis.

As paralysis extends beyond bulbar musculature, loss of head control, hy-

©2001 American Medical Association. All rights reserved.

Reprinted with permission from *JAMA*; February 28, 2001, Vol 285, No. 8

potonia, and generalized weakness become prominent. Dysphagia and loss of the protective gag reflex may require intubation and, usually, mechanical ventilation. Deep tendon reflexes may be present initially but diminish or disappear in the ensuing days, and constipation may occur. In untreated persons, death results from airway obstruction (pharyngeal and upper airway muscle paralysis) and inadequate tidal volume (diaphragmatic and accessory respiratory muscle paralysis).

Because botulism is an intoxication, patients remain afebrile unless they also have acquired a secondary infection (eg, aspiration pneumonia). The toxin does not penetrate brain parenchyma, so patients are not confused or obtunded. However, they often appear lethargic and have communication difficulties because of bulbar palsies (Figure 2). Botulism may be recognized by its classic triad: (1) symmetric, descending flaccid paralysis with prominent bulbar palsies in (2) an afebrile patient with (3) a clear sensorium. The prominent bulbar palsies can be summarized in part as "4 Ds": diplopia, dysarthria, dysphonia, and dysphagia.

EPIDEMIOLOGY

Early recognition of outbreaks of botulism, whether natural or intentional, depends on heightened clinical suspicion. Aerosol dissemination may not be difficult to recognize because a large number of cases will share a common temporal and geographical exposure and will lack a common dietary exposure. However, identification of the common exposure site initially may be difficult because of the mobility of persons exposed during the incubation period. Botulism and botulinum toxin are not contagious and cannot be transmitted from person to person. In contrast, a microbe intentionally modified to produce botulinum toxin might be contagious.

No instances of waterborne botulism have ever been reported.[42,49,50] Although the potency of botulinum toxin has led to speculation that it might be used to contaminate a municipal wa-

Table 2. Symptoms and Signs of Inhalational Botulism in Order of Onset

Humans (n = 3)[21]	Monkeys (n = 9)[39]*
Third day after exposure	12-18 hours after exposure
Mucus in throat	Mild muscular weakness
Difficulty swallowing solid food	Intermittent ptosis
Dizziness	Disconjugate gaze
Fourth day after exposure	Followed by
Difficulty moving eyes	Severe weakness of postural neck muscles
Mild pupillary dilation and nystagmus	Occasional mouth breathing
Indistinct speech	Serous nasal discharge
Unsteady gait	Salivation, dysphagia
Extreme weakness	Mouth breathing
	Rales
	Anorexia
	Severe generalized weakness
	Lateral recumbency
	Second to fourth day after exposure
	Death in some animals

*After exposure to 4 to 7 monkey median lethal doses of botulinum toxin. The time to onset and pace of paralysis were dose-dependent. Adapted from Middlebrook and Franz[48] with permission.

ter supply, this scenario is unlikely for at least 2 reasons.[51] First, botulinum toxin is rapidly inactivated by standard potable water treatments (eg, chlorination, aeration).[52] Second, because of the slow turnover time of large-capacity reservoirs, a comparably large (and technically difficult to produce and deliver) inoculum of botulinum toxin would be needed.[53] In contrast with treated water, botulinum toxin may be stable for several days in untreated water or beverages.[52,54] Hence, such items should be investigated in a botulism outbreak if no other vehicle for toxin can be identified.

If food were deliberately used as a vehicle for the toxin, the outbreak would need to be distinguished from naturally occurring foodborne botulism. During the past 20 years, the epidemiology of foodborne botulism has expanded beyond its traditional association with home-preserved foods and now includes nonpreserved foods and public eating places,[47] features that could make terrorist use of botulinum toxin more difficult to detect. Characteristics of outbreaks of botulism include:

Incubation Period

The rapidity of onset and severity of botulism depend on the rate and amount of toxin absorption. Symptoms of food-

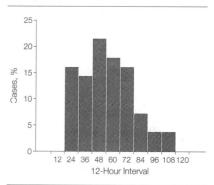

Figure 3. Fifty-Nine Cases of Botulism, by Interval Between Eating at a Restaurant and Onset of First Neurologic Symptom—Michigan, 1977

Reproduced from Terranova et al[57] with permission of Oxford University Press.

borne botulism may begin as early as 2 hours or as long as 8 days after ingestion of toxin.[55,56] Typically, cases present 12 to 72 hours after the implicated meal. In 1 large foodborne outbreak, new cases presented during the ensuing 3 days at a fairly even rate before decreasing (FIGURE 3).[57] The time to onset of inhalational botulism cannot be stated with certainty because so few cases are known. Monkeys showed signs of botulism 12 to 80 hours after aerosol exposure to 4 to 7 multiples of the monkey median lethal dose.[39] The 3 known human cases of inhalational botulism had

©2001 American Medical Association. All rights reserved.

Reprinted with permission from *JAMA*; February 28, 2001, Vol 285, No. 8

Box 1. Features of an Outbreak That Would Suggest a Deliberate Release of Botulinum Toxin

Outbreak of a large number of cases of acute flaccid paralysis with prominent bulbar palsies

Outbreak with an unusual botulinum toxin type (ie, type C, D, F, or G, or type E toxin not acquired from an aquatic food)

Outbreak with a common geographic factor among cases (eg, airport, work location) but without a common dietary exposure (ie, features suggestive of an aerosol attack)

Multiple simultaneous outbreaks with no common source

Note: A careful travel and activity history, as well as dietary history, should be taken in any suspected botulism outbreak. Patients should also be asked if they know of other persons with similar symptoms.

onset of symptoms approximately 72 hours after exposure to an unknown but probably small amount of reaerosolized toxin.[21]

Age and Sex

Persons of all ages are potentially susceptible to botulism. There are no sex differences in susceptibility.

Agent and Vehicles

Botulinum toxin in solution is colorless, odorless, and, as far as is known, tasteless. The toxin is readily inactivated by heat ($\geq 85°C$ for 5 minutes).[33,34,52] Thus, foodborne botulism is always transmitted by foods that are not heated, or not heated thoroughly, before eating. Almost every type of food has been associated with outbreaks of botulism, but the most commonly implicated foods in the United States are vegetables, particularly "low-acid" (ie, higher pH) vegetables such as beans, peppers, carrots, and corn.[42,50,58]

A novel epidemiological development is the occurrence of foodborne botulism after eating various nonpreserved foods in restaurants or delicatessens. Foil-wrapped baked potatoes are now known to be capable of causing restaurant-associated foodborne botulism[59] when held at room temperature after baking and then served plain,[60] as potato salad,[61,62] or as a Mediterranean-style dip.[59] Other outbreaks that originated in restaurants resulted from contaminated condiments such as sautéed onions,[63] garlic in oil,[64] and commercial cheese sauce.[65] Additional examples of notable commercial foods that have caused botulism outbreaks include inadequately eviscerated fish,[66] yogurt,[67] cream cheese,[68] and jarred peanuts.[69]

Incidence and Outbreak Size

Naturally occurring foodborne botulism is a rare disease. Approximately 9 outbreaks of foodborne botulism and a median of 24 cases occur annually in the United States.[42,47] The mean outbreak size has remained constant over the years at approximately 2.5 cases per outbreak. The largest outbreak of foodborne botulism in the United States in the last 100 years occurred in Michigan in 1977; 59 cases resulted from eating home-preserved jalapeño peppers at a restaurant.[57] However, only 45 of the 59 patients had clinically evident weakness and hypotonia.

Toxin Types

Of the 135 foodborne outbreaks in the 16 years from 1980 to 1996 in the United States, the toxin types represented were: type A, 54.1%; type B, 14.8%; type E, 26.7%; type F, 1.5%; and unknown, 3.0%.[42] Type F foodborne outbreaks are rare in the United States; a 1962 outbreak resulted from homemade venison jerky,[70] while other type F cases actually may have had intestinal botulism.[71] Toxin types C and D cause botulism in wildlife and domestic animals but have not caused human foodborne disease. However, humans are thought to be susceptible to these toxin types because they have caused botulism in primates when ingested.[72-74] Toxin type G is produced by a bacteria species discovered in South American soil in 1969 that has never caused recognized foodborne botulism.[75] Aerosol challenge studies in monkeys have established the susceptibility of primates to inhaled botulinum toxin types C, D, and G.[48]

Distribution

Although outbreaks of foodborne botulism have occurred in almost all states, more than half (53.8%) of the US outbreaks have occurred in just 5 western states (California, Washington, Oregon, Colorado, and Alaska). East of the Mississippi River, 60% of the foodborne outbreaks have resulted from type B toxin, while west of the Mississippi River, 85% have resulted from type A toxin. In the 46 years between 1950 and 1996, 20 states, mainly in the eastern United States, did not report any type A botulism outbreaks, while 24 states, mostly in the western United States, did not report any type B outbreaks.[42] In Canada and Alaska, most foodborne outbreaks resulted from type E toxin associated with native Inuit and Eskimo foods.[50,76]

Bioterrorism Considerations

Any outbreak of botulism should bring to mind the possibility of bioterrorism, but certain features would be particularly suggestive (BOX 1). The availability and speed of air transportation mandate that a careful travel and activity history, as well as a careful dietary history, be taken. Patients should also be asked whether they know of other persons with similar symptoms. Absence of a common dietary exposure among temporally clustered patients should suggest the possibility of inhalational botulism.

DIAGNOSIS AND DIFFERENTIAL DIAGNOSIS

Clinical diagnosis of botulism is confirmed by specialized laboratory test-

©2001 American Medical Association. All rights reserved.

Reprinted with permission from *JAMA*; February 28, 2001, Vol 285, No. 8

ing that often requires days to complete. Routine laboratory test results are usually unremarkable. Therefore, clinical diagnosis is the foundation for early recognition of and response to a bioterrorist attack with botulinum toxin.

Any case of suspected botulism represents a potential public health emergency because of the possibility that a contaminated food remains available to others or that botulinum toxin has been deliberately released. In these settings, prompt intervention by civil authorities is needed to prevent additional cases. Consequently, clinicians caring for patients with suspected botulism should notify their local public health department and hospital epidemiologist immediately to coordinate shipment of therapeutic antitoxin, laboratory diagnostic testing, and epidemiological investigation (BOX 2). In most jurisdictions of the United States, botulism suspected on clinical grounds alone by law must be reported immediately by telephone to local public health authorities. The attending clinician needs to be both prompt and persistent in accomplishing this notification.

Differential Diagnosis

Botulism is frequently misdiagnosed, most often as a polyradiculoneuropathy (Guillain-Barré or Miller-Fisher syndrome), myasthenia gravis, or a disease of the central nervous system (TABLE 3). In the United States, botulism is more likely than Guillain-Barré syndrome, intoxication, or poliomyelitis to cause a cluster of cases of acute flaccid paralysis. Botulism differs from other flaccid paralyses in its prominent cranial nerve palsies disproportionate to milder weakness and hypotonia below the neck, in its symmetry, and in its absence of sensory nerve damage.

A large, unintentional outbreak of foodborne botulism caused by a restaurant condiment in Canada provides a cautionary lesson about the potential difficulties in recognizing a covert, intentional contamination of food.[64] During a 6-week period in which the condiment was served, 28 persons

---

Box 2. Clinicians Caring for Patients With Suspected Botulism Should Immediately Contact Their:

(1) Hospital epidemiologist or infection control practitioner

and

(2) Local and state health departments

Consult your local telephone operator; the telephone directory under "government listings," or the Internet at: http://www.cdc.gov/other.htm#states or http://www.astho.org/state.html

If the local and state health departments are unavailable, contact the Centers for Disease Control and Prevention: (404) 639-2206; (404) 639-2888 [after hours].

Table 3. Selected Mimics and Misdiagnoses of Botulism*

Conditions	Features That Distinguish Condition From Botulism
Common Misdiagnoses	
Guillain-Barré syndrome† and its variants, especially Miller-Fisher syndrome	History of antecedent infection; paresthesias; often ascending paralysis; early areflexia; eventual CSF protein increase; EMG findings
Myasthenia gravis†	Recurrent paralysis; EMG findings; sustained response to anticholinesterase therapy
Stroke†	Paralysis often asymmetric; abnormal CNS image
Intoxication with depressants (eg, acute ethanol intoxication), organophosphates, carbon monoxide, or nerve gas	History of exposure; excessive drug levels detected in body fluids
Lambert-Eaton syndrome	Increased strength with sustained contraction; evidence of lung carcinoma; EMG findings similar to botulism
Tick paralysis	Paresthesias; ascending paralysis; tick attached to skin
Other Misdiagnoses	
Poliomyelitis	Antecedent febrile illness; asymmetric paralysis; CSF pleocytosis
CNS infections, especially of the brainstem	Mental status changes; CSF and EEG abnormalities
CNS tumor	Paralysis often asymmetric; abnormal CNS image
Streptococcal pharyngitis (pharyngeal erythema can occur in botulism)	Absence of bulbar palsies; positive rapid antigen test result or throat culture
Psychiatric illness†	Normal EMG in conversion paralysis
Viral syndrome†	Absence of bulbar palsies and flaccid paralysis
Inflammatory myopathy†	Elevated creatine kinase levels
Diabetic complications†	Sensory neuropathy; few cranial nerve palsies
Hyperemesis gravidarum†	Absence of bulbar palsies and acute flaccid paralysis
Hypothyroidism†	Abnormal thyroid function test results
Laryngeal trauma†	Absence of flaccid paralysis; dysphonia without bulbar palsies
Overexertion†	Absence of bulbar palsies and acute flaccid paralysis

*CSF indicates cerebrospinal fluid; EMG, electromyogram; CNS, central nervous system; and EEG, electroencephalogram.
†Misdiagnoses made in a large outbreak of botulism.[64]

---

in 2 countries became ill, but all were misdiagnosed (Table 3). The 28 were identified retrospectively only after correct diagnoses in a mother and her 2 daughters who had returned to their home more than 2000 miles away from the restaurant. Four (14%) of the cases had been misdiagnosed as having psychiatric disease, including "factitious" symptoms. It is possible that hysterical paralysis might occur as a conversion reaction in the anxiety that would

©2001 American Medical Association. All rights reserved.

Reprinted with permission from *JAMA*; February 28, 2001, Vol 285, No. 8

follow a deliberate release of botulinum toxin.

Diagnostic Testing

At present, laboratory diagnostic testing for botulism in the United States is available only at the CDC and approximately 20 state and municipal public health laboratories.[42] The laboratory should be consulted prospectively about specimen collection and processing. Samples used in diagnosis of botulism include serum ($\geq$30 mL of blood in "tiger"-top or red-top tubes from adults, less from children), stool, gastric aspirate, and, if available, vomitus and suspect foods. Serum samples must be obtained before therapy with antitoxin, which nullifies the diagnostic mouse bioassay. An enema may be required to obtain an adequate fecal sample if the patient is constipated. Sterile water should be used for this procedure because saline enema solution can confound the mouse bioassay. Gastric aspirates and, perhaps, stool may be useful for detecting inhaled aerosolized botulinum toxin released in a bioterrorist attack.[77] A list of the patient's medications should accompany the diagnostic samples because anticholinesterases, such as pyridostigmine bromide, and other medicines that are toxic to mice can be dialyzed from samples before testing. All samples should be kept refrigerated after collection.

The standard laboratory diagnostic test for clinical specimens and foods is the mouse bioassay,[42] in which type-specific antitoxin protects mice against any botulinum toxin present in the sample. The mouse bioassay can detect as little as 0.03 ng of botulinum toxin[10] and usually yields results in 1 to 2 days (range, 6-96 hours). Fecal and gastric specimens also are cultured anaerobically, with results typically available in 7 to 10 days (range, 5-21 days). Toxin production by culture isolates is confirmed by the mouse bioassay.

An electromyogram with repetitive nerve stimulation at 20 to 50 Hz can sometimes distinguish between causes of acute flaccid paralysis.[78,79] The char-

acteristic electromyographic findings of botulism include normal nerve conduction velocity, normal sensory nerve function, a pattern of brief, small-amplitude motor potentials, and, most distinctively, an incremental response (facilitation) to repetitive stimulation often seen only at 50 Hz. Immediate access to electrophysiological studies may be difficult to obtain in an outbreak of botulism.

Additional diagnostic procedures may be useful in rapidly excluding botulism as the cause of paralysis (Table 3). Cerebrospinal fluid (CSF) is unchanged in botulism but is abnormal in many central nervous system diseases. Although the CSF protein level eventually is elevated in Guillain-Barré syndrome, it may be normal early in illness. Imaging of the brain, spine, and chest may reveal hemorrhage, inflammation, or neoplasm. A test dose of edrophonium chloride briefly reverses paralytic symptoms in many patients with myasthenia gravis and, reportedly, in some with botulism.[64] A close inspection of the skin, especially the scalp, may reveal an attached tick that is causing paralysis.[80] Other tests that require days for results include stool culture for *Campylobacter jejuni* as a precipitant of Guillain-Barré syndrome and assays for the autoantibodies that cause myasthenia gravis, Lambert-Eaton syndrome, and Guillain-Barré syndrome.

Foods suspected of being contaminated should be refrigerated until retrieval by public health personnel. The US Food and Drug Administration and the US Department of Agriculture can assist other public health laboratories with testing of suspect foods by using methods similar to those applied to clinical samples.

THERAPY

The mortality and sequelae associated with botulism have diminished with contemporary therapy. In the United States, the percentage of persons who died of foodborne botulism decreased from 25% during 1950-1959 to 6% during 1990-1996, with a similar reduction for each botulinum toxin type.[42]

Despite this increase in survival, the paralysis of botulism can persist for weeks to months with concurrent requirements for fluid and nutritional support, assisted ventilation, and treatment of complications.

Therapy for botulism consists of supportive care and passive immunization with equine antitoxin. Optimal use of botulinum antitoxin requires early suspicion of botulism. Timely administration of passive neutralizing antibody will minimize subsequent nerve damage and severity of disease but will not reverse existent paralysis.[81,82] Antitoxin should be given to patients with neurologic signs of botulism as soon as possible after clinical diagnosis.[47] Treatment should not be delayed for microbiological testing. Antitoxin may be withheld at the time of diagnosis if it is certain that the patient is improving from maximal paralysis.

In the United States, botulinum antitoxin is available from the CDC via state and local health departments (Box 2). The licensed trivalent antitoxin contains neutralizing antibodies against botulinum toxin types A, B, and E, the most common causes of human botulism. If another toxin type was intentionally disseminated, patients could potentially be treated with an investigational heptavalent (ABCDEFG) antitoxin held by the US Army.[83] However, the time required for correct toxin typing and subsequent administration of heptavalent antitoxin would decrease the utility of this product in an outbreak.

The dose and safety precautions for equine botulinum antitoxin have changed over time. Clinicians should review the package insert with public health authorities before using antitoxin. At present, the dose of licensed botulinum antitoxin is a single 10-mL vial per patient, diluted 1:10 in 0.9% saline solution, administered by slow intravenous infusion. One vial provides between 5500 and 8500 IU of each type-specific antitoxin. The amount of neutralizing antibody in both the licensed and the investigational equine antitoxins far exceeds the highest serum toxin levels found in foodborne botu-

©2001 American Medical Association. All rights reserved.

Reprinted with permission from *JAMA*; February 28, 2001, Vol 285, No. 8

lism patients, and additional doses are usually not required. If a patient has been exposed to an unnaturally large amount of botulinum toxin as a biological weapon, the adequacy of neutralization by antitoxin can be confirmed by retesting serum for toxin after treatment.

There are few published data on the safety of botulinum antitoxins. From 1967 to 1977, when the recommended dose was larger than today, approximately 9% of recipients of equine botulinum antitoxin in the United States displayed urticaria, serum sickness, or other reactions suggestive of hypersensitivity.[84] Anaphylaxis occurred within 10 minutes of receiving antitoxin in 2% of recipients. When the US Army's investigational heptavalent antitoxin was given to 50 individuals in a large Egyptian outbreak of type E foodborne botulism in 1991, 1 recipient (2%) displayed serum sickness, and 9 (18%) had mild reactions.[83] To screen for hypersensitivity, patients are given small challenge doses of equine antitoxin before receiving a full dose. Patients responding to challenge with a substantial wheal and flare may be desensitized over 3 to 4 hours before additional antitoxin is given. During the infusion of antitoxin, diphenhydramine and epinephrine should be on hand for rapid administration in case of adverse reaction. Although both equine antitoxins have been partially despeciated by enzymatic cleavage of the allogenic F_c region, each contains a small residual of intact antibody that may sensitize recipients to additional doses.

Botulism patients require supportive care that often includes feeding by enteral tube or parenteral nutrition, intensive care, mechanical ventilation, and treatment of secondary infections. Patients with suspected botulism should be closely monitored for impending respiratory failure. In nonventilated infants with botulism, a reverse Trendelenburg positioning with cervical vertebral support has been helpful, but applicability of this positioning to adults with botulism remains untested. This tilted, flat-body positioning with neck support may improve

ventilation by reducing entry of oral secretions into the airway and by suspending more of the weight of the abdominal viscera from the diaphragm, thereby improving respiratory excursion (FIGURE 4). In contrast, placing a botulism patient in a supine or semirecumbent position (trunk flexed 45° at the waist) may impede respiratory excursion and airway clearance, especially if the patient is obese. The desired angle of the reverse Trendelenburg position is 20° to 25°.

Botulism patients should be assessed for adequacy of gag and cough reflexes, control of oropharyngeal secretions, oxygen saturation, vital capacity, and inspiratory force. Airway obstruction or aspiration usually precedes hypoventilation in botulism. When respiratory function deteriorates, controlled, anticipatory intubation is indicated. The proportion of patients with botulism who require mechanical ventilation has varied from 20% in a foodborne outbreak[64] to more than 60% in infant botulism.[85] In a large outbreak of botulism, the need for mechanical ventilators, critical care beds, and skilled personnel might quickly exceed local capacity and persist for weeks or months. Development of a reserve stockpile of mechanical ventilators in the United States is under way[86] and will require a complement of staff trained in their use.

Antibiotics have no known direct effect on botulinum toxin. However, secondary infections acquired during botulism often require antibiotic therapy. Aminoglycoside antibiotics and clindamycin are contraindicated because of their ability to exacerbate neuromuscular blockade.[87,88] Standard treatments for detoxification, such as activated charcoal,[89] may be given before antitoxin becomes available, but there are no data regarding their effectiveness in human botulism.

SPECIAL POPULATIONS

Based on limited information, there is no indication that treatment of children, pregnant women, and immunocompromised persons with botulism should differ from standard therapy.

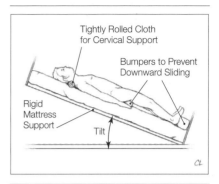

Figure 4. Preferred Positioning of Nonventilated Botulism Patients

Tightly Rolled Cloth for Cervical Support

Bumpers to Prevent Downward Sliding

Rigid Mattress Support

Tilt

Note flat, rigid mattress tilted at 20°, tightly rolled cloth to support cervical vertebrae, and bumpers to prevent downward sliding. Use of this position may postpone or avoid the need for mechanical ventilation in mildly affected patients because of improved respiratory mechanics and airway protection.

Despite the risks of immediate hypersensitivity and sensitization to equine proteins, both children[43,90] and pregnant women[91,92] have received equine antitoxin without apparent short-term adverse effects. The risks to fetuses of exposure to equine antitoxin are unknown. Treatment with human-derived neutralizing antibody would decrease the risk of allergic reactions posed by equine botulinum antitoxin, but use of the investigational product, Botulism Immune Globulin Intravenous (Human) (California Department of Health Services, Berkeley), is limited to suspected cases of infant botulism.[82,93]

PROPHYLAXIS

Botulism can be prevented by the presence of neutralizing antibody in the bloodstream. Passive immunity can be provided by equine botulinum antitoxin or by specific human hyperimmune globulin, while endogenous immunity can be induced by immunization with botulinum toxoid.

Use of antitoxin for postexposure prophylaxis is limited by its scarcity and its reactogenicity. Because of the risks of equine antitoxin therapy, it is less certain how best to care for persons who may have been exposed to botulinum toxin but who are not yet ill. In a small

©2001 American Medical Association. All rights reserved.

study of primates exposed to aerosolized toxin in which supportive care was not provided, all 7 monkeys given antitoxin after exposure but before the appearance of neurologic signs survived, while 2 of 4 monkeys treated with antitoxin only after the appearance of neurologic signs died.[39] Moreover, all monkeys infused with neutralizing antibody before exposure to toxin displayed no signs of botulism. In a balance between avoiding the potential adverse effects of equine antitoxin and needing to rapidly neutralize toxin, it is current practice in foodborne botulism outbreaks to closely monitor persons who may have been exposed to botulinum toxin and to treat them promptly with antitoxin at the first signs of illness.[47] To facilitate distribution of scarce antitoxin following the intentional use of botulinum toxin, asymptomatic persons who are believed to have been exposed should remain under close medical observation and, if feasible, near critical care services.

In the United States, an investigational pentavalent (ABCDE) botulinum toxoid is distributed by the CDC for laboratory workers at high risk of exposure to botulinum toxin and by the military for protection of troops against attack.[94] A recombinant vaccine is also in development.[95] The pentavalent toxoid has been used for more than 30 years to immunize more than 3000 laboratory workers in many countries. Immunization of the population with botulinum toxoid could in theory eliminate the hazard posed by botulinum toxins A through E. However, mass immunization is neither feasible nor desirable for reasons that include scarcity of the toxoid, rarity of natural disease, and elimination of the potential therapeutic benefits of medicinal botulinum toxin. Accordingly, preexposure immunization currently is neither recommended for nor available to the general population. Botulinum toxoid induces immunity over several months and, so, is ineffective as postexposure prophylaxis.

DECONTAMINATION

Despite its extreme potency, botulinum toxin is easily destroyed. Heating to an internal temperature of 85°C for at least 5 minutes will detoxify contaminated food or drink.[52] All foods suspected of contamination should be promptly removed from potential consumers and submitted to public health authorities for testing.

Persistence of aerosolized botulinum toxin at a site of deliberate release is determined by atmospheric conditions and the particle size of the aerosol. Extremes of temperature and humidity will degrade the toxin, while fine aerosols will eventually dissipate into the atmosphere. Depending on the weather, aerosolized toxin has been estimated to decay at between less than 1% to 4% per minute.[96] At a decay rate of 1% per minute, substantial inactivation ($\geq$13 logs) of toxin occurs by 2 days after aerosolization.

Recognition of a covert release of finely aerosolized botulinum toxin would probably occur too late to prevent additional exposures. When exposure is anticipated, some protection may be conferred by covering the mouth and nose with clothing such as an undershirt, shirt, scarf, or handkerchief.[97] In contrast with mucosal surfaces, intact skin is impermeable to botulinum toxin.

After exposure to botulinum toxin, clothing and skin should be washed with soap and water.[98] Contaminated objects or surfaces should be cleaned with 0.1% hypochlorite bleach solution if they cannot be avoided for the hours to days required for natural degradation.[33,52,98]

INFECTION CONTROL

Medical personnel caring for patients with suspected botulism should use standard precautions. Patients with suspected botulism do not need to be isolated, but those with flaccid paralysis from suspected meningitis require droplet precautions.

RESEARCH NEEDS

Additional research in diagnosis and treatment of botulism is required to minimize its threat as a weapon. Rapid diagnostic and toxin typing techniques currently under development would be useful for recognizing and responding to a bioterrorist attack. Although polymerase chain reaction assays can detect the botulinum toxin gene,[99] they are unable, as yet, to determine whether the toxin gene is expressed and whether the expressed protein is indeed toxic. Assays that exploit the enzymatic activity of botulinum toxin have the potential to supplant the mouse bioassay as the standard for diagnosis.[100] Detection of botulinum toxin in aerosols by enzyme-linked immunosorbent assay[101] is a component of the US military's Biological Integrated Detection System for rapid recognition of biological agents in the battlefield.[17]

The distribution of botulinum antitoxin to local hospitals from regional depots takes several hours. In contrast, standard detoxification techniques can be applied immediately. Studies are needed to assess whether activated charcoal and osmotic catharsis can prevent gastrointestinal tract absorption or reduce circulating levels of botulinum toxin. Enteral detoxification may be less useful in inhalational botulism than in foodborne disease.

The competing needs for immunity to weaponized botulinum toxin and for susceptibility to medicinal botulinum toxin could be reconciled by supplying human antibody that neutralizes toxin. With a half-life of approximately 1 month,[102] human antibody would provide immunity for long periods and avoid the reactogenicity of equine products. Existing in vitro technologies could produce the stockpiles of fully human antibody necessary both to deter terrorist attacks and to avoid the rationing of antitoxin that currently would be required in a large outbreak of botulism.[103-106] A single small injection of oligoclonal human antibodies could, in theory, provide protection against toxins A through G for many months. Until such a product becomes available, the possibilities for reducing the population's vulnerability to the intentional misuse of botulinum toxin remain limited.

Author Affiliations: Infant Botulism Treatment and Prevention Program (Drs Arnon and Schechter) and Viral and Rickettsial Diseases Laboratory (Dr Ascher),

©2001 American Medical Association. All rights reserved.

Reprinted with permission from *JAMA*; February 28, 2001, Vol 285, No. 8

California Department of Health Services, Berkeley; Center for Civilian Biodefense Studies, Johns Hopkins University Schools of Medicine (Drs Inglesby, Bartlett, and Perl) and Public Health (Drs Henderson, O'Toole, and Russell), Baltimore, Md; US Army Medical Research Institute of Infectious Diseases, Ft Detrick, Md (Drs Eitzen and Parker); Bureau of Communicable Disease, New York City Health Department, New York, NY (Drs Fine and Layton); Science Applications International Corp, McLean, Va (Mr Hauer); Centers for Disease Control and Prevention, Atlanta, Ga (Drs Lillibridge and Swerdlow); Infection Control Advisory Network Inc, Eden Prairie, Minn (Dr Osterholm); and Office of Emergency Preparedness, Department of Health and Human Services, Rockville, Md (Dr Tonat).

Ex Officio Participants in the Working Group on Civilian Biodefense: George Counts, MD, National Institutes of Health; Margaret Hamburg, MD, and Stuart Nightingale, MD, Office of Assistant Secretary for Planning and Evaluation; Robert Knouss, MD, Office of Emergency Preparedness; and Brian Malkin, US Food and Drug Administration.

Funding/Support: Funding for this study primarily was provided by each participant's institution or agency. The Johns Hopkins Center for Civilian Biodefense Studies provided travel funds for 6 members of the group.

Disclaimers: In some instances, the indications, dosages, and other information in this article are not consistent with current approved labeling by the US Food and Drug Administration (FDA). The recommendations on use of drugs and vaccine for uses not approved by the FDA do not represent the official views of the FDA nor of any of the federal agencies whose scientists participated in these discussions. Unlabeled uses of the products recommended are noted in the sections of this article in which these products are discussed. Where unlabeled uses are indicated, information used as the basis for the recommendation is discussed.

The views, opinions, assertions, and findings contained herein are those of the authors and should not be construed as official US Department of Defense or US Department of Army positions, policies, or decisions unless so designated by other documentation.

Additional Articles: This article is the fourth in a series entitled *Medical and Public Health Management Following the Use of a Biological Weapon: Consensus Statements of The Working Group on Civilian Biodefense.* See references 1 through 3.

Acknowledgment: The working group wishes to thank Christopher Davis, OBE, MD, PhD, for his participation in the consensus process; David Franz, DVM, PhD, for helpful information; Ellen Doyle, MPH, for epidemiological assistance; the reference librarians at the School of Public Health, University of California, Berkeley, for many years of superb help; and Molly D'Esopo, for administrative support.

REFERENCES

1. Inglesby TV, Henderson DA, Bartlett JG, et al, for the Working Group on Civilian Biodefense. Anthrax as a biological weapon: medical and public health management. *JAMA.* 1999;281:1735-1745.

2. Henderson DA, Inglesby TV, Bartlett JG, et al, for the Working Group on Civilian Biodefense. Smallpox as a biological weapon: medical and public health management. *JAMA.* 1999;281:2127-2137.

3. Inglesby TV, Henderson DA, Bartlett JG, et al, for the Working Group on Civilian Biodefense. Plague as a biological weapon: medical and public health management. *JAMA.* 2000;283:2281-2290.

4. Biological and chemical terrorism: strategic plan for preparedness and response: recommendations of the CDC Strategic Planning Workgroup. *MMWR Morb Mortal Wkly Rep.* 2000;49(RR-4):1-14.

5. Franz DR, Jahrling PB, Friedlander AM, et al. Clini-cal recognition and management of patients exposed to biological warfare agents. *JAMA.* 1997;278:399-411.

6. Gill MD. Bacterial toxins: a table of lethal amounts. *Microbiol Rev.* 1982;46:86-94.

7. National Institute of Occupational Safety and Health. *Registry of Toxic Effects of Chemical Substances (R-TECS).* Cincinnati, Ohio: National Institute of Occupational Safety and Health; 1996.

8. Montecucco C, ed. Clostridial neurotoxins: the molecular pathogenesis of tetanus and botulism. *Curr Top Microbiol Immunol.* 1995;195:1-278.

9. Scott AB. Botulinum toxin injection into extraocular muscles as an alternative to strabismus surgery. *J Pediatr Ophthalmol Strabismus.* 1980;17:21-25.

10. Schantz EJ, Johnson EA. Properties and use of botulinum toxin and other microbial neurotoxins in medicine. *Microbiol Rev.* 1992;56:80-99.

11. Jankovic J, Hallet M, eds. *Therapy With Botulinum Toxin.* New York, NY: Marcel Dekker Inc; 1994.

12. Silberstein S, Mathew N, Saper J, Jenkins S, for the Botox Migraine Clinical Research Group. Botulinum toxin type A as a migraine preventive treatment. *Headache.* 2000;40:445-450.

13. Foster L, Clapp L, Erickson M, Jabbari B. Botulinum toxin A and mechanical low back pain [abstract]. *Neurology.* 2000;54(suppl 3):A178.

14. Tucker JB, ed. *Toxic Terror: Assessing the Terrorist Use of Chemical and Biological Weapons.* Cambridge, Mass: MIT Press; 2000.

15. WuDunn S, Miller J, Broad WJ. How Japan germ terror alerted world. *New York Times.* May 26, 1998:A1, A10.

16. Geissler E, Moon JE, eds. *Biological and Toxin Weapons: Research, Development and Use From the Middle Ages to 1945.* New York, NY: Oxford University Press; 1999. Sipri Chemical & Biological Warfare Studies No. 18.

17. Smart JK. History of chemical and biological warfare: an American perspective. In: Sidell FR, Takafuji ET, Franz DR, eds. *Medical Aspects of Chemical and Biological Warfare.* Washington, DC: Office of the Surgeon General; 1997:9-86. *Textbook of Military Medicine;* part I, vol 3.

18. Hill EV. Botulism. In: *Summary Report on B. W. Investigations.* Memorandum to Alden C. Waitt, Chief Chemical Corps, United States Army, December 12, 1947; tab D. Archived at the US Library of Congress.

19. Cochrane RC. *History of the Chemical Warfare Service in World War II (1 July 1940–15 August 1945).* Historical Section, Plans, Training and Intelligence Division, Office of Chief, Chemical Corps, United States Army; November 1947. *Biological Warfare Research in the United States;* vol II. Archived at the US Army Medical Research Institute of Infectious Diseases, Ft Detrick, Md.

20. Bryden J. *Deadly Allies: Canada's Secret War, 1937-1947.* Toronto, Ontario: McClelland & Stewart; 1989.

21. Holzer VE. Botulism from inhalation [in German]. *Med Klin.* 1962;57:1735-1738.

22. United Nations Security Council. *Tenth Report of the Executive Chairman of the Special Commission Established by the Secretary-General Pursuant to Paragraph 9(b)(I) of Security Council Resolution 687 (1991), and Paragraph 3 of Resolution 699 (1991) on the Activities of the Special Commission.* New York, NY: United Nations Security Council; 1995. S/1995/1038.

23. Bozheyeva G, Kunakbayev Y, Yeleukenov D. *Former Soviet Biological Weapons Facilities in Kazakhstan: Past, Present and Future.* Monterey, Calif: Center for Nonproliferation Studies, Monterey Institute of International Studies; June 1999:1-20. Occasional paper No. 1.

24. Miller J. At bleak Asian site, killer germs survive. *New York Times.* June 2, 1999:A1, A10.

25. Alibek K, Handleman S. *Biohazard.* New York, NY: Random House; 1999.

26. Smithson AE. *Toxic Archipelago: Preventing Proliferation From the Former Soviet Chemical and Biological Weapons Complexes.* Washington, DC: The Henry L. Stimson Center; December 1999:7-21. Report No. 32. Available at: http://www.stimson.org/cwc/toxic.htm. Accessed January 16, 2001.

27. United States Department of State. *Patterns of Global Terrorism 1999.* Washington, DC: US Dept of State; April 2000. Department of State publication 10687. Available at: http://www.state.gov/global/terrorism/annual_reports.html. Accessed February 1, 2001.

28. Cordesman AH. *Weapons of Mass Destruction in the Gulf and Greater Middle East: Force Trends, Strategy, Tactics and Damage Effects.* Washington, DC: Center for Strategic and International Studies; November 9, 1998:18-52.

29. Bermudez JS. *The Armed Forces of North Korea.* London, England: IB Tauris; 2001.

30. Zilinskas RA. Iraq's biological weapons: the past as future? *JAMA.* 1997;278:418-424.

31. Hooper RR. The covert use of chemical and biological warfare against United States strategic forces. *Mil Med.* 1983;148:901-902.

32. Shapiro RL, Hatheway C, Becher J, Swerdlow DL. Botulism surveillance and emergency response: a public health strategy for a global challenge. *JAMA.* 1997;278:433-435.

33. Smith LDS. *Botulism: The Organism, Its Toxins, the Disease.* Springfield, Ill: Charles C. Thomas Publisher; 1977.

34. Hatheway CL, Johnson EA. *Clostridium:* the spore-bearing anaerobes. In: Collier L, Balows A, Sussman M, eds. *Topley & Wilson's Microbiology and Microbial Infections.* 9th ed. New York, NY: Oxford University Press; 1998:731-782.

35. Hall JD, McCroskey LM, Pincomb BJ, Hatheway CL. Isolation of an organism resembling *Clostridium baratii* which produces type F botulinal toxin from an infant with botulism. *J Clin Microbiol.* 1985;21:654-655.

36. Aureli P, Fenicia L, Pasolini B, Gianfranceschi M, McCroskey LM, Hatheway CL. Two cases of type E infant botulism caused by neurotoxigenic *Clostridium butyricum* in Italy. *J Infect Dis.* 1986;154:207-211.

37. Arnon SS. Botulism as an intestinal toxemia. In: Blaser MJ, Smith PD, Ravdin JI, Greenberg HB, Guerrant RL, eds. *Infections of the Gastrointestinal Tract.* New York, NY: Raven Press; 1995:257-271.

38. Lacy DB, Tepp W, Cohen AC, DasGupta BR, Stevens RC. Crystal structure of botulinum neurotoxin type A and implications for toxicity. *Nat Struct Biol.* 1998;5:898-902.

39. Franz DR, Pitt LM, Clayton MA, Hanes MA, Rose KJ. Efficacy of prophylactic and therapeutic administration of antitoxin for inhalation botulism. In: DasGupta BR, ed. *Botulinum and Tetanus Neurotoxins: Neurotransmission and Biomedical Aspects.* New York, NY: Plenum Press; 1993:473-476.

40. Herrero BA, Ecklung AE, Streett CS, Ford DF, King JK. Experimental botulism in monkeys: a clinical pathological study. *Exp Mol Pathol.* 1967;6:84-95.

41. Scott AB, Suzuki D. Systemic toxicity of botulinum toxin by intramuscular injection in the monkey. *Mov Disord.* 1988;3:333-335.

42. Centers for Disease Control and Prevention. *Botulism in the United States 1899-1996: Handbook for Epidemiologists, Clinicians, and Laboratory Workers.* Atlanta, Ga: Centers for Disease Control and Prevention; 1998. Available at: http://www.cdc.gov/ncidod/dbmd/diseaseinfo/botulism.pdf. Accessed January 16, 2001.

43. Weber JT, Goodpasture HC, Alexander H, Werner SB, Hatheway CL, Tauxe RV. Wound botulism in a patient with a tooth abscess: case report and literature review. *Clin Infect Dis.* 1993;16:635-639.

44. Hughes JM, Blumenthal JR, Merson MH, Lombard GL, Dowell VR Jr, Gangarosa EJ. Clinical fea-

©2001 American Medical Association. All rights reserved.

Reprinted with permission from *JAMA;* February 28, 2001, Vol 285, No. 8

tures of types A and B food-borne botulism. *Ann Intern Med.* 1981;95:442-445.

45. Duchen LW. Motor nerve growth induced by botulinum toxin as a regenerative phenomenon. *Proc R Soc Med.* 1972;65:196-197.

46. Mann JM, Martin S, Hoffman R, Marrazzo S. Patient recovery from type A botulism: morbidity assessment following a large outbreak. *Am J Public Health.* 1981;71:266-269.

47. Shapiro RL, Hatheway C, Swerdlow DL. Botulism in the United States: a clinical and epidemiologic review. *Ann Intern Med.* 1998;129:221-228.

48. Middlebrook JL, Franz DR. Botulinum toxins. In: Sidell FR, Takafuji ET, Franz DR, eds. *Medical Aspects of Chemical and Biological Warfare.* Washington, DC: Office of the Surgeon General; 1997:643-654. *Textbook of Military Medicine;* part I, vol 3.

49. Gangarosa EJ, Donadio JA, Armstrong RW, Meyer KF, Brachman PH, Dowell VR. Botulism in the United States, 1899-1969. *Am J Epidemiol.* 1971;93:93-101.

50. Hauschild AH. Epidemiology of human foodborne botulism. In: Hauschild AH , Dodds KL, eds. *Clostridium botulinum: Ecology and Control in Foods.* New York, NY: Marcel Dekker Inc; 1993:69-104.

51. Wannemacher RW Jr, Dinterman RE, Thompson WL, Schmidt MO, Burrows WD. Treatment for removal of biotoxins from drinking water. Frederick, Md: US Army Biomedical Research and Development Command; September 1993. Technical Report 9120.

52. Siegel LS. Destruction of botulinum toxin in food and water. In: Hauschild AH, Dodds KL, eds. *Clostridium botulinum: Ecology and Control in Foods.* New York, NY: Marcel Dekker Inc; 1993:323-341.

53. Burrows WD, Renner SE. Biological warfare agents as threats to potable water. *Environ Health Perspect.* 1999;107:975-984.

54. Kazdobina IS. Stability of botulin toxins in solutions and beverages [in Russian with English abstract]. *Gig Sanit.* January-February 1995:9-12.

55. Koenig MG, Drutz D, Mushlin AI, Schaffer W, Rogers DE. Type B botulism in man. *Am J Med.* 1967;42:208-219.

56. Geiger JC, Dickson EC, Meyer KF. *The Epidemiology of Botulism.* Washington, DC: US Government Printing Office; 1922. Public Health Bulletin 127.

57. Terranova W, Breman JG, Locey RP, Speck S. Botulism type B: epidemiological aspects of an extensive outbreak. *Am J Epidemiol.* 1978;109:150-156.

58. Meyer KF, Eddie B. *Sixty-Five Years of Human Botulism in the United States and Canada: Epidemiology and Tabulations of Reported Cases 1899 Through 1964.* San Francisco, Calif: G. W. Hooper Foundation and University of California San Francisco; 1965.

59. Angulo FJ, Getz J, Taylor JP, et al. A large outbreak of botulism: the hazardous baked potato. *J Infect Dis.* 1998;178:172-177.

60. MacDonald KL, Cohen ML, Blake PA. The changing epidemiology of adult botulism in the United States. *Am J Epidemiol.* 1986;124:794-799.

61. Mann JM, Hatheway CL, Gardiner TM. Laboratory diagnosis in a large outbreak of type A botulism: confirmation of the value of coproexamination. *Am J Epidemiol.* 1982;115:598-695.

62. Seals JE, Snyder JD, Kedell TA, et al. Restaurant-associated type A botulism: transmission by potato salad. *Am J Epidemiol.* 1981;113:436-444.

63. MacDonald KL, Spengler RF, Hatheway CL, Hargrett NT, Cohen ML. Type A botulism from sauteed onions: clinical and epidemiological observations. *JAMA.* 1985;253:1275-1278.

64. St. Louis ME, Peck SH, Bowering D, et al. Botulism from chopped garlic: delayed recognition of a major outbreak. *Ann Intern Med.* 1988;108:363-368.

65. Townes JM, Cieslak PR, Hatheway CL, et al. An outbreak of type A botulism associated with a commercial cheese sauce. *Ann Intern Med.* 1996;125:558-563.

66. Telzak EE, Bell EP, Kautter DA, et al. An international outbreak of type E botulism due to uneviscerated fish. *J Infect Dis.* 1990;161:340-342.

67. O'Mahony M, Mitchell E, Gilbert RJ, et al. An outbreak of foodborne botulism associated with contaminated hazelnut yoghurt. *Epidemiol Infect.* 1990;104:389-395.

68. Aureli P, Franciosa G, Pourshaban M. Foodborne botulism in Italy. *Lancet.* 1996;348:1594.

69. Chou JH, Hwant PH, Malison MD. An outbreak of type A foodborne botulism in Taiwan due to commercially preserved peanuts. *Int J Epidemiol.* 1988;17:899-902.

70. Midura TF, Nygaard GS, Wood RM, Bodily HL. *Clostridium botulinum* type F: isolation from venison jerky. *Appl Microbiol.* 1972;24:165-167.

71. McCroskey LM, Hatheway CL, Woodruff BA, Greenberg JA, Jurgenson P. Type F botulism due to neurotoxigenic *Clostridium baratii* from an unknown source in an adult. *J Clin Microbiol.* 1991;29:2618-2620.

72. Gunnison JB, Meyer KF. Susceptibility of monkeys, goats and small animals to oral administration of botulinum toxin types B, C and D. *J Infect Dis.* 1930;46:335-340.

73. Dolman CE, Murakami L. *Clostridium botulinum* type F with recent observations on other types. *J Infect Dis.* 1961;109:107-128.

74. Smart JL, Roberts TA, McCullagh KG, Lucke VM, Pearson H. An outbreak of type C botulism in captive monkeys. *Vet Rec.* 1980;107:445-446.

75. Giménez DF, Ciccarelli AS. Another type of *Clostridium botulinum. Zentralbl Bakteriol [Orig].* 1970;215:221-224.

76. Beller M, Gessner B, Wainwright R, Barrett DH. *Botulism in Alaska: A Guide for Physicians and Health Care Providers.* Anchorage: State of Alaska, Dept of Health and Social Services, Division of Public Health, Section of Epidemiology; 1993.

77. Woodruff BA, Griffin PM, McCroskey LM, et al. Clinical and laboratory comparison of botulism from toxin types A, B, and E in the United States, 1975-1988. *J Infect Dis.* 1992;166:1281-1286.

78. Maselli RA, Bakshi N. American Association of Electrodiagnostic Medicine case report 16: botulism. *Muscle Nerve.* 2000;23:1137-1144.

79. Cherington M. Clinical spectrum of botulism. *Muscle Nerve.* 1998;21:701-710.

80. Felz MW, Smith CD, Swift TR. A six-year-old girl with tick paralysis. *N Engl J Med.* 2000;342:90-94.

81. Tacket CO, Shandera WX, Mann JM, Hargrett NT, Blake PA. Equine antitoxin use and other factors that predict outcome in type A foodborne botulism. *Am J Med.* 1984;76:794-798.

82. Arnon SS. Infant botulism. In: Feigin RD, Cherry JD, eds. *Textbook of Pediatric Infectious Diseases.* 4th ed. Philadelphia, Pa: WB Saunders Co; 1998:1570-1577.

83. Hibbs RG, Weber JT, Corwin A, et al. Experience with the use of an investigational F(ab')₂ heptavalent botulism immune globulin of equine origin during an outbreak of type E botulism in Egypt. *Clin Infect Dis.* 1996;23:337-340.

84. Black RE, Gunn RA. Hypersensitivity reactions associated with botulinal antitoxin. *Am J Med.* 1980;69:567-570.

85. Schreiner MS, Field E, Ruddy R. Infant botulism: a review of 12 years' experience at the Children's Hospital of Philadelphia. *Pediatrics.* 1991;87:159-165.

86. Kahn AS, Morse S, Lillibridge S. Public-health preparedness for biological terrorism in the USA. *Lancet.* 2000;356:1179-1182.

87. Santos JI, Swensen P, Glasgow LA. Potentiation of *Clostridium botulinum* toxin by aminoglycoside antibiotics: clinical and laboratory observations. *Pediatrics.* 1981;68:50-54.

88. Schulze J, Toepfer M, Schroff KC, et al. Clindamycin and nicotinic neuromuscular transmission. *Lancet.* 1999;354:1792-1793.

89. Olson KR, ed. *Poisoning and Drug Overdose.* 3rd ed. Stamford, Conn: Appleton & Lange; 1999.

90. Keller MA, Miller VH, Berkowitz CD, Yoshimori RN. Wound botulism in pediatrics. *Am J Dis Child.* 1982;136:320-322.

91. Robin L, Herman D, Redett R. Botulism in a pregnant woman. *N Engl J Med.* 1996;335:823-824.

92. St. Clair EH, DiLiberti JH, O'Brien ML. Observations of an infant born to a mother with botulism. *J Pediatr.* 1975;87:658.

93. Arnon SS. Clinical trial of human botulism immune globulin. In: DasGupta BR, ed. *Botulinum and Tetanus Neurotoxins: Neurotransmission and Biomedical Aspects.* New York, NY: Plenum Press; 1993:477-482.

94. Siegel LS. Human immune response to botulinum pentavalent (ABCDE) toxoid determined by a neutralization test and by an enzyme-linked immunosorbent assay. *J Clin Microbiol.* 1988;26:2351-2356.

95. Byrne MP, Smith LA. Development of vaccines for prevention of botulism. *Biochimie.* 2000;82:955-966.

96. Dorsey EL, Beebe JM, Johns EE. Responses of airborne *Clostridium botulinum* toxin to certain atmospheric stresses. Frederick, Md: US Army Biological Laboratories; October 1964. Technical Memorandum 62.

97. Wiener SL. Strategies for the prevention of a successful biological warfare aerosol attack. *Mil Med.* 1996;161:251-256.

98. Franz DR. *Defense Against Toxin Weapons.* Ft Detrick, Md: US Army Medical Research Institute of Infectious Diseases; 1997.

99. Franciosa G, Ferreira JL, Hatheway CL. Detection of type A, B, and E botulism neurotoxin genes in *Clostridium botulinum* and other *Clostridium* species by PCR: evidence of unexpressed type B toxin genes in type A toxigenic organisms. *J Clin Microbiol.* 1994;32:1911-1917.

100. Wictome M, Newton K, Jameson K, et al. Development of an in vitro bioassay for *Clostridium botulinum* type B neurotoxin in foods that is more sensitive than the mouse bioassay. *Appl Environ Microbiol.* 1999;65:3787-3792.

101. Dezfulian M, Bartlett JG. Detection of *Clostridium botulinum* type A toxin by enzyme-linked immunosorbent assay with antibodies produced in immunologically tolerant animals. *J Clin Microbiol.* 1984;19:645-648.

102. Sarvas H, Seppala I, Kurikka S, Siegberg R, Makela O. Half-life of the maternal IgG1 allotype in infants. *J Clin Immunol.* 1993;13:145-151.

103. Amersdorfer P, Marks JD. Phage libraries for generation of anti-botulinum scFv antibodies. *Methods Mol Biol.* 2000;145:219-240.

104. Green LL, Hardy MC, Maynard-Currie CE, et al. Antigen-specific human monoclonal antibodies from mice engineered with human Ig heavy and light chain YACs. *Nat Genet.* 1994;7:13-21.

105. Bavari S, Pless DD, Torres ER, Lebeda FJ, Olson MA. Identifying the principal protective antigenic determinants of type A botulinum neurotoxin. *Vaccine.* 1998;16:1850-1856.

106. Marks C, Marks JD. Phage libraries: a new route to clinically useful antibodies. *N Engl J Med.* 1996;335:730-733.

CORRECTION

Incorrect Wording and Web Site Address: In the Consensus Statement entitled "Botulinum Toxin as a Biological Weapon: Medical and Public Health Management" published in the February 28, 2001, issue of THE JOURNAL (2001;285:1059-1070), 3 errors appeared. In the third introductory paragraph on page 69, the word "biological" should be "microbial." In the paragraph labeled "Toxin Types" on page 74, the word "bacteria" should be "bacterial." Finally, on page 79, the Web site address for reference 27 should be http://www.state.gov/www/global/terrorism/1999report/1999index.html.

©2001 American Medical Association. All rights reserved.

Reprinted with permission from *JAMA*; February 28, 2001, Vol 285, No. 8

Hemorrhagic Fever Viruses as Biological Weapons
Medical and Public Health Management

Luciana Borio, MD; Thomas
Inglesby, MD; C. J. Peters, MD;
Alan L. Schmaljohn, PhD; James M.
Hughes, MD; Peter B. Jahrling, PhD;
Thomas Ksiazek, DVM, PhD; Karl M.
Johnson, MD; Andrea Meyerhoff, MD;
Tara O'Toole, MD, MPH; Michael S.
Ascher, MD; John Bartlett, MD;
Joel G. Breman, MD, DTPH;
Edward M. Eitzen, Jr, MD, MPH;
Margaret Hamburg, MD; Jerry Hauer,
MPH; D. A. Henderson, MD, MPH;
Richard T. Johnson, MD; Gigi
Kwik, PhD; Marci Layton, MD;
Scott Lillibridge, MD; Gary J.
Nabel, MD, PhD; Michael T.
Osterholm, PhD, MPH; Trish M.
Perl, MD, MSc; Philip Russell, MD;
Kevin Tonat, DrPH, MPH

for the Working Group
on Civilian Biodefense

Objective To develop consensus-based recommendations for measures to be taken by medical and public health professionals if hemorrhagic fever viruses (HFVs) are used as biological weapons against a civilian population.

Participants The Working Group on Civilian Biodefense included 26 representatives from academic medical centers, public health, military services, governmental agencies, and other emergency management institutions.

Evidence MEDLINE was searched from January 1966 to January 2002. Retrieved references, relevant material published prior to 1966, and additional sources identified by participants were reviewed.

Consensus Process Three formal drafts of the statement that synthesized information obtained in the evidence-gathering process were reviewed by the working group. Each draft incorporated comments and judgments of the members. All members approved the final draft.

Conclusions Weapons disseminating a number of HFVs could cause an outbreak of an undifferentiated febrile illness 2 to 21 days later, associated with clinical manifestations that could include rash, hemorrhagic diathesis, and shock. The mode of transmission and clinical course would vary depending on the specific pathogen. Diagnosis may be delayed given clinicians' unfamiliarity with these diseases, heterogeneous clinical presentation within an infected cohort, and lack of widely available diagnostic tests. Initiation of ribavirin therapy in the early phases of illness may be useful in treatment of some of these viruses, although extensive experience is lacking. There are no licensed vaccines to treat the diseases caused by HFVs.

JAMA. 2002;287:2391-2405   www.jama.com

HEMORRHAGIC FEVER VIRUSES (HFVs) are the subject of the sixth article in a series on medical and public health management of civilian populations following use of biological weapons.[1-5] Historically, the term *viral hemorrhagic fever* (VHF) has referred to a clinical illness associated with fever and a bleeding diathesis caused by a virus belonging to 1 of 4 distinct families: Filoviridae, Arenaviridae, Bunyaviridae, and Flaviviridae (TABLE 1).

The HFVs are transmitted to humans via contact with infected animal reservoirs or arthropod vectors (the natural reservoirs and vectors of the Ebola and Marburg viruses are unknown). The mode of transmission, clinical course, and mortality of these illnesses vary with the specific virus, but

Author Affiliations: Johns Hopkins Center for Civilian Biodefense Strategies (Drs Borio, Inglesby, O'Toole, Henderson, and Kwik) and Departments of Microbiology and Neuroscience (Dr K. M. Johnson), Johns Hopkins Schools of Medicine and Public Health, and Division of Infectious Diseases, Johns Hopkins School of Medicine (Drs Bartlett and Perl), Baltimore, Md; Critical Care Medicine Department, Clinical Center (Dr Borio), Fogarty International Center (Dr Breman), and Vaccine Research Center (Dr Nabel), National Institutes of Health, Bethesda, Md; Center for Biodefense, University of Texas Medical Branch, Galveston (Dr Peters); US Army Medical Research Institute of Infectious Diseases, Frederick, Md (Drs Schmaljohn, Jahrling, and Eitzen); National Center for Infectious Diseases, Centers for Disease Control and Prevention, Atlanta, Ga (Drs Hughes and Ksiazek); Departments of Biology and Medicine, University of New Mexico, Albuquerque (Dr R. T. Johnson); Office of the Commissioner, US Food and Drug Administration (Dr Meyerhoff), and Office of Emergency Preparedness, Department of Health and Human Services (Dr Tonat), Rockville, Md; Office of Public Health Preparedness, Department of Health and Human Services (Drs Ascher, Lillibridge, and Russell and Mr Hauer), and Nuclear Threat Initiative (Dr Hamburg), Washington, DC; Bureau of Communicable Diseases, New York City Health Department, New York, NY (Dr Layton); and Center for Infectious Disease Research and Policy, University of Minnesota, Minneapolis (Dr Osterholm).
Corresponding Author and Reprints: Luciana Borio, MD, Johns Hopkins Center for Civilian Biodefense Strategies, Johns Hopkins Schools of Medicine and Public Health, 111 Market Pl, Suite 830, Baltimore, MD 21202 (e-mail: Lborio@jhsph.edu).

©2002 American Medical Association. All rights reserved.

Reprinted with permission from *JAMA*; May 8, 2002, Vol 287, No. 18

each is capable of causing a hemorrhagic fever syndrome. Clinical and epidemiological data are limited; outbreaks are sporadic and unanticipated, and there are few case series or clinical trials involving human subjects.

The Working Group on Civilian Biodefense previously established a list of key features that characterize biological agents that pose particularly serious risks if used as biological weapons against civilian populations: (1) high morbidity and mortality; (2) potential for person-to-person transmission; (3) low infective dose and highly infectious by aerosol dissemination, with a commensurate ability to cause large outbreaks; (4) effective vaccine unavailable or available only in limited supply; (5) potential to cause public and health care worker anxiety; (6) availability of pathogen or toxin; (7) feasibility of large-scale production; (8) environmental stability; and (9) prior research and development as a biological weapon. Some HFVs exhibit a significant number of these key characteristics and pose serious risk as biological weapons, including Ebola and Marburg viruses (Filoviridae), Lassa fever and New World arenaviruses (Arenaviridae), Rift Valley fever (Bunyaviridae), and yellow fever, Omsk hemorrhagic fever, and Kyasanur Forest disease (Flaviviridae).

Several viruses that can cause VHF will not be considered further in this analysis. Dengue is excluded because it is not transmissible by small-particle aerosol,[7] and primary dengue causes VHF only rarely. Crimean-Congo hemorrhagic fever (CCHF) and the agents of hemorrhagic fever with renal syndrome (HFRS) also have been excluded after much deliberation. Although these pathogens can cause VHF and may be transmissible by small-particle aerosol, the working group noted that technical difficulties (ie, barriers to large-scale production) currently preclude their development as mass casualty weapons. Crimean-Congo hemorrhagic fever and the agents of HFRS do not readily replicate to high concentrations in cell cultures, a prerequisite for weaponization of an infectious organism. However, CCHF, the agents of HFRS, and dengue may carry great morbidity and mortality in naturally occurring outbreaks. In particular, CCHF may be transmitted from person to person, has a high case-fatality rate, and is endemic in central Asia and southern Africa. We acknowledge that technical difficulties may be overcome with advances in technology and science, and these excluded viruses may become a greater threat in the future. Other sources provide information on the viruses not addressed herein.[8-12]

The consequences of an unannounced aerosol attack with an HFV are the primary focus of this analysis. A variety of attack scenarios with these agents are possible. This analysis does not attempt to forecast the most likely but focuses on perhaps the most serious scenario. Understanding and planning for a covert aerosol attack with HFVs will improve preparedness for other scenarios as well.

CONSENSUS METHODS

The working group for this article was composed of 26 professionals from academic medical centers, public health, military services, governmental agencies, and emergency management institutions. MEDLINE databases were searched from January 1966 to January 2002 for the Medical Subject Headings *viral hemorrhagic fever, Ebola, Marburg, Lassa, arenavirus, Junin, Guanarito, Machupo, Sabia, CCHF, Rift Valley fever, hantavirus, dengue, yellow fever, Omsk hemorrhagic fever, Kyasanur Forest disease, biological weapons, biological terrorism, biological warfare,* and *biowarfare.* The references were reviewed and relevant materials published prior to 1966 were identified. The working group also identified other published and unpublished references for review.

Table 1. Hemorrhagic Fever Viruses*

Family	Genus	Virus	Disease	Vector in Nature	Geographic Distribution
Filoviridae	Filovirus	**Ebola**†	Ebola hemorrhagic fever	Unknown	Africa
		Marburg	Marburg hemorrhagic fever	Unknown	Africa
Arenaviridae	Arenavirus	**Lassa**	Lassa fever	Rodent	West Africa
		New World Arenaviridae‡	New World hemorrhagic fever	Rodent	Americas
Bunyaviridae	Nairovirus	Crimean-Congo hemorrhagic fever	Crimean-Congo hemorrhagic fever	Tick	Africa, central Asia, eastern Europe, Middle East
	Phlebovirus	**Rift Valley fever**	Rift Valley fever	Mosquito	Africa, Saudi Arabia, Yemen
	Hantavirus	Agents of hemorrhagic fever with renal syndrome	Hemorrhagic fever with renal syndrome	Rodent	Asia, Balkans, Europe, Eurasia§
Flaviviridae	Flavivirus	Dengue	Dengue fever, Dengue hemorrhagic fever, and Dengue shock syndrome	Mosquito	Asia, Africa, Pacific, Americas
		Yellow fever	Yellow fever	Mosquito	Africa, tropical Americas
		Omsk hemorrhagic fever	Omsk hemorrhagic fever	Tick	Central Asia
		Kyasanur Forest disease	Kyasanur Forest disease	Tick	India

*Bold indicates hemorrhagic fever viruses that pose serious risk as biological weapons (addressed in this consensus statement).
†There are 4 subtypes of Ebola: Zaire, Sudan, Ivory Coast, and Reston.
‡The New World Arenaviridae include Machupo, the cause of Bolivian hemorrhagic fever; Junin, the cause of Argentine hemorrhagic fever; Guanarito, the cause of Venezuelan hemorrhagic fever; and Sabia, the cause of Brazilian hemorrhagic fever. An additional arenavirus has been isolated following 3 fatal cases of hemorrhagic fever in California, 1999-2000.[6]
§Additionally, the agents of hantavirus pulmonary syndrome have been isolated in North America.

©2002 American Medical Association. All rights reserved.

Reprinted with permission from *JAMA*; May 8, 2002, Vol 287, No. 18

A first draft resulted from the synthesis of information obtained during the evidence-gathering process. Members of the working group were convened to discuss the first draft of the formulated guidelines on January 10, 2002. Subsequently, a second draft was produced incorporating comments and judgments of the working group. They reviewed the second draft and submitted comments, which were incorporated into a third and final draft of the document.

HISTORY AND POTENTIAL AS BIOLOGICAL WEAPONS

Hemorrhagic fever viruses have been weaponized by the former Soviet Union, Russia, and the United States.[13-15] There are reports that yellow fever may have been weaponized by North Korea.[14] The former Soviet Union and Russia produced large quantities of Marburg, Ebola, Lassa, and New World arenaviruses (specifically, Junin and Machupo) until 1992.[13,15] Soviet Union researchers quantified the aerosol infectivity of Marburg virus for monkeys, determining that no more than a few virions are required to cause infection.[16] Yellow fever and Rift Valley fever viruses were developed as weapons by the US offensive biological weapons program prior to its termination in 1969.[14] The Japanese terrorist cult Aum Shinrikyo unsuccessfully attempted to obtain Ebola virus as part of an effort to create biological weapons.[17]

Several studies have demonstrated successful infection of nonhuman primates by aerosol preparations of Ebola,[18] Marburg,[19] Lassa,[20] and New World arenaviruses.[21] Arguments asserting that the absence of effective antiviral therapy and vaccines would make these viruses too dangerous to develop as weapons are not supported by the historical record.

In 1999, the Centers for Disease Control and Prevention (CDC) classified the HFVs as category A bioweapon agents, based on the potential to cause widespread illness and death, ease of dissemination or person-to-person transmission, potential for major public health impact, and requirement of special action for public health preparedness.[22]

EPIDEMIOLOGY OF DISEASE TRANSMISSION

In nature, HFVs reside in animal hosts or arthropod vectors. The natural reservoir of filoviruses is unknown. Humans are infected incidentally, acquiring the disease by the bite of an infected arthropod, via aerosol generated from infected rodent excreta, or by direct contact with infected animal carcasses.[23] With the exception of Rift Valley fever and the diseases caused by flaviviruses (yellow fever, Omsk hemorrhagic fever, and Kyasanur Forest disease), which are not transmissible from person to person, infected humans can spread the disease to close contacts, which may result in community outbreaks and nosocomial infections. Limited knowledge exists about transmission because outbreaks of these diseases are sporadic and unpredicted and often occur in areas without adequate medical and public health infrastructure. Outbreaks are usually well under way or have subsided by the time data gathering begins. The risks associated with various modes of transmission are not well defined because most persons who acquire these infections have a history of multiple contacts by multiple modes. Infections acquired percutaneously are associated with the shortest incubation period and highest mortality. Person-to-person airborne transmission appears to be rare but cannot be ruled out.

Filoviridae: Ebola and Marburg

Since 1967, when the first outbreak of VHF caused by Marburg virus occurred in Germany and Yugoslavia, there have been 18 reports of human outbreaks of VHF secondary to Ebola or Marburg viruses, resulting in approximately 1500 cases to date.[24] Most have occurred in Africa. Epidemiological investigation indicates that most cases occurred after direct contact with blood, secretions, or tissues of infected patients or nonhuman primates.

Several cases have followed needlestick injuries. During the 1976 Ebola epidemic in Zaire (now Democratic Republic of the Congo), 85 (26.7%) of 318 cases occurred in individuals who had received an injection, and every case of disease acquired by contaminated syringes resulted in death.[25] Mortality was substantially higher when the disease was acquired percutaneously. Evidence suggests that percutaneous exposure to very low inocula can result in infection.[26]

Filoviruses can also be transmitted by mucosal exposure. Experiments in nonhuman primates have documented transmission of infection after direct administration of Marburg virus into the mouths and noses of experimental animals[27] and after direct administration of Ebola virus into the mouths or conjunctiva[28] of experimental animals. Human infections might occur through contact of contaminated fingers with oral mucosa or conjunctiva,[29] but direct evidence is lacking.

Copious numbers of Ebola viral particles found in human skin and lumina of sweat glands have raised concern that disease transmission may occur from touching an infected patient or corpse.[30] In the 1995 Ebola outbreak in Kikwit, Democratic Republic of the Congo, several persons preparing bodies for burial acquired the infection.[31-33] According to local custom, burial practices may involve washing the body and cutting the hair and nails of the corpse.[34] However, a study using guinea pigs was unable to document Marburg virus transmission through intact skin, while infection through skin lesions did occur.[35]

A few cases of disease transmission by uncertain mechanisms described in 2 recent Ebola outbreaks,[36,37] and findings from animal studies[16,18,38] and 1 outbreak of Ebola in nonhuman primates,[39] raise concern about the potential for person-to-person transmission by way of small-droplet airborne nuclei. However, to date, Ebola epidemics in Africa were ultimately controlled and ended without use of specific airborne precautions. (HICPAC's definitions of standard, contact, droplet, and airborne precautions are at http://www.cdc.gov/ncidod/hip/isolat/isopart2.htm.)

Airborne transmission of Marburg virus was not observed in the 1967 outbreak in Germany and Yugoslavia fol-

©2002 American Medical Association. All rights reserved.

Reprinted with permission from *JAMA*; May 8, 2002, Vol 287, No. 18

lowing the importation of infected African green monkeys from eastern Africa.[40] In 1975, only 1 of 35 health care workers who cared for 2 patients with Marburg disease in South Africa without any barrier precautions became ill.[41] In 1979, an outbreak of Ebola in southern Sudan infected 34 people. Although direct physical contact could not be established in 2 instances, 29 cases resulted from direct physical contact with an infected person and there were no cases of illness among 103 persons who were exposed to cases in confined spaces without any physical contact.[42] In 1994, only 1 of 70 contacts of a patient with Ebola acquired the disease despite lack of airborne precautions.[43] In 1996, none of the 300 contacts of 2 patients with Ebola acquired the disease[44] despite involvement in numerous hazardous procedures prior to the patients' diagnosis, protected only by standard blood and bodily fluid precautions.

In 1995, 316 people became ill with Ebola in the Democratic Republic of the Congo; 25% of the cases involved health care workers. When barrier precautions were instituted, only 3 health care workers became infected. One was nonadherent to barrier precautions, the second had a needlestick injury, and it is speculated that the third, who always used protective equipment, became infected after touching her eyes with a contaminated glove.[45] None of the 78 household members who did not have direct physical contact with an infected person developed disease.[31] However, in this outbreak, the only risk factor identified for 5 patients was visiting an infected patient in the absence of physical contact. These few cases led researchers to conclude that airborne transmission could not be ruled out[37] but seemed to be, at most, a minor mode of transmission.

In 2000, 224 people died in Uganda during an Ebola outbreak.[37] Fourteen (64%) of 22 medical personnel were infected after institution of isolation wards and infection control measures[37] including donning gowns, gloves, and shoe covers, standard surgical masks, and either goggles or eye glasses.[46] It is not clear whether lack of adherence to guidelines contributed to nosocomial cases in this outbreak, but airborne transmission could not be ruled out.

Although Marburg virus has been isolated from healthy-appearing infected monkeys several days before clinical signs appear,[27] no transmission has been observed in this stage.[40] In humans, transmission of Ebola during the incubation period does not appear to be common.[31] Transmissibility of Ebola increases with the duration of disease, and direct physical contact with an ill person during the late phase of clinical illness confers an additional risk.[31] There has been only 1 reported case, during the outbreak in Zaire in 1976, in which the only possible source of infection was contact with an unconfirmed case hours before the patient developed symptoms.[25] The preponderance of evidence suggests that transmission of Ebola and Marburg virus rarely, if ever, occurs before the onset of signs and symptoms.

In several studies after the 1995 Kikwit outbreak, Ebola was detected in the seminal fluid of convalescing patients by reverse transcriptase polymerase chain reaction (RT-PCR) up to 101 days after disease onset,[47,48] and virus was isolated 82 days after disease onset in the seminal fluid of 1 patient.[48] Marburg has been isolated 83 days after disease onset from the seminal fluid of a patient who may have sexually transmitted the disease to his spouse.[40]

Arenaviridae: Lassa Fever and New World Arenaviruses

In nature, arenaviruses are transmitted to humans via inhalation of aerosols present in rodent urine and feces,[49] by ingestion of food contaminated with rodent excreta, or by direct contact of rodent excreta with abraded skin and mucous membranes.[50] Like filoviruses, person-to-person transmission of the arenaviruses occurs predominantly by direct contact with infectious blood and bodily fluids. A number of nosocomial outbreaks of Lassa fever[51-53] and of New World arenaviruses[54] have occurred via this mecha-

nism. As with filoviruses, person-to-person airborne transmission has been suspected in a few instances.

In 1969, during a nosocomial outbreak in Nigeria, an index patient with severe pulmonary involvement caused 16 secondary cases in persons who shared the same hospital ward with her. Airborne transmission was believed to have contributed to this outbreak, as there were no tertiary cases of Lassa fever in the hospital, despite the admission of Lassa fever–infected patients to other hospital wards.[51] However, there is no definitive evidence of airborne transmission and the exact mechanisms of disease transmission during that outbreak remain unknown. Conversely, in the case of 1 Lassa fever–infected individual who traveled from Sierra Leone to the United States, no cases were detected in 522 contacts, even prior to initiating additional barrier precautions beyond standard precautions.[55] In another instance, in which an infected individual originated in Nigeria and traveled to St Thomas in the US Virgin Islands, none of the 159 people who had direct contact with the patient developed clinical or serological evidence of infection, even though they attended to the patient, without barrier precautions, during a 5-day period before the diagnosis.[56]

Airborne transmission of Bolivian hemorrhagic fever has been implicated after a student became infected after watching a nursing instructor demonstrate the changing of bed linens of an infected patient, although the student did not touch the patient or any objects in the room and kept a distance of greater than 6 ft from the patient.[54] Conversely, approximately 80 involved health care workers who did not use airborne precautions remained healthy. Definitive evidence of person-to-person airborne transmission is lacking but, in these rare instances, there have been no plausible alternative explanations.

There have been no reports documenting transmission of arenaviruses by infected persons during the incubation period.[54,57] However, Lassa fever virus can be detected in semen up to 3 months

©2002 American Medical Association. All rights reserved.

Reprinted with permission from *JAMA*; May 8, 2002, Vol 287, No. 18

Table 2. Microbiology of Hemorrhagic Fever Viruses[71]

Family	Diameter, nm	Morphology	Presence of Envelope	Genome		
				Size, kbp	Nature*	Configuration*
Filoviridae	80	Bacilliform (filamentous)	Yes	19	Single-strand RNA (−)	Nonsegmented (1 − segment)
Arenaviridae	110-130	Spherical	Yes	11	Single-strand RNA (±)	2 ± Segments
Bunyaviridae	80-120	Spherical	Yes	11-19	Single-strand RNA (−)	3 − Segments
Flaviviridae	40-50	Isometric	Yes	10-12	Single-strand RNA (+)	Nonsegmented (1 + segment)

*Minus sign indicates negative-strand genome; plus sign, positive-strand genome; and plus/minus sign, ambisense genome.

after acute infection[58] and in urine 32 days after disease onset,[59] and Argentine hemorrhagic fever has been transmitted to spouses of convalescent patients 7 to 22 days after onset of illness.[60]

Bunyaviridae: Rift Valley Fever

Humans acquire Rift Valley fever from the bite of an infected mosquito, direct contact with infected animal tissues, or aerosolization of virus from infected animal carcasses.[61] Ingestion of contaminated raw animal milk has been implicated epidemiologically.[62] Despite high levels of viremia and isolation of low titers of virus from throat washings, there are no reported cases of person-to-person transmission of Rift Valley fever.[62] However, laboratory technicians are at risk of acquiring the disease by inhalation of infectious aerosols generated from specimens.[61,63]

If Rift Valley fever were used as a biological weapon, susceptible domestic livestock (sheep, cattle, buffalo, and goats) could also be infected. Infected livestock develop high levels of viremia, sufficient to infect susceptible mosquito vectors and lead to establishment of the disease in the environment[61] and large epizootic epidemics, as occurred in Egypt in 1977[64] and the Arabian peninsula in 2000.[65] Several genera of mosquitoes (eg, *Aedes*, *Anopheles*, and *Culex*) in the United States have the capacity to act as vectors of Rift Valley fever.[66,67]

Flaviviridae: Yellow Fever, Omsk Hemorrhagic Fever, and Kyasanur Forest Disease

Humans acquire yellow fever virus from the bite of an infected mosquito[68] and acquire Omsk hemorrhagic fever and Kyasanur Forest disease viruses from the bite of an infected tick.[69] There are no reported cases of person-to-person transmission or nosocomial spread of flaviviruses. Infection of laboratory personnel via inhalation of aerosols during cultivation of these viruses has been reported.[69,70] As with Rift Valley fever, there is a theoretical risk of flaviviruses becoming established in an environment following infection of susceptible arthropod vectors.

MICROBIOLOGY AND PATHOGENESIS

All of the HFVs are small RNA viruses with lipid envelopes. Specific microbiological characteristics of these viruses are listed in TABLE 2.

Information regarding the pathogenesis of these agents following infection in humans is incomplete. Most data have been derived from clinical observations and experimentally induced disease in nonhuman primates. Interpretation of data derived from animal studies may be confounded by a series of factors, such as the species of the animal, the route of inoculation, and the virus dose.[40]

All of the viruses of concern may lead to thrombocytopenia, and data suggest that platelet dysfunction is present in Ebola, Lassa fever, and Argentine hemorrhagic fever.[72] Reduced levels of coagulation factors may be secondary to hepatic dysfunction and/or disseminated intravascular coagulation and are most prominent in Rift Valley fever and yellow fever.[72] In addition, Ebola and Marburg viruses may lead to a hemorrhagic diathesis through direct damage of cells involved in hemostasis (such as platelets and endothelial cells) and/or indirectly through immunological and inflammatory pathways.[72]

Filoviruses are extremely virulent in nonhuman primates and humans.[73] Necrosis of visceral organs (such as liver, spleen, and kidneys) has been associated with both direct viral-induced cellular damage and impairment of the microcirculation. Filoviruses are cytotoxic to cells. In general, inflammatory infiltration is absent in the affected visceral organs.[74] Even when viral titers in the lungs of monkeys are elevated, the virus is not apparent in the alveoli or airways, occurring primarily in the vascular structures.[28] All experimentally infected monkeys develop disseminated intravascular coagulation. Ebola, but not Marburg virus, makes a secreted form of its glycoprotein that has been suggested to have a role in virulence.[73] Endothelial cells support Marburg virus replication, and their destruction may contribute to the associated hemorrhagic diathesis and shock.[75]

Infection with arenaviruses is initiated in nasopharyngeal mucosa.[76] Arenaviruses produce carrier states in rodents, their natural hosts, and viral multiplication is not associated with extensive cell damage. In vitro infections with Arenaviridae show that virus spreads throughout a variety of different cellular monolayers, with little or absent cytopathic effects[77]; hence, it is believed that these viruses may exert their effects (at least in part) by inducing the secretion of inflammatory mediators from macrophages. Following experimental infection of nonhuman primates with arenaviruses, virtually all tissues become infected, with little histologic evidence of damage.[78] Hemorrhage following arenavirus infection appears to be associated with the presence of a circulating inhibitor of platelet aggregation and thrombocytopenia.

©2002 American Medical Association. All rights reserved.

Reprinted with permission from *JAMA*; May 8, 2002, Vol 287, No. 18

However, disseminated intravascular coagulation does not appear to be a central pathogenic mechanism.[79] Lassa fever appears to be terminated by a cellular, not humoral, immune response,[77] whereas in New World arenaviruses, recovery is preceded by cellular and humoral immune responses.[80]

In contrast with arenaviruses, Rift Valley fever virus leads to destruction of infected cells.[77] The hemostatic derangements in Rift Valley fever are poorly understood, and a combination of vasculitis and hepatic necrosis has been postulated.[81,82] Interferon alfa given shortly before or after experimental infection with Rift Valley fever virus has been shown to protect rhesus monkeys from viremia and hepatocellular damage.[83] Clinical recovery is associated with appearance of neutralizing antibodies, and passive immunization prevented development of viremia in nonhuman primates inoculated with the virus.[83]

Like Rift Valley fever, yellow fever virus leads to destruction of infected cells. Hepatocyte infection and degeneration is a late event in the course of infection,[84] associated with virtually no inflammation.[68] Neutralizing antibodies correlate with clearance of viremia, and paradoxically, with the second phase of illness, when patients may develop hemorrhage and shock.[68]

Little is known about the pathogenesis of Omsk hemorrhagic fever and Kyasanur Forest disease viruses. Findings from postmortem examinations of 3 individuals who died of Kyasanur Forest disease showed degeneration of the larger visceral organs (especially liver and spleen) and hemorrhagic pneumonia.[85]

CLINICAL MANIFESTATIONS

Information on the clinical manifestations of these diseases is derived from naturally occurring outbreaks. Although data derived from experimentally infected animals do not support marked differences in the clinical presentation according to route of expo-

Table 3. Clinical Characteristics of Hemorrhagic Fever Viruses Noted in Past Case Series or Outbreaks

Virus	Distinctive Clinical Features	Person-to-Person Transmission	Incubation Period, d	Mortality, %	Treatment
Ebola[25,42-44,47,86,99]	High fever and severe prostration. A diffuse maculopapular rash may occur by day 5 of illness. Bleeding and disseminated intravascular coagulation are common.	Yes	2-21	50-90*	Supportive
Marburg[40,41,87,102]	High fever, myalgias. Nonpruritic maculopapular rash of the face, neck, trunk, and arms may develop. Bleeding and disseminated intravascular coagulation are common.	Yes	2-14	23-70†	Supportive
Lassa fever[52,88-91,100,101,110]	Gradual onset of fever, nausea, abdominal pain, severe sore throat, cough, conjunctivitis, ulceration of buccal mucosa, exudative pharyngitis, and cervical lymphadenopathy. Late signs include severe swelling of head and neck; pleural and pericardial effusions. Hemorrhagic complications less common.	Yes	5-16	15-20	Ribavirin, supportive
New World Arenaviruses[54,92,128]	Gradual onset of fever, myalgias, nausea, abdominal pain, conjunctivitis, flushing of face and trunk, and generalized lymphadenopathy. May develop petechiae, bleeding, and central nervous system dysfunction (tremors of the tongue and upper extremities, myoclonic movements, dysarthria, and generalized seizures).	Yes	7-14	15-30	Ribavirin, supportive
Rift Valley fever[61,93-96]	Fever, headache, retro-orbital pain, photophobia, and jaundice. Less than 1% develop hemorrhagic fever or encephalitis. Retinitis affects approximately 10%, which may occur at time of acute febrile illness or up to 4 weeks later.	No	2-6	<1	Ribavirin, supportive
Yellow fever[68,97]	Fever, myalgias, facial flushing, and conjunctival injection. Patients either recover or enter a short remission followed by fever, relative bradycardia, jaundice, renal failure, and hemorrhagic complications.	No	3-6	20	Supportive
Omsk hemorrhagic fever[69]‡	Fever, cough, conjunctivitis, papulovesicular eruption on the soft palate, marked hyperemia of the face and trunk (but no rash), generalized lymphadenopathy, and splenomegaly. Some patients may develop pneumonia and central nervous system dysfunction.	No	2-9	0.5-10	Supportive
Kyasanur Forest disease[69,98]	Similar to Omsk but biphasic illness: first phase lasts 6-11 days and is followed by an afebrile period of 9-21 days. Up to 50% of patients relapse and develop meningoencephalitis.	No	2-9	3-10	Supportive

*Reported Ebola data are for Sudan (50%) and Zaire (90%) subtypes. The Ivory Coast subtype has an indeterminate case-fatality rate, as there has been a single nonfatal human case. The Reston subtype causes subclinical infection in humans.
†Mortality ranges from 23% in the 1967 outbreak in Germany to 70% in the largest outbreak of 1999 in the Democratic Republic of the Congo.
‡Also Sergey Netesov, MD, written communication, February 27, 2002.

©2002 American Medical Association. All rights reserved.

Reprinted with permission from *JAMA*; May 8, 2002, Vol 287, No. 18

sure (parenteral vs aerosol),[18,21] it is not possible to be certain that the same manifestations would follow bioweapons attacks on humans.

There are a variety of potential clinical manifestations following infection with these viruses, and not all patients develop the classic VHF syndrome. Clinical manifestations are nonspecific and may include fever, myalgias, rash, and encephalitis. The propensity to cause the classic VHF syndrome also differs among agents. Therefore, in the event of a bioterrorist attack with one of these agents, infected patients may have a variety of clinical presentations, complicating early detection and management. It may not be possible to differentiate among these diseases on clinical grounds alone, although a number of specific clinical features may be useful clues to diagnosis (TABLE 3).

The overall incubation period for HFVs ranges from 2 to 21 days. Patients initially exhibit a nonspecific prodrome, which typically lasts less than 1 week. Symptoms typically include high fever, headache, malaise, arthralgias, myalgias, nausea, abdominal pain, and nonbloody diarrhea. Filoviruses, Rift Valley fever, and flaviviruses are characterized by an abrupt onset, while arenaviruses have a more insidious onset.[40,54,61,68,69,99,100]

Early signs typically include fever, hypotension, relative bradycardia, tachypnea, conjunctivitis, and pharyngitis. Most diseases are associated with cutaneous flushing or a skin rash (FIGURE 1 and FIGURE 2), but the specific characteristics of the rash vary with each disease (Table 3). Later, patients may show signs of progressive hemorrhagic diathesis, such as petechiae, mucous membrane and conjunctival hemorrhage (FIGURE 3); hematuria; hematemesis; and melena. Disseminated intravascular coagulation and circulatory shock may ensue. Central nervous system dysfunction may be present and manifested by delirium, convulsions, cerebellar signs, or coma and imparts a poor prognosis.

The differential diagnosis includes a variety of viral and bacterial diseases:

influenza, viral hepatitis, staphylococcal or gram-negative sepsis, toxic shock syndrome, meningococcemia, salmonellosis and shigellosis, rickettsial diseases (such as Rocky Mountain spotted fever), leptospirosis, borreliosis, psittacosis, dengue, hantavirus pulmonary syndrome, malaria, trypanosomiasis, septicemic plague, rubella, measles, and hemorrhagic smallpox. Noninfectious processes associated with bleeding diathesis that should be included in the differential diagnosis include idiopathic or thrombotic thrombocytopenic purpura, hemolytic uremic syndrome, acute leukemia, and collagen-vascular diseases.

Laboratory abnormalities include leukopenia (except in some cases of Lassa fever, in which leukocytosis occurs), anemia or hemoconcentration, thrombocytopenia, and elevated liver enzymes. Jaundice is typical in Rift Valley fever and yellow fever.[61,68] In addition, coagulation abnormalities may include prolonged bleeding time, prothrombin time, and activated partial thromboplastin time; elevated fibrin degradation products; and decreased fibrinogen. Urinalysis may reveal proteinuria and hematuria, and patients may develop oliguria and azotemia.[26,40,54,61,68,100,101]

Convalescence may be prolonged and complicated by weakness, fatigue, anorexia, cachexia, alopecia, and arthralgias.[43,45] Reported clinical sequelae include hearing or vision loss, impaired motor coordination, transverse myelitis, uveitis, pericarditis, orchitis, parotitis, and pancreatitis.[40,36,52,54,61,102]

The case-fatality rate varies markedly among these agents, ranging from as low as 0.5% for Omsk hemorrhagic fever[69] to as high as 90% for Ebola (subtype Zaire).[33] Death is typically preceded by hemorrhagic diathesis, shock, and multiorgan system failure 1 to 2 weeks following onset of symptoms.

DIAGNOSIS

A high index of suspicion will be required to diagnose VHF among persons exposed to a covert bioterrorist attack. In naturally occurring cases, patients are likely to have risk factors

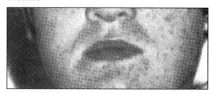

Figure 1. Maculopapular Rash in Marburg Disease

A nonpruritic maculopapular rash (resembling the rash of measles) may occur in up to 50% of patients infected with the Ebola or Marburg viruses within the first week of illness. The rash is more common in light-colored skin and desquamates on resolution. Reprinted with permission from Thieme (Martini GA, Knauff HG, Schmidt HA, et al. A hitherto unknown infectious disease contracted from monkeys. *Ger Med Mon.* 1968;13:457-470).

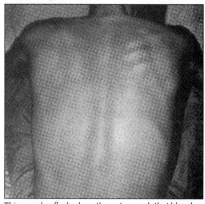

Figure 2. Erythematous Rash in Bolivian Hemorrhagic Fever

This macular, flushed, erythematous rash that blanches with pressure may be associated with infections caused by arenaviruses. The rash most commonly involves the face and thorax and may desquamate on convalescence. Reprinted with permission from Current Science/Current Medicine (Peters CJ, Zaki SR, Rollin PE. Viral hemorrhagic fevers. In: Fekety R, vol ed. *Atlas of Infectious Diseases, Volume VIII.* Philadelphia, Pa: Churchill Livingstone; 1997:10.1-10.26).

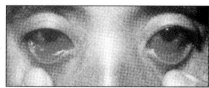

Figure 3. Ocular Manifestations in Bolivian Hemorrhagic Fever

Ocular manifestations associated with hemorrhagic fever viruses range from conjunctival injection to subconjunctival hemorrhage, as seen in this patient. Reprinted with permission from Current Science/Current Medicine (Peters CJ, Zaki SR, Rollin PE. Viral hemorrhagic fevers. In: Fekety R, vol ed. *Atlas of Infectious Diseases, Volume VIII.* Philadelphia, Pa: Churchill, Livingstone; 1997:10.1-10.26).

such as travel to Africa or Asia, handling of animal carcasses, contact with sick animals or people, or arthropod

©2002 American Medical Association. All rights reserved.

Reprinted with permission from *JAMA*; May 8, 2002, Vol 287, No. 18

Box 1. Key Medical and Public Health Interventions After Identification of Suspected Index Case of VHF

Identification

Identify suspected index case using these clinical criteria:* temperature ≥101°F (38.3°C) of <3 weeks' duration; severe illness, and no predisposing factors for hemorrhagic manifestations; and at least 2 of the following hemorrhagic symptoms: hemorrhagic or purple rash, epistaxis, hematemesis, hemoptysis, blood in stools, other, and no established alternative diagnosis.

Reporting

1. Report immediately to local and/or state health department.
2. Report immediately to infection control professional and laboratory personnel.

Treatment

1. Initiate supportive and ribavirin therapy (see Table 4) immediately while diagnostic confirmation is pending.
2. If infection with arenavirus or bunyavirus is confirmed, continue 10-day course of ribavirin.
3. If infection with filovirus or flavivirus is confirmed, or if the diagnosis of VHF is excluded or an alternative diagnosis is established, discontinue ribavirin.

Infection Control Measures

1. Initiate VHF-specific barrier precautions.
2. Initiate airborne precautions, with negative-pressure rooms if resources are available.

Public Health Measures

1. Confirm or exclude diagnosis via Laboratory Response Network.
2. Designated public health authority begins epidemiologic investigation.
3. Identify close and high-risk contacts and place under medical surveillance for 21 days from day of suspected/known exposure.
4. If contact does not have temperature ≥101°F (38.3°C) or signs or symptoms of VHF by the end of 21 days, discontinue medical surveillance.
5. If contact has temperature ≥101°F (38.3°C) or signs or symptoms consistent with VHF, initiate diagnostic workup and treatment, infection control, and public health interventions described for index case.

*Criteria are adapted from the World Health Organization's surveillance standards for acute hemorrhagic fever syndrome.[103]

---

bites within 21 days of onset of symptoms. No such risk factors would be associated with a bioterrorist attack. The variable clinical presentation of these diseases presents a major diagnostic challenge. Clinical microbiology and public health laboratories are not currently equipped to make a rapid diagnosis of any of these viruses, and clinical specimens would need to be sent to the CDC or the US Army Medical Research Institute of Infectious Diseases (USAMRIID; Frederick, Md), the only 2 level D laboratories in the Laboratory Response Network. There are future plans to decentralize the process required for the laboratory confirmation of these viruses by equipping selected US

public health laboratories in the Laboratory Response Network with standard diagnostic reagents. This would likely expedite laboratory confirmation of suspected cases in the event of an outbreak (Michael Ascher, MD, written communication, February 26, 2002).

All suspected cases of HFV disease should be immediately reported to local and/or state health departments (BOX 1), who would then notify the CDC. The World Health Organization has developed surveillance standards for acute VHF syndrome with the aim of early detection of naturally occurring outbreaks and notification of cases, even before identification of the causal agent.[103] This includes prompt reporting to public health authorities of any patient with acute onset of fever of less than 3 weeks' duration who is severely ill, has no known predisposing host factors for hemorrhagic manifestations, and has any 2 of the following: hemorrhagic or purpuric rash, epistaxis, hematemesis, hemoptysis, blood in stool, or other hemorrhagic symptom. This broad definition may be useful in the early period following a confirmed bioterrorist-related case of VHF as well. Public health authorities may develop more specific case definitions after the etiologic agent is identified.

Public health authorities, in consultation with the CDC, should provide assistance and detailed instructions to clinical laboratories and to clinicians for processing and transport of laboratory specimens required for diagnosis of these agents. (See "Packaging Protocols for Biological Agents/Diseases" at http://www.bt.cdc.gov/Agent/VHF/VHF.asp.)

Methods of diagnosis at specialized laboratories include antigen detection by antigen-capture enzyme-linked immunosorbent assay (ELISA), IgM antibody detection by antibody-capture ELISA, RT-PCR, and viral isolation. Antigen detection (by ELISA) and RT-PCR are the most useful diagnostic techniques in the acute clinical setting. Viral isolation is of limited value because it requires a biosafety level 4 (BSL-4) laboratory. (A full description of BSL-4 criteria is available at http://www.cdc.gov/od/ohs/biosfty/bmbl4/bmbl4s3.htm.) There are only 2 BSL-4 facilities in the United States, located at the CDC and the USAMRIID, with in-depth diagnostic capability. Either the presence of IgM or a 4-fold rise in titer of IgG antibody between acute- and convalescent-phase serum samples are diagnostic of these viral illnesses, but antibody-capture ELISA is of limited value in early diagnosis because antibodies to these viruses usually do not appear until onset of recovery, approximately at the second week of illness. The CDC requires approximately 1 working day (with prior notification of arrival) to offer a preliminary laboratory diagnosis following receipt of patient specimens.

©2002 American Medical Association. All rights reserved.

Reprinted with permission from *JAMA*; May 8, 2002, Vol 287, No. 18

The diagnosis of VHF should be based initially on clinical criteria and judgment, with laboratory testing used to confirm or exclude this clinical diagnosis. Laboratory testing will require time and, in the event of a large attack, may be delayed or perhaps not possible given current laboratory capacities.

TREATMENT

The mainstay of treatment of VHF is supportive, with careful maintenance of fluid and electrolyte balance, circulatory volume, and blood pressure. Because in some cases intravenous fluids have not reversed hypotension and may have contributed to pulmonary edema,[104] consideration should be given to early vasopressor support with hemodynamic monitoring. Mechanical ventilation, renal dialysis, and antiseizure therapy may be required. Intramuscular injections, aspirin, nonsteroidal anti-inflammatory drugs, and anticoagulant therapies are contraindicated. Steroids are not indicated.[9]

Drug Therapy

There are no antiviral drugs approved by the US Food and Drug Administration (FDA) for treatment of HFVs. Ribavirin, a nucleoside analog, has some in vitro and in vivo activity against Arenaviridae and Bunyaviridae (including CCHF) but no utility against Filoviridae or Flaviviridae. Oral ribavirin, in combination with interferon alfa, is FDA-approved for treatment of chronic hepatitis C virus infection. Intravenous ribavirin is of limited availability in the United States. It is produced by ICN Pharmaceuticals Inc (Costa Mesa, Calif) for compassionate use under an investigational new drug (IND) application. Although a risk of human teratogenicity has not been demonstrated for ribavirin, its pharmacologic action and its teratogenicity and embryolethality in several animal species raise concern that such a risk may exist with maternal therapy during pregnancy. Therefore, ribavirin is classified as a pregnancy category X drug, and is contraindicated in pregnancy.[105] The primary adverse effect caused by riba-

Table 4. Recommendations for Ribavirin Therapy in Patients With Clinically Evident Viral Hemorrhagic Fever of Unknown Etiology or Secondary to Arenaviruses or Bunyaviruses*

	Contained Casualty Setting	Mass Casualty Setting†
Adults	Loading dose of 30 mg/kg intravenously (IV) (maximum, 2 g) once, followed by 16 mg/kg IV (maximum, 1 g per dose) every 6 hours for 4 days, followed by 8 mg/kg IV (maximum, 500 mg per dose) every 8 hours for 6 days	Loading dose of 2000 mg orally once, followed by 1200 mg/d orally in 2 divided doses (if weight >75 kg), or 1000 mg/d orally in 2 doses (400 mg in AM and 600 mg in PM) (if weight ≤75 kg) for 10 days‡
Pregnant women§	Same as for adults	Same as for adults
Children	Same as for adults, dosed according to weight	Loading dose of 30 mg/kg orally once, followed by 15 mg/kg per day orally in 2 divided doses for 10 days

*Recommendations are not approved by the US Food and Drug Administration for any of these indications and should always be administered under an investigational new drug protocol. However, in a mass casualty setting, these requirements may need to be modified to permit timely administration of the drug.
†The threshold number of cases at which parenteral therapy becomes impossible depends on a variety of factors, including local health care resources.
‡Although a similar dosage (1000 mg/d in 3 divided doses) has been used in a small number of patients with Lassa fever,[106] this regimen would be impractical because the current formulation of oral ribavirin in the United States consists of 200-mg capsules, and ribavirin capsules may not be broken open.
§Refer to the section in text on treatment of pregnant women for details.

virin is a dose-related, reversible, hemolytic anemia. However, a range of cardiac and pulmonary events associated with anemia occurred in approximately 10% of patients treated with combination ribavirin-interferon therapy for hepatitis C.[105]

Small trials have shown that ribavirin may reduce mortality after infection with Lassa fever[106] and select New World arenaviruses.[57,107] Ribavirin does not penetrate the brain well; therefore, it is not expected to be particularly effective against the neurological effects of these pathogens.[57,108] Intravenous ribavirin given within the first 6 days of fever to patients with Lassa fever who had high levels of viremia decreased mortality from 76% to 9%.[107] A controlled trial of 18 patients with Argentine hemorrhagic fever resulted in 12.5% mortality in treated patients compared with 40% in untreated patients.[108]

Recommendations for drug therapy by the working group are not approved by the FDA for any of these indications and should always be administered under an IND protocol. In a mass casualty situation, these requirements may need to be modified to permit timely administration of the drug. In addition, treatment of other suspected possible causes, such as bacterial sepsis, should not be withheld while awaiting confirmation or exclusion of the diagnosis of VHF.

In a contained casualty situation (in which a modest number of patients require therapy), the working group recommends that an intravenous regimen of ribavirin be given as described in TABLE 4, in accordance with CDC's recommendations for treating patients with suspected VHF of unknown cause, pending identification of the agent.[109] A similar dose has been used in the treatment of Lassa fever.[106]

In a mass casualty situation (in which the number of persons requiring therapy is sufficiently high that delivery of intravenous therapy is no longer possible), an oral regimen of ribavirin as described in Table 4 is recommended. This dose is currently licensed for treatment of chronic hepatitis C infection in the United States.[105] Although it is substantially lower than that in the intravenous regimen, a similar dose has been used to treat a few patients with Lassa fever,[106] and there are no available studies on tolerability or efficacy of higher doses of oral ribavirin.

Ribavirin is contraindicated in pregnancy. However, in the context of infection with VHF of unknown cause or secondary to an arenavirus or Rift Valley fever, the working group believes that the benefits appear likely to outweigh

©2002 American Medical Association. All rights reserved.

Reprinted with permission from *JAMA*; May 8, 2002, Vol 287, No. 18

any fetal risk of ribavirin therapy, and ribavirin is therefore recommended. The associated mortality of VHF tends to be higher in pregnancy.[110]

The use of oral or intravenous ribavirin is not approved by the FDA for children, and proper doses have not been established. Only aerosolized ribavirin has been approved by the FDA for children, to treat respiratory syncytial virus infection. However, in the context of infection with VHF of unknown cause or secondary to an arenavirus or Rift Valley fever, the working group believes that the benefits likely outweigh the risks of ribavirin therapy, and it is therefore recommended as described in Table 4. Similar doses have been used to treat children with adenovirus pneumonia[111] and hepatitis C[112] and were well tolerated. Ribavirin capsules may not be broken open and are only available in 200-mg doses. However, Schering-Plough Corp (Kenilworth, NJ) produces a pediatric syrup formulation (which is not commercially available) for use under an IND application.

For infections caused by filoviruses or flaviviruses, the working group recommends supportive medical care only. Ribavirin has been shown to have no clinical utility against these groups of viruses.

Passive Immunization

Studies and case reports evaluating convalescent plasma as therapy (or prophylaxis) of the diseases caused by HFVs have yielded mixed results depending on the disease, with some reports suggesting clinical utility[26,80,82,101,113-117] and other studies showing no benefit.[52,106,118] Passive immunization has also been associated with enhanced viral replication in experimentally infected animals.[119] The logistics of collection, testing, and storing immune convalescent plasma are formidable. In the United States, the paucity of survivors of these diseases and the lack of a national program that collects and stores HFV immune plasma preclude its use in the initial response to a bioterrorist attack. Development of methods to manufacture monoclonal antibodies and recent advances in selecting highly effective human-derived or humanized products may provide new approaches to therapy in the future.

POSTEXPOSURE PROPHYLAXIS

Effective prophylaxis following exposure to an HFV is hampered by the absence of effective vaccines and antiviral medications. The working group does not recommend preemptive administration of ribavirin in the absence of signs of infection to persons with known or suspected exposures to the HFVs. Ribavirin has no utility against filoviruses or flaviviruses. For arenaviruses, there is limited experimental evidence that postexposure prophylaxis with ribavirin will delay onset of disease but not prevent it.[120,121] Furthermore, the effectiveness of ribavirin as postexposure prophylaxis for arenaviruses or Rift Valley fever virus has never been studied in humans. While 1995 CDC guidelines recommend ribavirin to high-risk contacts of patients with Lassa fever,[109] a review and possible revision of these recommendations is to be shortly undertaken (James Hughes, MD, oral communication, January 10, 2002). However, public health professionals suggest that stratification of risk groups into high-risk and close contacts may facilitate counseling and outbreak investigation. High-risk contacts are those who have had mucous membrane contact with a patient (such as during kissing or sexual intercourse) or have had a percutaneous injury involving contact with the patient's secretions, excretions, or blood. Close contacts are those who live with, shake hands with, hug, process laboratory specimens from, or care for a patient with clinical evidence of VHF prior to initiation of appropriate precautions.

Persons considered potentially exposed to HFVs in a bioterrorist attack and all known high-risk and close contacts of patients diagnosed with VHF should be placed under medical surveillance. All such individuals should be instructed to record their temperatures twice daily and report any temperature of 101°F (38.3°C) or higher (or any symptom noted in Table 3) to a clinician, hospital epidemiologist, or public health authority designated with surveillance. Surveillance should be continued for 21 days after the person's deemed potential exposure or last contact with the ill patient.

If a temperature of 101°F (38.3°C) or higher develops, ribavirin therapy should be initiated promptly as presumptive treatment of VHF, as described in Table 4, unless an alternative diagnosis is established or the etiologic agent is known to be a filovirus or a flavivirus. In the case of close and high-risk contacts of patients diagnosed with Rift Valley fever or a flavivirus, only those who process laboratory specimens from a patient prior to initiation of appropriate precautions require medical surveillance, as these specific viruses are not transmitted from person to person but may be transmitted in the laboratory setting.

VACCINE

With the exception of yellow fever live attenuated 17D vaccine, which is highly effective when administered to travelers to endemic areas,[68] there is no licensed vaccine for any of the HFVs. The yellow fever vaccine is produced in limited supply, and world stocks are not sufficient to meet a surge.[122] This vaccine would not be useful in preventing disease if given in the postexposure setting because yellow fever has a short incubation period of 3 to 6 days, and neutralizing antibodies take longer to appear following vaccination.[68]

INFECTION CONTROL

Given the lack of licensed or effective therapies and vaccines against the HFVs, efforts to prevent transmission of infection must rely on the meticulous implementation of and compliance with strict infection control measures. Filoviruses and arenaviruses are highly infectious after direct contact with infected blood and bodily secretions. A suspected case of VHF must be immediately reported to the hospital epidemiologist (or infection control professional) and to the local or state health department. The epi-

©2002 American Medical Association. All rights reserved.

Reprinted with permission from *JAMA*; May 8, 2002, Vol 287, No. 18

demiologist (or infection control professional) should, in turn, notify the clinical laboratory (so that additional precautions are put in place) as well as other clinicians and public health authorities.

Isolation Precautions

Direct contact with infected blood and bodily fluids has accounted for the majority of person-to-person transmission of filoviruses and arenaviruses. Therefore, we recommend that in the case of any patient with suspected or documented VHF, VHF-specific barrier precautions should be implemented immediately (Box 2). These precautions do not reflect HICPAC's isolation guidelines terminology and are defined here as strict hand hygiene plus use of double gloves, impermeable gowns, face shields, eye protection, and leg and shoe coverings (given the copious amounts of infected material, such as vomitus and liquid stool, that may be present in the environment).

Airborne transmission of HFVs appears to be a rare event but cannot be conclusively excluded. Given the inability to completely exclude this potential, the lack of preventive vaccines, and, in the case of filoviruses, the lack of effective drug therapy, we recommend that in addition to VHF-specific barrier precautions, airborne precautions also be instituted. Airborne precautions entail the use of a high-efficiency particulate respirator for any person entering the room and, as required by HICPAC standards,[123] the patient should be placed in a room with negative air pressure, 6 to 12 air changes per hour, air exhausted directly to the outdoors or passage through a high-efficiency particulate air (HEPA) filter before recirculation, and doors kept closed. There are many circumstances in which the use of negative-pressure rooms may not be possible, including mass casualty situations. In such conditions, all other infection control measures should be taken (ie, VHF-specific barrier precautions and a HEPA respirator for any person entering the room), which would, in combination, substantially reduce the risk of nosoco-

---

Box 2. Recommendations for Protective Measures Against Nosocomial Transmission of Hemorrhagic Fever Viruses

Strict adherence to hand hygiene:
> Health care workers should clean their hands prior to donning personal protective equipment for patient contact. After patient contact, health care workers should remove gown, leg and shoe coverings, and gloves and immediately clean their hands. Hands should be clean prior to the removal of facial protective equipment (ie, personal respirators, face shields, and goggles) to minimize exposure of mucous membranes with potentially contaminated hands, and once again after the removal of all personal protective equipment

Double gloves

Impermeable gowns

N-95 masks or powered air-purifying respirators, and a negative isolation room with 6-12 air changes per hour, as required by Healthcare Infection Control Practices Advisory Committee standards for airborne precautions*

Leg and shoe coverings

Face shields†

Goggles for eye protection†

Restricted access of nonessential staff and visitors to patient's room

Dedicated medical equipment, such as stethoscopes, glucose monitors, and, if available, point-of-care analyzers

Environmental disinfection with an Environmental Protection Agency–registered hospital disinfectant or a 1:100 dilution of household bleach

If there are multiple patients with viral hemorrhagic fever in one health care facility, they should be cared for in the same part of the hospital to minimize exposures to other patients and health care workers

*These resources may not be possible in many health care facilities or in a mass casualty situation. In this case, all other measures should be taken and would, in combination, be expected to substantially diminish the risk of nosocomial spread.

†Face shields and eye protection may be already incorporated in certain personal protective equipment, such as powered air-purifying respirators.

---

mial transmission. Available evidence suggests that in the great preponderance of historical cases, these measures were sufficient to prevent transmission of disease to health care workers, family members, and other patients. Nonessential staff and visitors should have restricted access to patients' rooms. If there are multiple patients with VHF in a health care facility, they should be cared for in the same part of the hospital to minimize exposure to other persons.

All persons, including health care workers and laboratory personnel who have had a close or high-risk contact with a patient infected with a filovirus or an arenavirus within 21 days of the patient's onset of symptoms, prior to the institution of appropriate infection control precautions, should be placed under medical surveillance and managed as described in the section on postex-

posure prophylaxis. Laboratory personnel who have processed laboratory specimens from a patient with any HFVs (including Rift Valley fever and the flaviviruses) within 21 days of the patient's onset of symptoms, prior to the institution of appropriate infection control precautions, should also be placed under medical surveillance.

Because some of these viruses may remain present in bodily fluids for long periods following clinical recovery, convalescent patients continue to pose a risk of disease transmission.[40,60] Therefore, patients convalescing from a filoviral or an arenaviral infection should refrain from sexual activity for 3 months after clinical recovery.

Personal Protective Equipment

Powered air-purifying respirators (PAPRs) are theoretically more effica-

©2002 American Medical Association. All rights reserved.

Reprinted with permission from *JAMA*; May 8, 2002, Vol 287, No. 18

cious than N-95 disposable masks in providing respiratory protection from small-particle aerosols, mostly due to issues related to proper fitting of the masks.[124] However, no data exist to support higher efficacy of PAPRs over N-95 masks in preventing airborne transmission of infection in the health care setting.[125] PAPRs are more expensive ($300-$600 vs less than $1 for disposable N-95 masks), are bulky, require maintenance, and impair voice communication to a higher degree than disposable N-95 masks.[126] One study has shown that PAPRs are associated with a higher incidence of needlestick injuries.[127] Disadvantages of the N-95 masks include the difficulty in ensuring a reliable face-mask seal with each use and impossibility of effective use by bearded individuals. The theoretical advantage of PAPRs over N-95 masks may be offset by the danger of increased needlestick or sharp injuries to those using PAPRs in these settings. The N-95 masks (in combination with face shields and goggles) are likely equivalent in protection to PAPRs in the health care setting.

Therefore, we recommend that clinicians caring for patients with a VHF use either N-95 masks or PAPRs, depending on their familiarity with one or the other, the suitability for the individual, and availability at a given institution. Some experts have advocated that PAPRs be used during cough-inducing procedures (ie, endotracheal intubations, bronchoscopies), autopsies, and centrifugation or pipetting of laboratory specimens. While there are no data to support this recommendation, we would concur as long as the health care workers are familiar with the use of PAPRs and are not subjecting themselves to the risk of inadvertent needlestick injury.

Laboratory Testing

The HFVs described herein (including Rift Valley fever and the flaviviruses) are highly infectious in the laboratory setting and may be transmitted to laboratory personnel via small-particle aerosols. The risk is especially high during aerosol-generating procedures, such as centrifugation. To minimize the possibility of small-particle aerosol generation, all laboratory staff must be alerted to any suspected diagnosis of VHF. Designated laboratory workers should receive training in handling specimens from any suspected VHF patients in advance of such an event. Laboratory workers should wear personal protective equipment that ensures VHF-specific barrier and airborne precautions (Box 2). All specimens should be handled, at a minimum, in a class 2 biological safety cabinet following BSL-3 practices.[127] (A detailed description of class 2 biological safety cabinets is available at http://www.cdc.gov/od/ohs/biosfty/bmbl4/b4aa.htm, and a detailed description of BSL-3 practices is available at http://www.cdc.gov/od/ohs/biosfty/bmbl4/bmbl4s3.htm.) Most clinical facilities are not equipped with a BSL-3 laboratory. Virus isolation should only be attempted in a BSL-4 laboratory.

Potential hazards associated with handling of clinical specimens from patients infected with an HFV pose great problems in hospital facilities. Laboratory tests should be limited to critical diagnostic tests. If adequate resources are available, point-of-care analyzers for routine laboratory analysis of infected patients should be used. Point-of-care analyzers are small, portable devices that may be used at the bedside, require only a few drops of fresh whole blood, display test results in a few minutes, limit the exposure of laboratory personnel to infectious clinical specimens, do not disrupt the clinical laboratory routine, and do not contaminate clinical laboratory equipment.

If point-of-care analyzers are not available, clinical specimens need to be processed in a clinical laboratory. Precautions that parallel those of a US hospital's successful efforts to care for a patient infected with a New World arenavirus should be followed.[128] Laboratory specimens should be clearly identified, double bagged, and hand carried to the laboratory at prescheduled times, preferably prior to equipment maintenance to enable decontamination of instruments af-ter testing. Specimens should never be transported in pneumatic tube systems. Only dedicated, trained laboratory personnel should process clinical specimens from patients with VHF, wearing protective equipment to ensure airborne and VHF-specific barrier precautions. Serum should be pretreated with the detergent Triton X-100 (10 µL of 10% Triton X-100 per 1 mL of serum for 1 hour). Pretreatment with Triton X-100 may reduce the titers of these enveloped viruses, but efficacy has not been tested.[109] Pretreatment with Triton X-100 does not significantly alter serum electrolytes, urea nitrogen, creatinine, and glucose or liver function test results.[128] Additional guidelines for clinical specimen transport, processing, and disposal have been described by Armstrong et al.[128]

Postmortem Practices

In the event of an outbreak of VHF, special provisions will be required for burial practices. Contact with cadavers has been implicated as a source of transmission in the Kikwit Ebola outbreak of 1995[36] and in Uganda in 2000.[37] We recommend that trained personnel, using the same infection control precautions as those used to transport ill patients, handle the bodies of patients who die of VHF. Autopsies should be performed only by specially trained persons using VHF-specific barrier precautions and HEPA-filtered respirators (N-95 masks or PAPRs) and negative-pressure rooms, as would be customary in cases in which contagious biological aerosols, such as *Mycobacterium tuberculosis*, are deemed a possible risk.[129] We recommend prompt burial or cremation of the deceased, with minimal handling. Specifically, no embalming should be done. Surgery or postmortem examinations are associated with increased risks of transmission and should be done only when absolutely indicated and after consultation with experts.

Environmental Decontamination

Linen handlers and workers involved in environmental decontamination should wear personal protective equipment that

©2002 American Medical Association. All rights reserved.

Reprinted with permission from *JAMA*; May 8, 2002, Vol 287, No. 18

ensures VHF-specific barrier precautions (Box 2). We recommend that contaminated linens be placed in double bags and washed without sorting in a normal hot water cycle with bleach. Alternatively, they may be autoclaved or incinerated.[109] Detailed instructions on handling and disinfection of contaminated linens are available from the CDC.[109] Environmental surfaces in patients' rooms and contaminated medical equipment should be disinfected with an Environmental Protection Agency–registered hospital disinfectant or a 1:100 dilution of household bleach.[109]

It has been suggested that excreta should be disinfected with 0.6% sodium hypochlorite before disposal.[130] Although a theoretical concern remains that the disposal of contaminated human excreta may contaminate sewage systems, the working group does not recommend the addition of disinfectants to human excreta prior to disposal. Disinfectants are not effective in sterilizing solid waste, the indiscriminate addition of hypochlorite may damage septic tanks, and these viruses are not likely to survive standard sewage treatment in the United States.

In general, in their natural state, these lipid-enveloped viruses are not environmentally stable and are not expected to persist in the environment for prolonged periods.[7] Decisions regarding the need for and methods of decontamination following an attack with an HFV should be made following expert analysis of the contaminated environment and the weapons used in the attack, in consultation with experts in environmental remediation.

ONGOING RESEARCH AND PROPOSED AGENDA

Mechanisms of disease transmission in human outbreaks of HFVs are still poorly understood. Clarification of the role of airborne transmission is vital. Rapid diagnostic methods need to be developed for all of the HFVs, including those that have been excluded from this article and made available to selected state health departments for the expedient diagnosis of suspected cases. Meth-

ods to safely handle potentially infected specimens in a clinical laboratory should be developed.

The diagnostic and therapeutic armamentarium urgently needs to be augmented. There also is an urgent need to develop vaccines and drug therapy. A live attenuated vaccine against Argentine hemorrhagic fever (candid No. 1) developed at the USAMRIID[131] is available as an IND. This vaccine has been shown to be safe and effective in protecting agricultural workers in South America[132] and may provide cross-protection against Bolivian hemorrhagic fever.[9] There are 2 vaccines against Rift Valley fever also available as INDs. One is formalin inactivated and appears to be safe and effective when administered to laboratory workers. However, it is available only in limited supply, and the manufacturing capacity for producing additional vaccine no longer exists in the United States.[133,134] Lastly, a formalin-inactivated Kyasanur Forest disease vaccine exists and has been shown to be protective in field trials in India.[135] There are several promising vaccines in development for prevention of filoviruses and Lassa fever, some in nonhuman primate models.[136-139] Passive immunization strategies using recombinant human monoclonal antibodies should be pursued, given the potential benefit of passive immunization in a series of reports.[80,114,116,117,140] Research with these agents is hampered by the requirement of conducting experiments in BSL-4 laboratories. More BSL-4 laboratories would expand research opportunities.

Ribavirin is the only potentially effective drug available for selected hemorrhagic fever because it is approved by the FDA for another indication. However, it is not effective against all of the HFVs and it is not widely available. The supply of ribavirin should be rapidly augmented, and studies to demonstrate its efficacy and safety against selected HFVs should be conducted to support an FDA approval for those indications. We also recommend the addition of intravenous and oral formulations of ribavirin to the US National Pharmaceutical Stockpile (a reposi-

tory of antibiotics, chemical antidotes, and other medical supplies managed by the CDC that may be emergently sent to the site of a disaster anywhere in the United States). New antiviral therapies should be pursued for the treatment of all HFVs, including those excluded from this article. The effects of any developed therapy in pediatric populations should also be evaluated.

Disclaimer: The views, opinions, assertions, and findings contained herein are those of the authors and should not be construed as official US Department of Health and Human Services, US Department of Defense, or US Department of Army positions, policies, or decisions unless so designated by other documentation. The recommendations on the use of drugs for uses not approved by the FDA do not represent the official views of the FDA or of any of the federal agencies whose scientists participated in these discussions. Unlabeled uses of the products recommended are noted in the sections of this article in which these products are discussed. Where unlabeled uses are indicated, information used as the basis for the recommendation is discussed.

Additional Articles: This article is the sixth in a series entitled *Medical and Public Health Management Following the Use of a Biological Weapon: Consensus Statements of the Working Group on Civilian Biodefense.* See references 1 through 5.

Acknowledgment: We thank those who generously provided invaluable assistance in the preparation of this article: Julie Gerberding, MD, MPH, Jim LeDuc, PhD, Steve Ostroff, MD, Duane Gubler, ScD, Denise Cardo, MD, and Lynn Steele, MS, CDC; Anthony Suffredini, MD, National Institutes of Health; Elin Gursky, ScD, and Paul Pham, PharmD, Johns Hopkins University; and Lauren Iacono-Connors, PhD, Karen Midthun, MD, Joanne Holmes, MBA, Jerry Weir, PhD, Kathleen Uhl, MD, Diane Kennedy, RPh, MPH, Dianne Murphy, MD, Harry Haverkos, MD, Brad Leissa, MD, Sandra Folkendt, Lewis Markoff, MD, and Karen Oliver, MSN, FDA.

REFERENCES

1. Inglesby TV, Henderson DA, Bartlett JG, et al, for the Working Group on Civilian Biodefense. Anthrax as a biological weapon. *JAMA.* 1999;281:1735-1745.
2. Henderson DA, Inglesby TV, Bartlett JG, et al, for the Working Group on Civilian Biodefense. Smallpox as a biological weapon. *JAMA.* 1999;281:2127-2137.
3. Inglesby TV, Dennis DT, Henderson DA, et al, for the Working Group on Civilian Biodefense. Plague as a biological weapon. *JAMA.* 2000;283:2281-2290.
4. Arnon SS, Schechter R, Inglesby TV, et al, for the Working Group on Civilian Biodefense. Botulinum toxin as a biological weapon. *JAMA.* 2001;285:1059-1070.
5. Dennis DT, Inglesby TV, Henderson DA, et al, for the Working Group on Civilian Biodefense. Tularemia as a biological weapon. *JAMA.* 2001;285:2763-2773.
6. Fatal illnesses associated with a new world arenavirus—California, 1999-2000. *MMWR Morb Mortal Wkly Rep.* 2000;49:709-711.
7. Peters CJ, Jahrling PB, Khan AS. Patients infected with high-hazard viruses. *Arch Virol Suppl.* 1996;11: 141-168.
8. Solomon T, Mallewa M. Dengue and other emerging flaviviruses. *J Infect.* 2001;42:104-115.
9. Jahrling P. Viral hemorrhagic fevers. In: *Textbook of Military Medicine.* Vol 1. Falls Church, Va: Office of the Surgeon General; 1989.
10. Mandell GL, Douglas RG, Bennett JE, Dolin R. *Mandell, Douglas, and Bennett's Principles and Practice of Infectious Diseases.* 5th ed. Philadelphia, Pa: Churchill Livingstone; 2000.

©2002 American Medical Association. All rights reserved.

11. Swanepoel R, Shepherd AJ, Leman PA, et al. Epidemiologic and clinical features of Crimean-Congo hemorrhagic fever in southern Africa. *Am J Trop Med Hyg.* 1987;3:120-132.

12. Peters CJ, Simpson GL, Levy H. Spectrum of hantavirus infection: hemorrhagic fever with renal syndrome and hantavirus pulmonary syndrome. *Annu Rev Med.* 1999;50:531-545.

13. Alibek K, Handelman S. *Biohazard: The Chilling True Story of the Largest Covert Biological Weapons Program in the World, Told From the Inside by the Man Who Ran It.* New York, NY: Random House; 1999.

14. Center for Nonproliferation Studies. Chemical and biological weapons: possession and programs past and present. November 2000. Available at: http://cns.miis.edu/research/cbw/possess.htm. Accessed January 10, 2002.

15. Miller J, Engelberg S, Broad WJ. *Germs: Biological Weapons and America's Secret War.* Waterville, Me: GK Hall; 2002.

16. Bazhutin NB, Belanov EF, Spiridonov VA, et al. The effect of the methods for producing an experimental Marburg virus infection on the characteristics of the course of the disease in green monkeys [in Russian]. *Vopr Virusol.* 1992;37:153-156.

17. *Global Proliferation of Weapons of Mass Destruction: Hearings Before the Permanent Subcommittee on Investigations of the Committee on Governmental Affairs, United States Senate,* 104th Cong, 1st-2nd Sess (1996).

18. Johnson E, Jaax N, White J, Jahrling P. Lethal experimental infections of rhesus monkeys by aerosolized Ebola virus. *Int J Exp Pathol.* 1995;76:227-236.

19. Lub M, Sergeev AN, P'Iankov OV, P'Iankova OG, Petrishchenko VA, Kotliarov LA. Certain pathogenetic characteristics of a disease in monkeys in infected with the Marburg virus by an airborne route [in Russian]. *Vopr Virusol.* 1995;40:158-161.

20. Stephenson EH, Larson EW, Dominik JW. Effect of environmental factors on aerosol-induced Lassa virus infection. *J Med Virol.* 1984;14:295-303.

21. Kenyon RH, McKee KT Jr, Zack PM, et al. Aerosol infection of rhesus macaques with Junin virus. *Intervirology.* 1992;33:23-31.

22. Centers for Disease Control and Prevention. Category A agents. Available at: http://www.bt.cdc.gov/Agent/Agentlist.asp. Accessed January 10, 2002.

23. LeDuc JW. Epidemiology of hemorrhagic fever viruses. *Rev Infect Dis.* 1989;11(suppl 4):S730-S735.

24. Schou S, Hansen AK. Marburg and Ebola virus infections in laboratory nonhuman primates: a literature review. *Comp Med.* 2000;50:108-123.

25. Ebola haemorrhagic fever in Zaire, 1976. *Bull World Health Organ.* 1978;56:271-293.

26. Emond RT, Evans B, Bowen ET, Lloyd G. A case of Ebola virus infection. *BMJ.* 1977;2:541-544.

27. Simpson DI. Marburg agent disease. *Trans R Soc Trop Med Hyg.* 1969;63:303-309. Cited by: Schou S, Hansen AK. Marburg and Ebola virus infections in laboratory nonhuman primates. *Comp Med.* 2000;50:2108-2123.

28. Jaax NK, Davis KJ, Geisbert TJ, et al. Lethal experimental infection of rhesus monkeys with Ebola-Zaire (Mayinga) virus by the oral and conjunctival route of exposure. *Arch Pathol Lab Med.* 1996;120:140-155.

29. Colebunders R, Borchert M. Ebola haemorrhagic fever—a review. *J Infect.* 2000;40:16-20.

30. Zaki SR, Shieh WJ, Greer PW, et al. A novel immunohistochemical assay for the detection of Ebola virus in skin. *J Infect Dis.* 1999;179(suppl 1):S36-S47.

31. Dowell SF, Mukunu R, Ksiazek TG, Khan AS, Rollin PE, Peters CJ. Transmission of Ebola hemorrhagic fever: a study of risk factors in family members, Kikwit, Democratic Republic of the Congo, 1995. *J Infect Dis.* 1999;179(suppl 1):S87-S91.

32. Khan AS, Tshioko FK, Heymann DL, et al. The reemergence of Ebola hemorrhagic fever, Democratic Republic of the Congo, 1995. *J Infect Dis.* 1999;179(suppl 1):S76-S86.

33. Muyembe-Tamfum JJ, Kipasa M, Kiyungu C, Colebunders R. Ebola outbreak in Kikwit, Democratic Republic of the Congo: discovery and control measures. *J Infect Dis.* 1999;179(suppl 1):S259-S262.

34. Butler JC, Kilmarx PH, Jernigan DB, Ostroff SM. Perspectives in fatal epidemics. *Infect Dis Clin North Am.* 1996;10:917-937.

35. Shu HL, Siegert R, Slenczka W. The pathogenesis and epidemiology of the "Marburg-virus" infection. *Ger Med Mon.* 1969;14:7-10.Cited by: Schou S, Hansen AK. Marburg and Ebola virus infections in laboratory nonhuman primates. *Comp Med.* 2000;50:2108-2123.

36. Roels TH, Bloom AS, Buffington J, et al. Ebola hemorrhagic fever, Kikwit, Democratic Republic of the Congo, 1995: risk factors for patients without a reported exposure. *J Infect Dis.* 1999;179(suppl 1):S92-S97.

37. Outbreak of Ebola hemorrhagic fever, Uganda, August 2000–January 2001. *MMWR Morb Mortal Wkly Rep.* 2001;50:73-77.

38. Jaax N, Jahrling P, Geisbert T, et al. Transmission of Ebola virus (Zaire strain) to uninfected control monkeys in a biocontainment laboratory. *Lancet.* 1995;346:1669-1671.

39. Dalgard DW, Hardy RJ, Pearson SL, et al. Combined simian hemorrhagic fever and Ebola virus infection in cynomolgus monkeys. *Lab Anim Sci.* 1992;42:152-157.

40. Slenczka WG. The Marburg virus outbreak of 1967 and subsequent episodes. *Curr Top Microbiol Immunol.* 1999;235:49-75.

41. Gear JS, Cassel GA, Gear AJ, et al. Outbreak of Marburg virus disease in Johannesburg. *BMJ.* 1975;4:489-493.

42. Baron RC, McCormick JB, Zubeir OA. Ebola virus disease in southern Sudan. *Bull World Health Organ.* 1983;61:997-1003.

43. Formenty P, Hatz C, Le Guenno B, Stoll A, Rogenmoser P, Widmer A. Human infection due to Ebola virus, subtype Cote d'Ivoire. *J Infect Dis.* 1999;179(suppl 1):S48-S53.

44. Richards GA, Murphy S, Jobson R, et al. Unexpected Ebola virus in a tertiary setting. *Crit Care Med.* 2000;28:240-244.

45. Guimard Y, Bwaka MA, Colebunders R, et al. Organization of patient care during the Ebola hemorrhagic fever epidemic in Kikwit, Democratic Republic of the Congo, 1995. *J Infect Dis.* 1999;179(suppl 1):S268-S273.

46. Centers for Disease Control and Prevention and World Health Organization. Infection control for viral hemorrhagic fevers in the African health care setting. Atlanta, Ga: Centers for Disease Control and Prevention. Available at: http://www.cdc.gov/ncidod/dvrd/spb/mnpages/vhfmanual.htm. Accessed January 10, 2002.

47. Rowe AK, Bertolli J, Khan AS, et al. Clinical, virologic, and immunologic follow-up of convalescent Ebola hemorrhagic fever patients and their household contacts, Kikwit, Democratic Republic of the Congo. *J Infect Dis.* 1999;179(suppl 1):S28-S35.

48. Rodriguez LL, De Roo A, Guimard Y, et al. Persistence and genetic stability of Ebola virus during the outbreak in Kikwit, Democratic Republic of the Congo, 1995. *J Infect Dis.* 1999;179(suppl 1):S170-S176.

49. Johnson KM, Mackenzie RB, Webb PA, Kuns ML. Chronic infection of rodents by Machupo virus. *Science.* 1965;150:1618-1619.

50. Johnson KM, Kuns ML, Mackenzie RB, Webb PA, Yunker CE. Isolation of Machupo virus from wild rodent *Calomys callosus. Am J Trop Med Hyg.* 1966;15:103-106.

51. Carey DE, Kemp GE, White HA, et al. Lassa fever: epidemiological aspects of the 1970 epidemic, Jos, Nigeria. *Trans R Soc Trop Med Hyg.* 1972;66:402-408.

52. White HA. Lassa fever: a study of 23 hospital cases. *Trans R Soc Trop Med Hyg.* 1972;66:390-401.

53. Monath TP, Mertens PE, Patton R, et al. A hospital epidemic of Lassa fever in Zorzor, Liberia, March-April 1972. *Am J Trop Med Hyg.* 1973;22:773-779.

54. Peters CJ, Kuehne RW, Mercado RR, Le Bow RH, Spertzel RO, Webb PA. Hemorrhagic fever in Cochabamba, Bolivia, 1971. *Am J Epidemiol.* 1974;99:425-433.

55. Zweighaft RM, Fraser DW, Hattwick MA, et al. Lassa fever: response to an imported case. *N Engl J Med.* 1977;297:803-807.

56. Cooper CB, Gransden WR, Webster M, et al. A case of Lassa fever: experience at St Thomas's Hospital. *BMJ.* 1982;285:1003-1005.

57. Kilgore PE, Ksiazek TG, Rollin PE, et al. Treatment of Bolivian hemorrhagic fever with intravenous ribavirin. *Clin Infect Dis.* 1997;24:718-722.

58. World Health Organization. Fact sheet 179: Lassa fever. April 2000. Available at: http://www.who.int/inf-fs/en/fact179.html. Accessed January 10, 2002.

59. Buckley SM, Casals J. Lassa fever, a new virus disease of man from West Africa, III: isolation and characterization of the virus. *Am J Trop Med Hyg.* 1970;19:680-691.

60. Briggiler AM, Enria DA, Feuillade MR, Maiztegui JI. Contagio interhumano e infeccion clinical con virus Junin en matrimonios residentes en el area endemica de fiebre hemorragica Argentina. *Medicina (B Aires).* 1987;47:565.

61. Swanepoel R, Coetzer JA. Rift Valley fever. In: *Infectious Diseases of Livestock With Special Reference to Southern Africa.* Vol 1. New York, NY: Oxford University Press; 1994.

62. Jouan A, Coulibaly I, Adam F, et al. Analytical study of a Rift Valley fever epidemic. *Res Virol.* 1989;140:175-186.

63. Smithburn KC, Mahaffy AF, Haddow AJ, Kitchen SF, Smith JF. Rift Valley fever: accidental infections among laboratory workers. *J Immunol.* 1949;62:213-227.

64. Meegan JM. The Rift Valley fever epizootic in Egypt 1977-78, I: description of the epizootic and virological studies. *Trans R Soc Trop Med Hyg.* 1979;73:618-623.

65. Shawky S. Rift valley fever. *Saudi Med J.* 2000;21:1109-1115.

66. Turell MJ, Kay BH. Susceptibility of selected strains of Australian mosquitoes (Diptera: Culicidae) to Rift Valley fever virus. *J Med Entomol.* 1998;35:132-135.

67. Gargan TP II, Clark GG, Dohm DJ, Turell MJ, Bailey CL. Vector potential of selected North American mosquito species for Rift Valley fever virus. *Am J Trop Med Hyg.* 1988;38:440-446.

68. Monath TP. Yellow fever: an update. *Lancet Infect Dis.* 2001;1:11-20.

69. Cunha BA. *Tickborne Infectious Diseases: Diagnosis and Management.* New York, NY: Marcel Dekker; 2000.

70. Banerjee K, Gupta NP, Goverdhan MK. Viral infections in laboratory personnel. *Indian J Med Res.* 1979;69:363-373.

71. International Committee on Taxonomy of Viruses. *Seventh Report of the International Committee on Taxonomy of Viruses.* San Diego, Calif: Academic Press; 2000.

72. Chen JP, Cosgriff TM. Hemorrhagic fever virus-induced changes in hemostasis and vascular biology. *Blood Coagul Fibrinolysis.* 2000;11:461-483.

73. Feldmann H, Volchkov VE, Volchkova VA, Klenk HD. The glycoproteins of Marburg and Ebola virus and their potential roles in pathogenesis. *Arch Virol Suppl.* 1999;15:159-169.

74. Ryabchikova EI, Kolesnikova LV, Luchko SV. An analysis of features of pathogenesis in 2 animal models of Ebola virus infection. *J Infect Dis.* 1999;179(suppl 1):S199-S202.

75. Schnittler HJ, Mahner F, Drenckhahn D, Klenk HD, Feldmann H. Replication of Marburg virus in human endothelial cells. *J Clin Invest.* 1993;91:1301-1309.

76. Samoilovich SR, Carballal G, Weissenbacher MC. Protection against a pathogenic strain of Junin virus by mucosal infection with an attenuated strain. *Am J Trop Med Hyg.* 1983;32:825-828.

77. Peters CJ, Liu CT, Anderson GW Jr, Morrill JC, Jahrling PB. Pathogenesis of viral hemorrhagic fevers. *Rev Infect Dis.* 1989;11(suppl 4):S743-S749.

©2002 American Medical Association. All rights reserved.

Reprinted with permission from *JAMA*; May 8, 2002, Vol 287, No. 18

78. Jahrling PB, Hesse RA, Eddy GA, Johnson KM, Callis RT, Stephen EL. Lassa virus infection of rhesus monkeys. *J Infect Dis.* 1980;141:580-589.

79. Cummins D, Molinas FC, Lerer G, Maiztegui JI, Faint R, Machin SJ. A plasma inhibitor of platelet aggregation in patients with Argentine hemorrhagic fever. *Am J Trop Med Hyg.* 1990;42:470-475.

80. Enria DA, Briggiler AM, Fernandez NJ, Levis SC, Maiztegui JI. Importance of dose of neutralising antibodies in treatment of Argentine haemorrhagic fever with immune plasma. *Lancet.* 1984;2:255-256.

81. Cosgriff TM, Morrill JC, Jennings GB, et al. Hemostatic derangement produced by Rift Valley fever virus in rhesus monkeys. *Rev Infect Dis.* 1989;11(suppl 4):S807-S814.

82. Peters CJ, Jones D, Trotter R, et al. Experimental Rift Valley fever in rhesus macaques. *Arch Virol.* 1988;99:31-44.

83. Morrill JC, Jennings GB, Cosgriff TM, Gibbs PH, Peters CJ. Prevention of Rift Valley fever in rhesus monkeys with interferon-alpha. *Rev Infect Dis.* 1989;11(suppl 4):S815-S825.

84. Monath TP, Brinker KR, Chandler FW, Kemp GE, Cropp CB. Pathophysiologic correlations in a rhesus monkey model of yellow fever with special observations on the acute necrosis of B cell areas of lymphoid tissues. *Am J Trop Med Hyg.* 1981;30:431-443.

85. Iyer CG, Laxmana Rao R, Work TH, Narasimha Murthy DP. Pathological findings in 3 fatal human cases of Kyasanur Forest disease. *Indian J Med Sci.* 1959;13:1011-1022. Cited by: Pavri K. Clinical, clinicopathologic, and hematological features of Kyasanur Forest disease. *Rev Infect Dis.* 1989;11(suppl 4):S854-S859.

86. Ebola haemorrhagic fever in Sudan, 1976. *Bull World Health Organ.* 1978;56:247-270.

87. Smith DH, Johnson BK, Isaacson M, et al. Marburgvirus disease in Kenya. *Lancet.* 1982;1:816-820.

88. Monson MH, Frame JD, Jahrling PB, Alexander K. Endemic Lassa fever in Liberia, I: clinical and epidemiological aspects at Curran Lutheran Hospital, Zorzor, Liberia. *Trans R Soc Trop Med Hyg.* 1984;78:549-553.

89. Keane E, Gilles HM. Lassa fever in Panguma Hospital, Sierra Leone, 1973-6. *BMJ.* 1977;1:1399-1402.

90. Mertens PE, Patton R, Baum JJ, Monath TP. Clinical presentation of Lassa fever cases during the hospital epidemic at Zorzor, Liberia, March-April 1972. *Am J Trop Med Hyg.* 1973;22:780-784.

91. McCormick JB, King IJ, Webb PA, et al. A case-control study of the clinical diagnosis and course of Lassa fever. *J Infect Dis.* 1987;155:445-455.

92. Re-emergence of Bolivian hemorrhagic fever. *Epidemiol Bull.* 1994;15:4-5.

93. Gear JH. Haemorrhagic fevers of Africa: an account of 2 recent outbreaks. *J S Afr Vet Assoc.* 1977;48:5-8. As cited in: Gear JH. Clinical aspects of African viral hemorrhagic fevers. *Rev Infect Dis.* 1989;11(suppl 4):S777-S782.

94. Abd el-Rahim IH, Abd el-Hakim U, Hussein M. An epizootic of Rift Valley fever in Egypt in 1997. *Rev Sci Tech.* 1999;18:741-748.

95. Laughlin LW, Meegan JM, Strausbaugh LJ, Morens DM, Watten RH. Epidemic Rift Valley fever in Egypt. *Trans R Soc Trop Med Hyg.* 1979;73:630-633.

96. Strausbaugh LJ, Laughlin LW, Meegan JM, Watten RH. Clinical studies on Rift Valley fever, I: acute febrile and hemorrhagic-like diseases. *J Egypt Public Health Assoc.* 1978;53:181-182.

97. Craven RB. Flaviviruses. In: *Textbook of Human Virology.* 2nd ed. St Louis, Mo: Mosby–Year Book Medical; 1991.

98. Adhikari Prabha MR, Prabhu MG, Raghuveer CV, Bai M, Mala MA. Clinical study of 100 cases of Kyasanur Forest disease with clinicopathological correlation. *Indian J Med Sci.* 1993;47:124-130.

99. Bwaka MA, Bonnet MJ, Calain P, et al. Ebola hemorrhagic fever in Kikwit, Democratic Republic of the Congo: clinical observations in 103 patients. *J Infect Dis.* 1999;179(suppl 1):S1-S7.

100. Frame JD, Baldwin JM Jr, Gocke DJ, Troup JM. Lassa fever, a new virus disease of man from West Africa, I: clinical description and pathological findings. *Am J Trop Med Hyg.* 1970;19:670-676.

101. Monath TP, Maher M, Casals J, Kissling RE, Cacciapuoti A. Lassa fever in the Eastern Province of Sierra Leone, 1970-1972, II: clinical observations and virological studies on selected hospital cases. *Am J Trop Med Hyg.* 1974;23:1140-1149.

102. Kuming BS, Kokoris N. Uveal involvement in Marburg virus disease. *Br J Ophthalmol.* 1977;61:265-266.

103. World Health Organization. Acute haemorrhagic fever syndrome. Available at: http://www.who.int/emc-documents/surveillance/docs/whocdscsrisr992.html/41Acute%20haemorrhagic%20fever%20syndrome.htm. Accessed February 10, 2002.

104. Franz DR, Jahrling PB, Friedlander AM, et al. Clinical recognition and management of patients exposed to biological warfare agents. *JAMA.* 1997;278:399-411.

105. Rebetol product information. Available at: http://www.hepatitisinnovations.com/pro/rebetol/rebetol_pi.html. Accessed January 10, 2002.

106. McCormick JB, King IJ, Webb PA, et al. Lassa fever: effective therapy with ribavirin. *N Engl J Med.* 1986;314:20-26.

107. Enria DA, Maiztegui JI. Antiviral treatment of Argentine hemorrhagic fever. *Antiviral Res.* 1994;23:23-31.

108. Huggins JW. Prospects for treatment of viral hemorrhagic fevers with ribavirin, a broad-spectrum antiviral drug. *Rev Infect Dis.* 1989;11(suppl 4):S750-S761.

109. Update: management of patients with suspected viral hemorrhagic fever—United States. *MMWR Morb Mortal Wkly Rep.* 1995;44:475-479.

110. Frame JD. Clinical features of Lassa fever in Liberia. *Rev Infect Dis.* 1989;11(suppl 4):S783-S789.

111. Shetty AK, Gans HA, So S, Millan MT, Arvin AM, Gutierrez KM. Intravenous ribavirin therapy for adenovirus pneumonia. *Pediatr Pulmonol.* 2000;29:69-73.

112. Kelly DA, Bunn, SK, Apelian D, et al. Safety, efficacy, and pharmacokinetics of interferon alfa-2b plus ribavirin in children with chronic hepatitis C. *Hepatology.* 2001;342A:abstract 680.

113. Mupapa K, Massamba M, Kibadi K, et al. Treatment of Ebola hemorrhagic fever with blood transfusions from convalescent patients. *J Infect Dis.* 1999;179(suppl 1):S18-S23.

114. Stille W, Bohle E, Helm E, van Rey W, Siede W. On an infectious disease transmitted by *Cercopithecus aethiops* ("green monkey disease") [in German]. *Dtsch Med Wochenschr.* 1968;93:572-582. Cited by: Slenczka WG. The Marburg virus outbreak of 1967 and subsequent episodes. *Curr Top Microbiol Immunol.* 1999;235:49-75.

115. Leifer E, Gocke DJ, Bourne H. Lassa fever, a new virus disease of man from West Africa, II: report of a laboratory-acquired infection treated with plasma from a person recently recovered from the disease. *Am J Trop Med Hyg.* 1970;19:677-679.

116. Frame JD, Verbrugge GP, Gill RG, Pinneo L. The use of Lassa fever convalescent plasma in Nigeria. *Trans R Soc Trop Med Hyg.* 1984;78:319-324.

117. Maiztegui JI, Fernandez NJ, de Damilano AJ. Efficacy of immune plasma in treatment of Argentine haemorrhagic fever and association between treatment and a late neurological syndrome. *Lancet.* 1979;2:1216-1217.

118. Clayton AJ. Lassa immune serum. *Bull World Health Organ.* 1977;55:435-439.

119. Halstead SB. In vivo enhancement of dengue virus infection in rhesus monkeys by passively transferred antibody. *J Infect Dis.* 1979;140:527-533.

120. Kenyon RH, Canonico PG, Green DE, Peters CJ. Effect of ribavirin and tributylribavirin on argentine hemorrhagic fever (Junin virus) in guinea pigs. *Antimicrob Agents Chemother.* 1986;29:521-523.

121. Seiler P, Senn BM, Klenerman P, Kalinke U, Hengartner H, Zinkernagel RM. Additive effect of neutralizing antibody and antiviral drug treatment in preventing virus escape and persistence. *J Virol.* 2000;74:5896-5901.

122. Nathan N, Barry M, Van Herp M, Zeller H. Shortage of vaccines during a yellow fever outbreak in Guinea. *Lancet.* 2001;358:2129-2130.

123. Garner JS. Guideline for isolation precautions in hospitals. *Infect Control Hosp Epidemiol.* 1996;17:53-80.

124. National Institute for Occupational Safety and Health. *NIOSH Guide to the Selection and Use of Particulate Respirators.* Cincinnati, Ohio: National Institute for Occupational Safety and Health; January 1996. Publication 96-101.

125. Fennelly KP. Personal respiratory protection against *Mycobacterium tuberculosis. Clin Chest Med.* 1997;18:1-17.

126. Eck EK, Vannier A. The effect of high-efficiency particulate air respirator design on occupational health. *Infect Control Hosp Epidemiol.* 1997;18:122-127.

127. Richmond JY, McKinney RW. *Biosafety in Microbiological and Biomedical Laboratories.* 4th ed. Washington, DC: US Government Printing Office; 1999.

128. Armstrong LR, Dembry LM, Rainey PM, et al. Management of a Sabia virus-infected patients in a US hospital. *Infect Control Hosp Epidemiol.* 1999;20:176-182.

129. Gershon RR, Vlahov D, Escamilla-Cejudo JA, et al. Tuberculosis risk in funeral home employees. *J Occup Environ Med.* 1998;40:497-503.

130. Management of patients with suspected viral hemorrhagic fever. *MMWR Morb Mortal Wkly Rep.* 1988;37(suppl 3):1-16.

131. McKee KT Jr, Oro JG, Kuehne AI, Spisso JA, Mahlandt BG. Candid No. 1 Argentine hemorrhagic fever vaccine protects against lethal Junin virus challenge in rhesus macaques. *Intervirology.* 1992;34:154-163.

132. Maiztegui JI, McKee KT Jr, Barrera Oro JG, et al. Protective efficacy of a live attenuated vaccine against Argentine hemorrhagic fever. *J Infect Dis.* 1998;177:277-283.

133. Niklasson B, Peters CJ, Bengtsson E, Norrby E. Rift Valley fever virus vaccine trial. *Vaccine.* 1985;3:123-127.

134. Pittman PR, Liu CT, Cannon TL, et al. Immunogenicity of an inactivated Rift Valley fever vaccine in humans. *Vaccine.* 1999;18:181-189.

135. Dandawate CN, Desai GB, Achar TR, Banerjee K. Field evaluation of formalin inactivated Kyasanur forest disease virus tissue culture vaccine in 3 districts of Karnataka state. *Indian J Med Res.* 1994;99:152-158.

136. Sullivan NJ, Sanchez A, Rollin PE, Yang ZY, Nabel GJ. Development of a preventive vaccine for Ebola virus infection in primates. *Nature.* 2000;408:605-609.

137. Vanderzanden L, Bray M, Fuller D, et al. DNA vaccines expressing either the GP or NP genes of Ebola virus protect mice from lethal challenge. *Virology.* 1998;246:134-144.

138. Hevey M, Negley D, Pushko P, Smith J, Schmaljohn A. Marburg virus vaccines based upon alphavirus replicons protect guinea pigs and nonhuman primates. *Virology.* 1998;251:28-37.

139. Fisher-Hoch SP, Hutwagner L, Brown B, McCormick JB. Effective vaccine for Lassa fever. *J Virol.* 2000;74:6777-6783.

140. Gupta M, Mahanty S, Bray M, Ahmed R, Rollin PE. Passive transfer of antibodies protects immunocompetent and immunodeficient mice against lethal Ebola virus infection without complete inhibition of viral replication. *J Virol.* 2001;75:4649-4654.

©2002 American Medical Association. All rights reserved.

Reprinted with permission from *JAMA*; May 8, 2002, Vol 287, No. 18

SECTION TWO, **SEGMENT TWO**

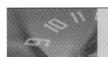 Chemical Terrorism Agents

INTRODUCTION

Most of the United States' terrorism preparedness is being focused on biological terrorism. Congress and the president have appropriated significant funds to the states to develop biological preparedness plans. This work is proceeding, but scant attention has been paid to preparedness for a chemical terrorism event. Granted, biological terrorism is more of an enigma than chemical terrorism, and this response may be related to the tragic anthrax-induced fatalities in 2001.

However, successful biological terrorism is more difficult to achieve than chemical terrorism, especially given the ease of obtaining potential chemical terrorism agents. The production of biological agents requires technological sophistication, whereas toxic organophosphate insecticides are available quite readily from home improvement and agricultural supply stores. The ease of procurement makes chemical nerve agents (organophosphate insecticides) likely candidates as terrorism agents. A multitude of hazardous industrial chemicals and commercial products are all potential terrorism agents. The proactive health-system pharmacist should consider the impending danger that chemicals pose and be prepared accordingly. Development of a hazardous materials preparedness plan will assist the pharmacist in the management of terrorism events that involve atypical chemical agents. Consultation with the Local Emergency Planning Committee (LEPC) will help to identify hazardous chemicals in your region and assist in the preparation of a hazardous materials preparedness response plan.

A key to the recognition of chemical terrorism is the rapid development of symptoms after exposure. Most chemical agents produce their toxic effects within seconds, to minutes, to hours, rather than days as in the case of a bacterial or viral terrorism agent. Patient decontamination and supportive care are essential if a favorable patient outcome is to be achieved. With some chemical poisons, such as the nerve agents, there are viable pharmacological antagonists to reverse the toxic effects. However, there are few effective antidotes.

This section addresses four classes of potential chemical terrorism agents: pulmonary agents, cyanide, vesicants (mustard), and nerve agents. These substances are emphasized in the literature as likely chemical terrorism agents. The nerve agents were used in Japanese terrorist events in 1994 and 1995 and are probably the most likely of the four classes to be redeployed. Each agent is summarized in the following sections. For detailed information the reader is referred to pages 10 through 74 of the *Medical Management of Chemical Casualties Handbook*, 3rd edition, which is reproduced following this summary.

In developing guidelines or policies and in directing patient care, it is important to be aware of the contemporary literature and standards of care and not to rely solely on this work to make those decisions.

Pulmonary Agents

It has been suggested that most chemical terrorism attacks will involve the aerosolization of a chemical agent. An explosive device or aircraft could be used to disseminate the chemical agent. Therefore, inhalation is likely to be a significant route of exposure during a chemical attack, making nearly every agent a "pulmonary agent." However, true pulmonary agents are those that are designed specifically to be inhaled as the primary route of exposure, and the target of their adverse effects is the lungs. Chlorine and phosgene are prime examples of pulmonary agents with the capability of producing significant respiratory dysfunction. Chlorine and phosgene were used extensively during World War I (WWI). The agents

have been part of subsequent warfare arsenals but have not been traditional battlefield agents since WWI.

While a truck or train that is transporting chlorine could be sabotaged, chlorine is not a likely candidate to be used as a chemical terrorism agent. Chlorine is an atypical terrorism agent because the element of surprise is greatly reduced. Chlorine gas, while devastating in high concentrations, has a characteristic odor (strong bleach) and low threshold for identification, thus allowing the potential victims to vacate the terrorism scene prior to experiencing a significant exposure. Ocular and upper-respiratory irritation also provoke a flight response. Furthermore, it is difficult to conceal the chlorine containers unless the target is a small and confined area. Upon contact with moisture in the lungs, chlorine is converted to hypochlorous and hydrochloric acid. These by-products of chlorine are associated with the evolution of profound pulmonary pathology, which includes interstitial edema and bronchospasm.

Phosgene is included as a potential chemical terrorism agent because it has been weaponized and the possibility that terrorists may secure phosgene must always be considered. Phosgene is not removed by secretions in the upper-respiratory tract, and once it comes into contact with moisture in the upper-respiratory tract, bronchioles, and alveoli, it hydrolyzes to form hydrochloric acid. Additionally, the acylation product of phosgene's carbonyl group compromises the alveolar capillary membranes and results in the development of pronounced pulmonary edema. Unlike chlorine, phosgene's odor (freshly mown hay!) may be mild or unnoticeable and result in excessive exposure by the victim—and this is further complicated by the fact that phosgene is twice as toxic as chlorine.

The management of those exposed to pulmonary agents involves termination of the exposure and, if necessary, decontamination of the skin and clothing. First, care providers should take proper precautions to protect themselves from victim-transmitted exposure. Aggressive supportive care and the anticipation of the delayed onset of pulmonary edema are key to a good patient outcome.

Summarized in part from U.S. Army Medical Research Institute of Chemical Defense–Chemical Casualty Care Division. Medical management of chemical casualties handbook. *3rd ed. Aberdeen Proving Ground–Edgewood Area, MD, 1999, 1-8.*

Cyanide

Few are unaware of cyanide's lethality. The use of cyanide in Nazi death camps, the Jonestown, Guyana massacre/

suicides, and the Tylenol®-tampering incidents are evidence of the mortality associated with its use. Cyanide lethality is directly proportional to the amount of cyanide that is ingested or inhaled—the larger the dose the more rapidly death occurs. Death can occur in minutes, which imposes significant treatment limitations. The lethal nature of cyanide and the fear associated with exposure to cyanide mandate that it be considered a potential chemical terrorism agent.

As a military weapon, cyanide can be vaporized when bombs explode and affect nearby troops. In a chemical terrorism incident the threat is more likely to involve the liberation of cyanide gas (e.g., the gas chamber in capital punishment) from a mixture of an acid with a cyanide salt (e.g., potassium or sodium cyanide). Therefore, it is unlikely that large numbers of individuals will perish from cyanide-related chemical terrorism. However, fatalities are likely to occur.

Cyanide interferes with aerobic metabolism and prohibits cells from utilizing oxygen. In essence, cyanide produces cellular suffocation. While the biochemistry of cyanide toxicity is more complex, cellular hypoxia initiates a cascade of adverse events that lead to the demise of the cyanide-exposed victim. The expression of toxicity is dose related. A high concentration of cyanide vapor may produce flushing, tachypnea, vomiting, and tachycardia that progress to seizure activity, coma, and death. The clinical presentation varies with the extent and duration of exposure. The evolution of symptoms takes longer with lower doses. Only patients exposed to low to moderate amounts of cyanide are likely to be salvageable with aggressive supportive care and pharmacological intervention.

The medical management of cyanide poisoning involves aggressive intervention to support respirations (assisted ventilation and 100 percent oxygen), hemodynamic stabilization, and correction of metabolic acidosis. Benzodiazepines may be necessary to control seizure activity. The cornerstone of pharmacological therapy is the administration of the cyanide antidote kit components. This is also the major limitation of successful therapy since first responders rarely stock a sufficient number of kits to treat more than one or two patients and this is often true of emergency departments as well. The cyanide antidote kit contains three components: amyl nitrite for inhalation and sodium nitrite and sodium thiosulfate for intravenous administration. Nitrites are administered to produce a relative degree of methemoglobinemia. Methemoglobin has a high affinity for cyanide. The sequestration of cyanide by methemoglobin allows cellular respiration to resume.

Following the administration of the nitrites, sodium thiosulfate is administered. Sodium thiosulfate serves as a sulfur donor and catalyzes the rhodanese conversion of cyanide to thiocyanate, which is nontoxic. Hydroxocobalamin (vitamin B$_{12}$) is used as a cyanide antidote in Europe but is neither approved nor available in the proper solution in the United States. Hydroxocobalamin combines with cyanide to form cyanocobalamin, another nontoxic variant of vitamin B$_{12}$.

Summarized in part from U.S. Army Medical Research Institute of Chemical Defense–Chemical Casualty Care Division. Medical management of chemical casualties handbook. *3rd ed. Aberdeen Proving Ground–Edgewood Area, MD, 1999:9-19.*

Vesicants

Sulfur mustard gained infamy as a WWI chemical warfare agent. Mustard was responsible for a high number of the WWI chemical warfare casualties. There have been a limited number of battlefield uses in recent history, but there is no evidence that sulfur mustard has been used as an agent of chemical terrorism. However, given its known toxic potential and the fact that a number of nations still retain munitions that contain mustard, it should be considered as a low-risk but potential chemical terrorism threat. Other known vesicants include Lewisite and phosgene oxime, but they are not considered to be high priority agents.

Mustard has physical characteristics that offer both advantages and disadvantages to the chemical terrorist. The oily nature of mustard makes it a persistent agent that does not dissipate easily. This same characteristic limits the ability to aerosolize mustard and affect large numbers of individuals—mustard freezes at 57°F and vaporizes at 100°F. Unlike the biologicals anthrax and smallpox, the aerosolization of mustard would most likely affect a smaller number of people. For example, mustard gas could be released into a crowd (e.g., sporting event, cultural gathering, airport) and affect only those who were exposed directly, whereas anthrax spores could travel for miles downwind and affect a large number of people.

Following exposure to mustard, the onset of symptoms will depend upon the degree of volatilization and the mustard's concentration. Victims who are exposed to a high concentration may note skin and mucous membrane irritation hours prior to those who are exposed to a low concentration. Mustard is absorbed efficiently through the skin, binding to the skin and reaching systemic circulation.

The dermal manifestations are impressive, first appearing as sunburnlike erythema that evolves into huge coalesced blisters. The blisters are thought to be due to the destruction of the epidermal–dermal junction and are pathognomonic of mustard exposure. Pulmonary (e.g., sore throat, cough, dyspnea) and ocular effects (e.g., pain, lacrimation, conjunctivitis) are also consistent with exposure to a mustard aerosol.

The treatment of patients who are exposed to mustard is challenging because the victims are not likely to be aware of the exposure and tissue damage begins to occur within minutes of the exposure. Immediate removal of contaminated clothing and external decontamination of exposed areas are the only ways to prevent mustard-related damage. Following decontamination, supportive care and meticulous skin care (similar to the treatment of burns) are the foundations of therapy. First care providers should take proper precautions to protect themselves from victim-transmitted exposure.

Summarized in part from U.S. Army Medical Research Institute of Chemical Defense–Chemical Casualty Care Division. Medical management of chemical casualties handbook. 3rd ed. Aberdeen Proving Ground–Edgewood Area, MD, 1999:20-43.

Nerve Agents

Nerve agents may be the most feared of all potential chemical terrorism agents. Like the biological agents, the nerve agents are mysterious and unfamiliar to the lay public and many medical professionals. The cinema has portrayed nerve agents as substances that produce instant collapse and death. However, the fatalities and casualties that resulted from the Matsumoto and Tokyo sarin releases by the Aum Shinrikyo cult were the events that motivated the U.S. government to develop a national preparedness program for chemical terrorism. The National Pharmaceutical Stockpile Program recognizes the gravity of nerve agent chemical terrorism by including the key pharmacological antagonists (e.g., atropine, pralidoxime, diazepam) in the stockpile. Many of the preparedness exercises that are conducted throughout the United States include the simulated release of a nerve agent.

Nerve agent is a broad term that applies more specifically to chemicals that interfere with the *in vivo* balance of the neurotransmitter acetylcholine. Traditional nerve agents are organophosphate compounds that inhibit the action of acetylcholinesterase. The enzymatic inhibition produces an excessive imbalance of endogenous acetylcholine, and

a cholinergic crisis occurs. The cholinergic effects are manifest as stimulation of both muscarinic and nicotinic neuroreceptors. These pharmacological actions are the basis for using organophosphate compounds as agricultural pesticides and household/commercial insect-control agents. Prior to their use as pesticides, organophosphates were developed as chemical warfare agents preceding, during, and following World War II (WWII). Organophosphate nerve agents were developed by the Germans and deemed the "G" agents:

- GA-tabun
- GB-sarin
- GD-soman

These agents are not known to have been used on the battlefield. When vaporized and inhaled, they are highly toxic and cause the rapid development of symptoms. Following WWII, the British and Americans developed VX, an agent even more deadly than tabun, sarin, and soman. Sarin is the most easily volatilized of the agents, which may account for its use by the Aum Shinrikyo in 1994 and 1995. VX is difficult to aerosolize due to it physical properties. While less toxic on a mg/kg basis, commercial organophosphate pesticides have the potential (available without restriction in hardware stores, agricultural chemical stores, etc.) to be used as chemical terrorism agents if an adequate dispersal system is used. Regardless of the agent used, the clinical symptom complex or toxidrome is common to all of the agents.

The clinical manifestations are those of a cholinergic crisis:

- Miosis
- Excessive secretions
  - Bronchial
  - Lacrimal
  - Dermal
  - Nasal
  - Salivary
- Bradycardia
- Skeletal muscle fasciculations
- Seizures

The presence, onset, and severity of symptoms will depend on the route of exposure and the dose. For example, miosis is often a presenting symptom following a nerve agent vapor exposure but is unlikely to occur via other routes of exposure unless the dose is high.

Organophosphate nerve agents attach to acetylcholinesterase, and over time (within the first 24–48 hours, but within two minutes with soman) the binding becomes permanent. This is referred to as "aging." The anticholinergic, antimuscarinic agent atropine is the first-line pharmacological antagonist to reverse the muscarinic effects of the chemical terrorism nerve agent. Atropine is used in amounts that exceed customary dosing. An initial adult dose may be 2 to 6 mg, and additional doses should be titrated to the resolution of the patient's life-threatening symptoms, such as excessive bronchial secretions. Do not use the resolution of miosis as the indicator.

The combined treatment of several hundred victims suffering from nerve agent poisoning may require that the pharmacy stock several grams of atropine. A possible alternative to storing hundreds of doses of parenteral atropine is to stock a modest supply to respond to the initial emergency and then to compound larger amounts extemporaneously from pharmaceutical-grade atropine sulfate powder.

However, atropine does not restore the innate enzymatic activity of acetylcholinesterase, and pralidoxime must be administered prior to aging to reactivate the enzyme. Early administration of pralidoxime will reduce morbidity, mortality, and the length of hospitalization. Depending upon the exposure, a considerable amount of diazepam may be needed to control seizure activity. Atropine and pralidoxime are the foundation of pharmaceutical care. Decontamination and aggressive supportive care are likewise critical to the successful management of the nerve agent-poisoned patient. First care providers should take proper precautions to protect themselves from victim-transmitted exposure.

Summarized in part from U.S. Army Medical Research Institute of Chemical Defense–Chemical Casualty Care Division. Medical management of chemical casualties handbook. *3rd ed. Aberdeen Proving Ground–Edgewood Area, MD, 1999:44-63.*

READINGS

MEDICAL MANAGEMENT OF CHEMICAL CASUALTIES HANDBOOK

UNITED STATES ARMY MEDICAL RESEARCH INSTITUTE OF CHEMICAL DEFENSE-CHEMICAL CASUALTY CARE DIVISION, THIRD EDITION

PULMONARY AGENTS, CG

OVERVIEW

Inhalation of selected organohalides, oxides of nitrogen (NOx), and other compounds can result in varying degrees of pulmonary edema, usually after a symptom-free period that varies in duration with the amount inhaled. Chemically induced, acute lung injury by these groups of agents involves a permeability defect in the blood-air barrier (the alveolar-capillary membrane); however, the precise mechanisms of toxicity remain an enigma. The United States produces over a billion pounds of phosgene (CG) per year for industrial uses; however, we do not stockpile this agent for military use.

Perfluoroisobutylene (PFIB) is a toxic pyrolysis product of tetrafluoroethylene polymers encountered in military materiel (e.g., Teflon®, found in the interior of many military vehicles). The oxides of nitrogen (NOx) are components of blast weapons or may be toxic decomposition products. Smokes (e.g., HC) contain toxic compounds that cause the same effects as phosgene. The remainder of this chapter will deal solely with phosgene because it is the prototype of this class of agents; however, the principles of medical management of phosgene exposure also apply to casualties from compounds such as PFIB or NOx.

PHYSICOCHEMICAL CHARACTERISTICS

Phosgene is transported as a liquid. Military dispersion during World War I followed the explosion of liquid filled shells with subsequent rapid vaporization and formation of a white cloud due to its slight solubility in an aqueous environment. It spontaneously converted to a colorless, low-lying gas four times as dense as air. Because of its relatively low boiling point (7.5°C), phosgene was often mixed with other substances. It has a characteristic odor of sweet, newly-mown hay.

MECHANISM OF TOXICITY

The pulmonary agents are absorbed almost exclusively by inhalation. Because they are gases, they readily penetrate to the level of the respiratory bronchioles and the alveoli, that is, to the peripheral compartment of the respiratory tree. However, most of these agents are essentially consumed by reactions occurring at the alveolar-capillary membrane or more proximally in the respiratory tract and are not systemically distributed to a clinically significant extent.

TOXICITY

The odor threshold for phosgene is about 1.5 mg/m³, and phosgene irritates mucous membranes at 4 mg/m³. The LCt$_{50}$ of phosgene is approximately 3200 mg-min/m³, which is half the LCt$_{50}$ (6,000 mg-min/m³) of chlorine, the first gas used on a large scale in World War I. Since only half as much phosgene is required to kill half of an exposed group, phosgene is thus twice as potent as chlorine. That it is less potent than almost all of the subsequently developed chemical warfare agents should not lead to an underestimation of its danger; deaths have occurred after the inhalation of only a few breaths of high concentrations of phosgene. Perfluoroisobutylene is ten times more toxic than phosgene.

TOXICODYNAMICS (MECHANISM OF ACTION)

Chemicals that are highly reactive or highly soluble in aqueous solutions (or both) tend to act in the conducting, or central compartment, of the respiratory tract. Most of the pulmonary agents are relatively insoluble and nonreactive compared to centrally acting irritants such as ammonia and hydrochloric acid, which cause pronounced irritation of the epithelial cells lining the upper airway on inhalation. Additionally, at low concentrations, they are essentially consumed by deposition and reaction in the conducting airways before having the chance to reach the peripheral portion of the respiratory tract. Peripherally acting agents such as phosgene, oxides of nitrogen, and PFIB are still largely unreacted by the time they reach the alveoli and the alveolar-capillary membranes, where they then undergo acylation reactions and are essentially consumed at that site, causing the damage that may eventually lead to pulmonary edema (see the section on toxicodynamics). However, it should be emphasized that the distinction between centrally and peripherally acting agents is not a strict either/or dichotomy. Centrally acting irritants such as hydrochloric acid (and the chemical warfare vesicants sulfur mustard and Lewisite, to be discussed in a subsequent chapter) when administered in high enough concentrations will not be entirely used up by reactions in the nasopharynx, trachea, bronchi, and large to medium-sized bronchioles. Enough of these agents may remain to act peripherally to cause pulmonary edema. Similarly, high concentrations of peripherally acting agents can release enough hydrochloric acid to cause significant central airway irritation and epithelial damage. Moreover, agents such as chlorine are approximately midway between the two poles of this spectrum. Chlorine-exposed soldiers in World War I usually exhibited both central

Adapted and reprinted with permission from the United States Army Medical Research Institute of Chemical and Defense–Chemical Casualty Care Division; 1999

airway damage and pulmonary edema, even from moderate concentrations of the gas.

Phosgene is only slightly soluble in water and aqueous solutions; however, once dissolved, it rapidly hydrolyzes to form carbon dioxide and hydrochloric acid. The early onset ocular, nasopharyngeal, and central airway irritation from high concentrations of phosgene results from the release of hydrochloric acid during phosgene hydrolysis by water in the upper airways. However, the carbonyl group (C=O) of phosgene can undergo acylation reactions with amino (-NH2), hydroxyl (-OH), and sulfhydryl (-SH) groups, and these reactions account for the major pathophysiological effects of phosgene. Acylation occurs at alveolar-capillary membranes and leads to leakage of fluid from those capillaries into the interstitial portions of the lung. This effect is from direct contact of phosgene with these membranes; phosgene exposure by other routes, e.g., intravenous administration, does not cause this damage.

Phosgene-induced leakage of fluid from capillaries into the pulmonary interstitium is normally opposed by lymphatic drainage from the parenchyma, but as the fluid leakage increases, normal drainage mechanisms become progressively overwhelmed. After an asymptomatic or latent period of 20 minutes to 24 hours or longer, fluid eventually reaches alveoli and peripheral airways, leading to increasingly severe dyspnea and clinically evident pulmonary edema.

CLINICAL EFFECTS

Phosgene produces pulmonary edema following a clinical latent period of variable length that depends primarily on the intensity of exposure (i.e., the Ct), but also partly on the physical activity of the exposed individual. After the latent period, the patient experiences worsening respiratory distress that at first is unaccompanied by objectively verifiable signs of pulmonary damage, but may progress relentlessly to pulmonary edema and death.

During the time preceding the appearance of shortness of breath, individuals exposed to particularly high concentrations of organohalides may report symptoms associated with mucous membrane irritation. Exposure to large quantities of phosgene may irritate moist mucous membranes, presumably because of the generation of hydrochloric acid from the hydrolysis of phosgene. Transient burning sensation in the eyes with lacrimation and chemical conjunctivitis may coexist with mild, early onset cough and a substernal ache with a sensation of pressure. Irritation of the larynx by very large concentrations of the agent may lead to sudden laryngeal spasm and death.

A clinical latent period during which the patient is asymptomatic may follow low Ct exposure or the transient irritation associated with substantial phosgene exposure. This asymptomatic period may persist up to 24 hours after organohalide inhalation. The duration of this latent period is shorter following high Cts and is shortened by physical exertion following exposure.

The most prominent symptom following the clinical latent period is dyspnea, perceived as shortness of breath, with or without chest tightness. These sensations reflect hypoxemia, increased ventilatory drive, and decreased lung compliance, all of which result from the accumulation of fluid in the pulmonary interstitium and peripheral airways. Fine crackles appear at the lung bases, but these may not be clearly audible unless auscultation is conducted after a forced expiration. Later, auscultation reveals coarse crackles and râles in all lung fields, and increasing quantities of thin, watery secretions are noted. The buildup of fluid in the lungs has two clinically pertinent effects. First, developing pulmonary edema interferes with oxygen delivery to alveolar capillaries and may lead to hypoxemia, and if a sufficient percentage of hemoglobin is unoxygenated, cyanosis will become apparent. Secondly, the sequestration of plasma-derived fluid (up to one liter per hour) in the lungs may lead to hypovolemia and hypotension, interfering with oxygen delivery to the brain, kidneys, and other crucial organs. Death results from respiratory failure, hypoxemia, hypovolemia, or a combination of these factors. Hypoxia and hypotension may progress particularly rapidly and suggest a poor prognosis. The development of symptoms and signs of pulmonary edema within four hours of exposure is an especially accurate indicator of a poor prognosis; in the absence of immediately available intensive medical support, such patients are at high risk of death. Complications include infection of damaged lungs and delayed deaths following such respiratory infections.

DIFFERENTIAL DIAGNOSIS

Phosgene is distinguished by its odor, its generalized mucous membrane irritation in high concentrations, dyspnea, and *pulmonary edema of delayed onset.*

Riot-control agents produce a burning sensation predominantly in the eyes and upper airways. This irritation is typically more intense than that caused by phosgene and is unaccompanied by the distinctive odor of phosgene.

Nerve agents induce the production of watery secretions as well as respiratory distress; however, their other characteristic effects distinguish nerve agent toxicity from organohalide inhalation injury.

The respiratory toxicity associated with vesicants is usually delayed but predominantly affects the central, rather than the peripheral airways. Vesicant inhalation severe enough to cause dyspnea typically causes signs of airway necrosis, often with pseudomembrane formation and partial or complete upper airway obstruction. Finally, pulmonary parenchymal damage following vesicant exposure usually manifests itself as hemorrhage rather than pulmonary edema.

LABORATORY FINDINGS

No commonly available laboratory tests exist for the specific identification or quantification of phosgene inhalation; however, an increase in the hematocrit may reflect the hemoconcentration induced by transudation of fluid into the pulmonary parenchyma. Arterial blood gases may show a low PaO_2 or $PaCO_2$, which are early, nonspecific warnings of increased interstitial fluid in the lung.

Peak expiratory flow rate may decrease early after a massive phosgene exposure. This nonspecific test helps to assess the degree of airway damage and the effect of bronchodilator therapy. Decreased lung compliance and carbon monoxide diffusing capacity are particularly sensitive indicators of interstitial fluid volume in the lung, but are complex tests for hospital use only.

Early findings on chest x-ray are hyperinflation, followed later

---

Adapted and reprinted with permission from the United States Army Medical Research Institute of Chemical and Defense–Chemical Casualty Care Division; 1999

by pulmonary edema without cardiovascular changes of redistribution or cardiomegaly. Ventilation profusion ratio (V/Q) scanning is very sensitive but is nonspecific and for hospital use only.

MEDICAL MANAGEMENT

Terminate exposure as a vital first measure. This may be accomplished by physically removing the casualty from the contaminated environment or by isolating him from surrounding contamination by supplying a properly fitting mask. Decontamination of liquid agent on clothing or skin terminates exposure from that source.

Execute the ABCs of resuscitation as required. Establishing an airway is especially crucial in a patient exhibiting hoarseness or stridor; such individuals may face impending laryngeal spasm and require intubation. Establishing a clear airway also aids in interpretation of auscultatory findings. Steps to minimize the work of breathing must be taken. Because of the always present danger of hypotension induced by pulmonary edema or positive airway pressure, accurate determination of the casualty's circulatory status is vital not just initially, but also at regularly repeated intervals and whenever indicated by the clinical situation.

Enforce rest. Even minimal physical exertion may shorten the clinical latent period and increase the severity of respiratory symptoms and signs in an organohalide casualty, and physical activity in a symptomatic patient may precipitate acute clinical deterioration and even death. Strict limitation of activity (i.e., forced bed rest) and litter evacuation are mandatory for patients suspected of having inhaled any of the edematogenic agents. This is true whether or not the patient has respiratory symptoms and whether or not objective evidence of pulmonary edema is present.

Prepare to manage airway secretions and prevent/treat bronchospasm. Unless superinfection is present, secretions present in the airways of phosgene casualties are usually copious and watery. They may serve as an index to the degree of pulmonary edema and do not require specific therapy apart from suctioning and drainage. Antibiotics should be reserved for those patients with an infectious process documented by sputum gram staining and culture. Bronchospasm may occur in individuals with reactive airways, and these patients should receive theophylline, or beta-adrenergic bronchodilators. Steroid therapy is also indicated for bronchospasm as long as parenteral administration is chosen over topical therapy, which may result in inadequate distribution to damaged airways. Methylprednisolone, 700-1000 mg or its equivalent, may be given intravenously in divided doses during the first day and then tapered during the duration of the clinical illness. The increased susceptibility to bacterial infection during steroid therapy mandates careful surveillance of the patient. No human studies have shown any benefit from steroids. Thus, steroids are not recommended in individuals without evidence of overt or latent reactive airway disease.

Prevent/treat pulmonary edema. Positive airway pressure provides some control over the clinical complications of pulmonary edema. Early use of a positive pressure mask may be beneficial. Positive airway pressure may exacerbate hypotension by decreasing thoracic venous return, necessitating intravenous fluid administration and perhaps judicious use of the pneumatic anti-shock garment.

Prevent/treat hypoxia. Oxygen therapy is definitely indicated and may require supplemental positive airway pressure administered via one of several available devices for generating intermittent or continuous positive pressure. Intubation with or without ventilatory assistance may be required, and positive pressure may need to be applied during at least the end-expiratory phase of the ventilator cycle.

Prevent/treat hypotension. Sequestration of plasma-derived fluid in the lungs may cause hypotension that may be exacerbated by positive airway pressure. Urgent intravenous administration of either crystalloid or colloid (which in this situation appear equally effective) may need to be supplemented by the judicious application of the pneumatic anti-shock garment. The use of vasopressors is a temporary measure until fluids can be replaced.

TRIAGE

Patients seen within 12 hours of exposure. A patient with pulmonary edema only is classified *immediate* if intensive pulmonary care is immediately available. In general, a shorter latent period portends a more serious illness. A *delayed* patient is dyspneic without objective signs and should be observed closely and retriaged hourly. An asymptomatic patient with known exposure should be classified *minimal* and observed and retriaged every two hours. If this patient remains asymptomatic 24 hours after exposure, discharge the patient. If exposure is doubtful and the patient remains asymptomatic 12 hours following putative exposure, consider discharge. An *expectant* patient presents with pulmonary edema, cyanosis, and hypotension. A casualty who presents with these signs within six hours of exposure generally will not survive; a casualty with the onset of these signs six hours or longer after exposure may survive with immediate, intensive medical care.

Patients seen more than 12 hours after exposure. A patient with pulmonary edema is classified *immediate* provided he will receive intensive care within several hours. If cyanosis and hypotension are also present, triage the patient as expectant. A *delayed* patient is dyspneic and should be observed closely and retriaged every two hours. If the patient is recovering, discharge him 24 hours after exposure. An asymptomatic patient or patient with resolving dyspnea is classified *minimal*. If the patient is asymptomatic 24 hours after exposure, discharge him. A patient with persistent hypotension despite intensive medical care is *expectant*.

CYANIDE AC, CK

OVERVIEW

Cyanide is a rapidly acting lethal agent that is limited in its military usefulness by its high LCt_{50} and high volatility. Death occurs within six to eight minutes after inhalation of a high Ct. Sodium nitrite and sodium thiosulfate are effective antidotes.

Terms. The term cyanide refers to the anion CN^-, or to its acidic form, hydrocyanic acid (HCN). Cyanogen (C_2N_2) is formed by the oxidation of cyanide ions; however, the term cyanogen has also come to refer to a substance that forms cyanide upon metab-

Adapted and reprinted with permission from the United States Army Medical Research Institute of Chemical and Defense–Chemical Casualty Care Division; 1999

olism and produces the biological effects of free cyanide (the term cyanogen is from "cyano" and "gennan," Greek meaning "to produce"). A simple *cyanide* (HCN, NaCN) is a compound that dissociates to the cyanide anion (CN^-) and a cation (H^+, Na^+). A *nitrile* is an organic compound that contains cyanide. A *cyanogen* usually refers to a nitrile that liberates the cyanide anion during metabolism and produces the biological effects of the cyanide anion. Cyanogens may be simple (cyanogen chloride) or complex (sodium nitroprusside).

Cyanides are also called "blood agents," an antiquated term still used by many in the military. At the time of the introduction of cyanide in World War I, the other chemical agents in use caused mainly local effects. Riot-control agents injured the skin and mucous membranes from direct contact, and phosgene damaged the lungs after inhalation. In contrast, inhaled cyanide produces systemic effects and was thought to be carried in the blood; hence the term "blood agent" The widespread distribution of absorbed nerve agents and vesicants via the blood invalidates this term as a specific designator for cyanide. Also, the use of "blood agent" also carries the connotation that the main site of action of cyanide is in the blood, whereas cyanide acts primarily outside the bloodstream.

Materials of interest as chemical agents are the cyanide **hydrogen cyanide (hydrocyanic acid, AC)** and the simple cyanogen, **cyanogen chloride (CK)**. Cyanogen bromide was used briefly in World War I, but is of no present interest.

Sources other than military. The cyanide ion is ubiquitous in nearly all living organisms that tolerate and even require the ion in low concentrations. The fruits and seeds (especially pits) of many plants, such as cherries, peaches, almonds, and lima beans contain cyanogens capable of releasing free cyanide following enzymatic degradation. The edible portion (the roots) of the cassava plant (widely used as a food staple in many parts of the world) is also cyanogenic. The combustion of any material containing carbon and nitrogen has the potential to form cyanide; some plastics (particularly acrylonitriles) predictably release clinically significant amounts when burned. Industrial concerns in the U.S. manufacture over 300,000 tons of hydrogen cyanide annually. Cyanides find widespread use in chemical syntheses, electroplating, mineral extraction, dyeing, printing, photography, and agriculture, and in the manufacture of paper, textiles, and plastics.

PHYSICOCHEMICAL CHARACTERISTICS

The cyanides exist as liquids in munitions but rapidly vaporize upon detonation of the munitions. The major threat is from the vapor. The liquid toxicity is approximately that of mustard (see toxicity, below).

The preferred way to deliver cyanide is by large munitions (bombs, large shells), because smaller weapons will not provide the concentrations needed for effects.

MECHANISM OF TOXICITY

Cyanide salts in solid form or in solution are readily absorbed from the gastrointestinal tract when ingested. Moreover, the lower the pH in the stomach, the more hydrogen cyanide is released as gas from ingested salts. Liquid cyanide and cyanide in solution can be absorbed even through intact skin, but this route

of entry is usually not clinically significant. Parenteral absorption of liquid cyanide can also occur from wounds. Cyanide is readily absorbed through the eyes, but the most important route of entry in a battlefield or terrorist scenario would likely be by inhalation. Following absorption, cyanide is quickly and widely distributed to all organs and tissues of the body. Ingestion leads to particularly high levels in the liver when compared with inhalation exposure, but both routes lead to high concentrations in plasma and erythrocytes and in the heart, lungs, and brain.

An example of the ability of cyanide to react with metals in the body is its reaction with the cobalt in hydroxycobalamin (vitamin B_{12a}) to form cyanocobalamin (vitamin B_{12}). The reactions of cyanide with metals are reversible and exhibit concentration-dependent equilibria, but he reactions of cyanide with sulfur-containing compounds are catalyzed by the enzyme rhodanese (EC 2.8.I.1) and are essentially one-way and irreversible. The rate-limiting factor in the rhodanese-mediated reactions is usually the availability of sulfur donors in the body. These reactions can be accelerated therapeutically by providing a sulfane such as sodium thiosulfate. The reaction products, thiocyanates and sulfites, are significantly less toxic than cyanide itself and are eliminated in the urine. Cyanide also reacts with carbonyl and sulfhydryl groups (directly or via 3-MPST and other enzymes). However, the two most important kinds of reactions from the perspective of understanding the classical mechanism of action of cyanide and its response to specific antidotal therapy are the reactions with metals and the enzyme-catalyzed reactions with sulfur-containing compounds.

Cyanide is eliminated unchanged from the body in breath, sweat, and urine—as sodium thiocyanate in the urine and as iminothiocarboxyllic acid (ITCA) from reaction with sulfhydryl groups. High concentrations of cyanide in the body will also lead to measurable increases in urinary elimination of cyanocobalamin (vitamin B_{12}).

TOXICITY

Cyanide is the least toxic of the "lethal" chemical agents. The $LCt_{50}s$ of AC and CK by inhalation have been estimated to be **2500-5000 mg-min/m³** for AC and about *11,000 mg-min/m³* for CK. $LD_{50}s$ for hydrogen cyanide have been estimated to be 1.1 mg/kg for IV administration and 100 mg/kg after skin exposure. The oral $LD_{50}s$ for sodium and potassium cyanide are about 100 and 200 mg/kg, respectively.

Cyanide is unique among military chemical agents because it is detoxified at a rate that is of practical importance, about 17 mcg/kg·min. As a result the LCt_{50} is greater for a long exposure (e.g., 60 minutes) than for a short exposure (e.g., 2 minutes).

TOXICODYNAMICS (MECHANISM OF ACTION)

Cyanide has a high affinity for certain sulfur compounds (sulfanes, which contain two covalently bonded but unequally charged sulfur atoms) and for certain metallic complexes, particularly those containing cobalt and the trivalent form of iron (Fe^{3+}). The cyanide ion can rapidly combine with iron in cytochrome a_3 (a component of the cytochrome aa_3 or cytochrome oxidase complex in mitochondria) to inhibit this enzyme, thus preventing intra-

Adapted and reprinted with permission from the United States Army Medical Research Institute of Chemical and Defense–Chemical Casualty Care Division; 1999

cellular oxygen utilization. The cell then utilizes anaerobic metabolism, creating excess lactic acid and a metabolic acidosis. Cyanide also has a high affinity for the ferric iron of methemoglobin, and one therapeutic stratagem induces the formation of methemoglobin to which cyanide preferentially binds.

The small quantity of cyanide always present in human tissues is metabolized at the approximate rate of 17 mcg/kg·min, primarily by the hepatic enzyme rhodanese, which catalyzes the irreversible reaction of cyanide and a sulfane to produce thiocyanate, a relatively nontoxic compound excreted in the urine. (An elevated concentration of thiocyanate in either blood or urine is evidence of cyanide exposure.) The limiting factor under normal conditions is the availability of a sulfane as a substrate for rhodanese, and sulfur is administered therapeutically as sodium thiosulfate to accelerate this reaction. The lethal dose of cyanide is time dependent because of the ability of the body to detoxify small amounts of cyanide via the rhodanese-catalyzed reaction with sulfane. A given amount of cyanide absorbed slowly may cause no biological effects even though the same amount administered over a very short period of time may be lethal. In contrast, the LCt_{50} of each of the other chemical agents, which are not metabolized to the same extent as is cyanide, is relatively constant over time. A lethal amount causes death whether administered within minutes or over several hours.

CLINICAL EFFECTS

The organs most susceptible to cyanide are the central nervous system (CNS) and the heart. Most clinical effects are of CNS origin and are nonspecific.

Approximately 15 seconds after inhalation of a high concentration of cyanide, there is a transient hyperpnea, followed within in 15 to 30 seconds by the onset of convulsions. Respiratory activity stops two to three minutes later, and cardiac activity ceases several minutes later still, or approximately six to eight minutes after exposure.

The onset and progression of signs and symptoms after ingestion of cyanide or after inhalation of a lower concentration of vapor are slower. The first effects may not occur until several minutes after exposure, and the time course of these effects depends on the amount absorbed and the rate of absorption. The initial transient hyperpnea may be followed by feelings of anxiety or apprehension, agitation, vertigo, a feeling of weakness, nausea with or without vomiting, and muscular trembling. Later, consciousness is lost, respiration decreases in rate and depth, and convulsions, apnea, and cardiac dysrhythmias and standstill follow. Because this cascade of events is prolonged, diagnosis and successful treatment are possible.

The effects of cyanogen chloride include those described for hydrogen cyanide. Cyanogen chloride is also similar to the riot-control agents in causing irritation to the eyes, nose, and airways, as well as marked lacrimation, rhinorrhea, and bronchosecretions.

Physical Findings. Physical findings are few and nonspecific. The two that are said to be characteristic are in fact not always observed. The first is severe respiratory distress in an acyanotic individual. When seen, "cherry-red" skin suggests either circulating carboxyhemoglobin from carbon monoxide poisoning or high venous oxygen content from failure of extraction of oxygen by tissues poisoned by cyanide or hydrogen sulfide. However, cyanide victims may have normal appearing skin and may even be cyanotic, although cyanosis is not classically associated with cyanide poisoning.

In addition to the preceding effects, CK causes intense irritation of the eyes, nose, and airways.

The second classic sign is the odor of bitter almonds; however, approximately 50% of the population are genetically unable to detect the odor of cyanide.

TABLE: CYANIDE (AC AND CK) *Effects from Vapor Exposure*

Moderate, from low concentration	Transient increase in rate and depth of breathing, dizziness, nausea, vomiting, headache.	These may progress to severe effects if exposure continues.	The time of onset of these effects depends on the concentration but is often within minutes after onset of exposure.
Severe, from high concentration	Transient increase in rate and depth of breathing – 15 seconds. Convulsions – 30 seconds. Cessation of respiration – 2 to 4 minutes. Cessation of heartbeat – 4 to 8 minutes.		

Adapted and reprinted with permission from the United States Army Medical Research Institute of Chemical and Defense–Chemical Casualty Care Division; 1999

The casualty may be diaphoretic with normal sized or large pupils. A declining blood pressure and tachycardia follow an initial hypertension and compensatory bradycardia. Terminal hypotension is accompanied by bradyarrhythmias before asystole.

TIME COURSE OF EFFECTS

Effects begin 15 seconds following inhalation of a lethal Ct; death ensues in 6 to 8 minutes. The onset of effects following inhalation of lower Cts may be as early as minutes after the onset of exposure. After exposure is terminated by evacuation to fresh air or by masking, there is little danger of delayed onset of effects.

DIFFERENTIAL DIAGNOSIS

Battlefield inhalation exposure to either cyanide or a nerve agent may precipitate the sudden onset of loss of consciousness followed by convulsions and apnea. The nerve agent casualty has miosis (until shortly before death), copious oral and nasal secretions, and muscular fasciculations. The cyanide casualty has normal sized or dilated pupils, few secretions, and muscular twitching, but no fasciculations. In addition, the nerve agent casualty may be cyanotic, and the cyanide casualty usually is not.

LABORATORY FINDINGS

1. *An elevated blood cyanide concentration.* Mild effects may be apparent at concentrations of 0.5-1.0 mcg/ml, and concentrations of 2.5 mcg/ml and higher are associated with coma, convulsions and death.

2. *Acidosis.* Metabolic acidosis with a high concentration of lactic acid (lactic acidosis) or a metabolic acidosis with an unexplained high anion gap (if the means to measure lactic acid are not available) may be present. Because oxygen cannot be utilized, anaerobic metabolism with the production of lactic acid replaces aerobic metabolism. Lactic acidosis, however, may reflect other disease states and is not specific for cyanide poisoning.

3. *Oxygen content of venous blood greater than normal.* This also is a result of poisoning of the intramitochondrial respiratory chain and the resulting failure of cells to extract oxygen from arterial blood. This finding is also not specific for cyanide poisoning.

MEDICAL MANAGEMENT

Management of cyanide poisoning begins with removal to fresh air. Dermal decontamination is unnecessary if exposure has been only to vapor, but wet clothing should be removed and the underlying skin should be washed with soap and water or water alone if liquid on the skin is a possibility. Attention to the basics of intensive supportive care is critical and includes mechanical ventilation as needed, circulatory support with crystalloids and vasopressors, correction of metabolic acidosis with IV sodium bicarbonate, and seizure control with benzodiazepine administration. The fact that cyanide inhibits cellular utilization of oxygen would lead to the expectation that supplemental oxygen would not be of use in cyanide poisoning. However, in fact, administration of 100% oxygen has been found empirically to exert a beneficial effect and should be a part of general supportive care for every cyanide-poisoned patient.

Symptomatic patients, especially those with severe manifestations, may further benefit from specific antidotal therapy. This is provided in a two-step process. First, a methemoglobin-forming agent such as amyl nitrite (available in civilian antidote kits, but not in military kits, as crushable ampoules for inhalation) or sodium nitrite (for IV use) is administered, since the ferric ion (Fe^{3+}) in methemoglobin has an even higher affinity for cyanide than does cytochrome a_3. The equilibrium of this reaction causes dissociation of bound cyanide from cytochrome a_3 and frees the enzyme to help produce ATP again. The orthostatic hypotension produced by nitrite administration is not usually a concern in a severely intoxicated and prostrate cyanide casualty, but overproduction of methemoglobin may compromise oxygen-carrying capacity. Thus, nitrite is relatively contraindicated in, for example, smoke-inhalation victims. The initial adult dose, equivalent to one of the two sodium nitrite vials in the standard Pasadena (formerly Lilly) Cyanide Antidote Kit, is 10 ml. Pediatric nitrite dosing (in the case of a military response to a civilian terrorist incident) is dependent on body weight and hemoglobin concentration. The recommended pediatric dose, assuming a methemoglobin concentration of 12 g/dl, is 0.33 ml/kg of the standard 3% solution given slowly, IV, over 5 to 10 minutes.

The second step is provision of a sulfur donor, typically sodium thiosulfate, which is utilized as a substrate by rhodanese for its conversion of cyanide to thiocyanate. Sodium thiosulfate itself is efficacious, relatively benign, and also synergistic with oxygen administration and thus may be used without nitrites empirically in situations such as smoke inhalation with high carboxyhemoglobin levels. The initial adult dose, equivalent to one of the two large bottles in the Pasadena Kit, is 50 ml. The initial thiosulfate dose for pediatric patients is 1.65 ml/kg of the standard 25% solution, IV. Second treatments with each of the two antidotes may be given at up to half the original dose if needed.

It is important to realize that, although the combination of sodium nitrite and sodium thiosulfate may save victims exposed to 10 to 20 lethal doses of cyanide and are effective even after breathing has stopped, many patients will recover even without specific antidotal treatment if vigorous general supportive care is emphasized. Lack of availability of antidotes is therefore not a reason to consider even apneic cyanide casualties expectant. It is also important to realize that administration of antidotes, especially if not given slowly enough or if given in extremely large doses, is also associated with morbidity and even mortality. Antidotes should not be withheld in a patient in whom cyanide poisoning is suspected, but infusion rates should be slow and the drugs should be titrated to effect. Overdosage should be avoided.

Several alternative therapies are experimental antidotes are used in other NATO countries. Germany uses dimethylaminophenol (DMAP), a rapid methemoglobin former developed for intramuscular (IM) use. However, muscle necrosis at the site of injection occurs, and only the IV route of administration is recommended.

Certain cobalt compounds directly chelate cyanide to reduce its toxicity. Because cobalt compounds do not depend upon the

Adapted and reprinted with permission from the United States Army Medical Research Institute of Chemical and Defense–Chemical Casualty Care Division; 1999

formation of methemoglobin, they may exert their antidotal activity more quickly than do methemoglobin formers. Great Britain and France use cobalt edetate (Kelocyanor), but clear superiority to the methemoglobin formers has not been demonstrated, and cobalt toxicity is occasionally seen, particularly if the patient has only a mild exposure. The other cobalt compound sometimes used in France is hydroxycobalamin (vitamin B_{12a}), which complexes with cyanide on a molar basis. Clinical trials of this compound are underway in the U.S.

Ongoing research is examining whether slow methemoglobin formers can be used as pretreatment to induce clinically asymptomatic methemoglobinemia in troops at high risk for cyanide exposure.

TRIAGE

An **immediate** casualty is one who presents within minutes of inhalation exposure with convulsions or the recent onset of apnea, but with circulation intact. Immediate antidote administration will be lifesaving.

A **minimal** casualty is one who has inhaled less than a lethal amount and has mild effects. The antidotes may reduce his symptoms, but are not lifesaving.

The **delayed** casualty is one recovering from mild effects or successful therapy. Generally, it will be hours before full recovery. Evacuation is not necessary but might be considered until full recovery takes place.

An **expectant** casualty is apneic with circulatory failure.

Generally, a casualty who has had inhalation exposure and survives long enough to reach medical care will need little treatment.

VESICANTS HD, H, L, CX

OVERVIEW

Sulfur mustard has posed a military threat since its introduction on the battlefield in World War I. Most of this chapter concerns this agent. Unless otherwise noted, the term "mustard" refers to sulfur mustard.

The nitrogen mustards (HN1, HN2, and HN3) were synthesized in the 1930s, but were not produced in large amounts for warfare. Mechlorethamine (HN2, Mustargen) became the prototypical cancer chemotherapeutic compound and remained the standard compound for this purpose for many years.

Lewisite (L) was synthesized during the late stages of World War I, but probably has not been used on a battlefield. The Lewisite antidote, British-Anti-Lewisite (BAL), finds medicinal use today as a heavy-metal chelator.

Although classified as a vesicant, phosgene oxime (CX) is a corrosive urticant that also has not seen battlefield use.

Lewisite and phosgene oxime pose only minor potential military threats and will be discussed briefly at the end of this chapter.

MUSTARD HD, H

OVERVIEW

Vesicant agents, specifically sulfur mustard (H, HD), have been major military threat agents since their introduction in World War I. They constitute both a vapor and a liquid threat to all exposed skin and mucous membranes. Mustard's effects are delayed, appearing hours after exposure. Organs most commonly affected are the skin (with erythema and vesicles), eyes (with mild conjunctivitis to severe eye damage), and airways (with mild irritation of the upper respiratory tract, to severe bronchiolar damage leading to necrosis and hemorrhage of the airway mucosa and musculature). Following exposure to large quantities of mustard, precursor cells of the bone marrow are damaged, leading to pancytopenia and increased susceptibility to infection. The GI tract may be damaged, and there are sometimes central nervous system signs. There is no specific antidote, and management is symptomatic therapy. Immediate decontamination is the only way to reduce damage.

PHYSICOCHEMICAL CHARACTERISTICS

Mustard is an oily liquid with a color ranging from light yellow to brown (description). Its odor is that of garlic, onion, or mustard (hence its name), but because of accommodation of the sense of smell, odor should not be relied on for detection. Under temperate conditions, mustard evaporates slowly and is primarily a liquid hazard, but its vapor hazard increases with increasing temperature. At 100°F or above, it is a definite vapor hazard. Mustard freezes at 57°F, and since a solid is difficult to disperse, mustard is often mixed with substances with a lower freezing point, e.g., Lewisite (the mixture is HL), or agent T, a closely related vesicant (the mixture is HT) so that the mixture will remain liquid at lower temperatures. The mixture HT also refers to mustard that has been thickened with small quantities of newer thickening agents.

MECHANISM OF TOXICITY

Mustard vapor and liquid readily penetrate thin layers of most fabrics (but not the chemical protective ensemble) to reach underlying skin. Although mustard dissolves relatively slowly in aqueous solutions such as sweat, the lipophilicity of mustard guarantees effective absorption through even intact skin. Penetration is rapid (1 to 4 mcg/cm²-min) and is enhanced by moisture, heat, and thin skin. This explains the otherwise baffling observation that World War I mustard burns involved the scrotum in 42% of cases, but the presumably more readily exposed hands in only 4% of cases. Ocular and respiratory routes of entry are also important, as is parenteral absorption in casualties with conventional wounds. Ingestion (enteral absorption) was an important route of entry for mustard in the sailors exposed outside Bari in World War II. Approximately 10% of the amount of mustard that begins to penetrate the skin will bind to the skin as "fixed" (reacted) mustard; the remaining 90% of the dose reaches the circulation and is systemically distributed as "free" (unreacted and hydrolyzed) mustard. Distribution to almost all organs and tissues including the kidneys, liver, intestines, and lungs occurs; although, because of dilutional effects and reactions of mustard in the bloodstream,

Adapted and reprinted with permission from the United States Army Medical Research Institute of Chemical and Defense–Chemical Casualty Care Division; 1999

clinical effects from systemic distribution are seen only at high doses. After intravenous administration, mustard disappears from the blood within seconds to minutes. Because of the rapid fixation of mustard to tissue, the fluid inside the blisters that eventually develop at the sites of skin contact contains no free mustard and does not pose a contamination hazard to health care providers. Mustard participates in a variety of biotransformative (metabolic) reactions in the body. Some of these reactions are catalyzed by enzymes, but most absorbed mustard reacts directly by forming covalent bonds (via alkylation) with DNA, RNA, proteins, components of cell membranes, and other macromolecules in the body. Mustard is eliminated primarily in the urine as by-products of alkylation.

TOXICITY

The LCt_{50} of sulfur mustard dispersed as a vapor is 1500 mg-min/m³ in an unprotected group and 10,000 mg-min/m³ in a group with respiratory protection. This demonstrates not only the importance of respiratory protection, but also the fact that sufficient concentrations of vapor and sufficient exposure times render mustard vapor lethal, even in masked individuals. The LD_{50} of liquid mustard on the skin is 100 mg/kg. Thus, administration of 7 g (about a teaspoon) of liquid mustard to each member of a group of individuals weighing 70 kg would be expected to cause the death of half of those exposed. Although 7 g of a liquid applied evenly to the surface of the skin may cover approximately 20 to 25% of the total body surface area (BSA), the correlation between BSA involvement and deaths from mustard in the field is poor. One plausible reason for this discrepancy is that using BSA figures by themselves ignore the inhalational component of mustard exposure. Another conceivable explanation is that measurement solely of affected BSA neglects factors such as the thickness of coverage, subsequent spread, contact time, and continued exposure. A 10 mcg droplet of sulfur mustard can produce a small vesicle on exposed skin.

TOXICODYNAMICS (MECHANISM OF ACTION)

Absorbed mustard must first dissolve in aqueous solution such as sweat or extracellular fluid. Although mustard molecules dissolve slowly in such solutions, once they dissolve they rapidly (within seconds to a minute or two) rearrange to form extremely reactive cyclic ethylene sulfonium ions that immediately bind to intracellular and extracellular enzymes, proteins, and other cellular components. Mustard has many biological actions, but the exact mechanism by which it produces tissue injury is not known. According to one prominent hypothesis, biological damage from mustard results from DNA alkylation and crosslinking in rapidly dividing cells, such as basal keratinocytes, mucosal epithelium, and bone marrow precursor cells. This leads to cellular death and inflammatory reaction, and, in the skin, protease digestion of anchoring filaments at the epidermal-dermal junction and the formation of blisters.

Mustard also possesses mild cholinergic activity, which may be responsible for effects such as early GI symptoms and miosis.

It should be re-emphasized that mustard reacts with tissue within minutes of entering the body and that blood, tissue, and blister fluid do not contain free mustard, nor do they represent a contamination risk for medical personnel.

CLINICAL EFFECTS

Topical effects of mustard occur in the eye, airways, and skin. Systemically absorbed mustard may produce effects in the bone marrow, GI tract, and CNS. Direct injury to the GI tract may also occur following ingestion of the compound.

Combined data from United States forces in World War I and Iranians in the Iraq-Iran conflict suggest equal incidence of eye, airway, and skin involvement (between 80 and 90% for each). However, there were higher incidences of eye and lung damage in Iranian casualties than in World War I casualties, probably because of the larger amount of evaporation of the agent in the hot climate.

Skin. Erythema is the mildest and earliest form of skin injury after exposure to mustard. It resembles sunburn and is associated with pruritus or burning, stinging pain. Erythema begins to appear in 2 to 48 hours after vapor exposure with time of onset dependent on Ct, ambient temperature and humidity, and skin site exposed. The skin sites most sensitive are the warm, moist locations with thinner skin such as the perineum, external genitalia, axillae, antecubital fossae, and neck.

Within the erythematous areas, small vesicles can develop which may later coalesce to form bullae. The typical bulla, or blister, is large, dome-shaped, thin-walled, translucent, yellowish, and surrounded by erythema. The blister fluid is clear, at first thin and straw-colored, but later yellowish and tending to coagulate. The fluid does not contain mustard and is not a vesicant.

At extremely high doses such as those from liquid exposure, lesions may develop a central zone of coagulation necrosis with blister formation at the periphery. These lesions take longer to heal and are more prone to secondary infection than the uncomplicated lesions seen at lower exposure levels.

Pulmonary. The primary airway lesion from mustard is necrosis of the mucosa with later damage to the musculature of the airways if the amount of agent is large. The damage begins in the upper airways and descends to the lower airways in a dose-dependent manner. Usually the terminal airways and alveoli are affected only as a terminal event. Pulmonary edema is not usually present unless the damage is very severe, and then it usually is hemorrhagic.

The earliest effects from mustard, perhaps the only effects from a low Ct, involve the nose, sinuses, and pharynx. There may be irritation or burning of the nares, epistaxis, sinus pain or irritation, and irritation or soreness of the pharynx. As the Ct increases, other effects occur—laryngitis with voice changes and a nonproductive cough. Damage to the trachea and upper bronchi leads to a cough productive of sputum. Lower airway involvement causes dyspnea and an increasingly severe cough with increased quantities of sputum. Terminally, there may be necrosis of the smaller airways with hemorrhagic edema into surrounding alveoli. This hemorrhagic pulmonary edema is rarely a feature.

Necrosis of the airway mucosa with resulting inflammation can cause pseudomembrane formation. Pseudomembranes may occur from the most proximal parts of the airways to the most distal portions. These membranes may cause local airway obstruc-

Adapted and reprinted with permission from the United States Army Medical Research Institute of Chemical and Defense–Chemical Casualty Care Division; 1999

tion at the sites of formation, and detachment may lead to obstruction of lower airways.

The cause of death in mustard poisoning is commonly respiratory failure. Mechanical obstruction by pseudomembranes and agent-induced laryngospasm are important causes of death in the first 24 hours after exposure. Deaths occurring from the third to the sixth day after exposure result from secondary bacterial pneumonia caused by bacterial invasion of denuded respiratory mucosa and necrotic debris. Agent-induced bone marrow suppression is a contributory factor in later, septic deaths from pneumonia.

Eyes. The eyes are the organs most sensitive to mustard vapor injury. The latent period is shorter for eye injury than for skin injury and is also Ct dependent.

After low-dose vapor exposure, irritation evidenced by reddening of the eyes may be the only effect. As the dose increases, the spectrum of injury includes progressively more severe conjunctivitis, photophobia, blepharospasm, pain, and corneal damage.

Blisters do not normally form in the eyes. Instead, swelling and loosening of corneal epithelial cells lead to corneal edema and clouding with leukocytes (which affects vision). Corneal vascularization with secondary edema may last for weeks. Scarring between the iris and lens may follow severe effects; this scarring may restrict pupillary movements and may predispose victims to glaucoma.

The most severe damage is caused by liquid mustard from airborne droplets or by self-contamination. After extensive eye exposure, severe corneal damage with possible perforation of the cornea and loss of the eye can occur. Eye loss also results from panophthalmitis if appropriate therapy is not instituted.

During World War I, mild conjunctivitis accounted for 75% of eye injuries, with recovery in one to two weeks. Moderate conjunctivitis with minimal corneal involvement, blepharospasm, edema of the lids and conjunctivae, and orange-peel roughening of the cornea accounted for 15% of the cases, with recovery in four to six weeks. Severe corneal involvement accounted for 10% of the cases. Those with permanent corneal damage accounted for less than 1% of cases. About 0.1% of these severe casualties would meet the criteria for legal blindness today.

Miosis noted after mustard exposure in both humans and experimental animals is probably from the cholinomimetic activity of mustard.

Gastrointestinal (GI) tract. The mucosa of the GI tract is very susceptible to mustard damage, either from systemic absorption or ingestion of the agent. However, reports of severe GI effects from mustard poisoning are relatively infrequent.

Mustard exposure, even exposure to a small amount, will often cause nausea, with or without vomiting, lasting 24 hours or less. The nausea and vomiting appear not to be a direct effect of the agent on the GI tract, but rather they are from a stress reaction, a nonspecific reaction to the odor, or cholinergic stimulation by mustard. Further GI symptoms are usually minimal unless the exposure was severe (even then, GI signs are not common) or exposure resulted from ingestion of contaminated food or drink. Diarrhea has been reported; constipation is equally common. Diarrhea (rarely bloody) and vomiting beginning days after a high-dose exposure imply a poor prognosis.

Central nervous system (CNS). The CNS effects of mustard remain poorly defined. Animal work demonstrated that mustards (particularly the nitrogen mustards) are convulsants, and there are several human case reports describing victims who were exposed to very large amounts and had neurological effects within several hours after exposure just prior to death. Reports from World War I, and again from Iran, described people exposed to small amounts of mustard who appeared sluggish, apathetic, and lethargic. These reports suggest that minor psychological problems could linger for a year or longer.

TIME COURSE OF EFFECTS

Mustard binds irreversibly to tissue within several minutes after contact. If decontamination is not done immediately after exposure, there is no way to prevent injury, although later decontamination might prevent a more severe lesion.

The clinical effects of mustard are delayed. Signs and symptoms may appear as early as 2 hours after a high-dose exposure, whereas following a low-dose vapor exposure, the latent or asymptomatic period may extend to 48 hours. There are several reports of individuals exposed to very large amounts who died within hours; this type of occurrence is extremely rare. The typical onset time is between four and eight hours. The concentration (C) of the mustard vapor, time (t) of exposure, ambient weather, and body site exposed are factors in the onset time.

It must be emphasized that **mustard causes tissue damage within several minutes after contact without causing any concomitant clinical effects,** e.g., burning or erythema. Because of the lack of immediate effects, the contaminated person is often unaware of the exposure and does not decontaminate. **To prevent injury, decontamination must be done immediately after contact.** Later decontamination may prevent further damage, absorption, or spread of the agent.

DIFFERENTIAL DIAGNOSIS

Of the three vesicant agents, mustard is the only one that does not cause immediate pain. The casualty is asymptomatic until the lesion becomes apparent hours later.

Lewisite and phosgene oxime, in contrast, cause immediate pain or irritation to the eye, skin, or respiratory tract. This causes sufficient stimulus to decontaminate immediately or to mask.

Isolated small blisters or a small group of blisters suggest possible exposure to mustard, to plants such as poison ivy or poison oak, drugs, or other substances. The physical characteristics of the lesion are not distinctive; therefore, the history of exposure is invaluable.

Although the blisters of mustard and Lewisite are slightly different (there is less erythema around the Lewisite blister), this information is of little value in individual cases.

LABORATORY FINDINGS

Leukocytosis occurs during the first day, and the magnitude of increase in leukocytes during the subsequent days correlates roughly with the amount of tissue injury, primarily to skin or

Adapted and reprinted with permission from the United States Army Medical Research Institute of Chemical and Defense–Chemical Casualty Care Division; 1999

TABLE: *Effects of Mustard Vapor*

ORGAN	SEVERITY	EFFECTS	ONSET OF FIRST EFFECT
Eye	Mild	Tearing, itchy, burning, gritty feeling	4-12 hours
	Moderate	Above, plus reddening, swelling of lids, moderate pain	3-6 hours
	Severe	Marked swelling of lids, possible cornea damage, severe pain	1-2 hours
Airways	Mild	Runny nose, sneezing, nosebleed, hoarseness, hacking cough	12-24 hours
	Severe	Above, plus severe productive cough, shortness of breath	2-4 hours
Skin	Mild to Severe	Erythema (redness), blisters	2-24 hours

pulmonary tissue. If systemic absorption is large, leukocytes in the peripheral blood will decrease beginning on day three to day five; this decrease indicates damage to precursor cells in the blood-forming organs. The fall may be precipitate, e.g., a decrease of 5000 to 10,000 cells/day. If the marrow damage is severe, erythrocytes and thrombocytes may later decrease, but the casualty usually recovers or dies before this is apparent. A leukocyte count of 500 or fewer is a sign of an unfavorable prognosis.

Signs of a chemical pneumonitis may appear within the first two to three days after inhalation exposure. Leukocytosis, fever, and sputum production suggest a bacterial process, but within this time period sputum cultures are usually negative for pathogens. Organisms commonly invade the damaged airway tissue at days three to five. A change in the fever pattern, an increase in leukocytosis, and a change in the character of the sputum in this time period suggest a bacterial process. Sputum Gram Stain and culture should be done for identification of the specific organism.

Damaged skin should be cultured routinely, particularly if there is an increase in the exudate or in the inflammatory reaction.

Although GI bleeding is unusual, declining hematocrit values should prompt serial analyses of stool for occult blood.

Thiodiglycol, a urinary metabolite of sulfur mustard, can be measured by the Theater Army Medical Laboratory (TAML), which will be deployed. There is no clinical laboratory test for mustard in blood or tissue, nor is one expected, as mustard is biotransformed and bound to tissues within minutes after absorption. However, ways to measure blood and tissue adducts produced in the body after reaction with sulfur mustard are being studied.

MEDICAL MANAGEMENT

The management of a patient exposed to mustard may be simple, as in the provision of symptomatic care for a sunburn-like erythema, or extremely complex, as providing total management for a severely ill patient with burns, immunosuppression, and multi-system involvement. Suggested therapeutic measures for each organ system are provided below. Guidelines for general patient care are not intended to take the place of sound clinical judgment, especially in the management of complicated cases.

Skin. Erythema should be treated with calamine or other soothing lotion or cream (e.g., 0.25% camphor and menthol, calamine) to reduce burning and itching. Small blisters (under 1-2 cm) should be left intact, but because larger ones will eventually break (the blister fluid does not contain mustard), they should be carefully unroofed. Denuded areas should be irrigated three to four times daily with saline, another sterile solution, or soapy water and then liberally covered with a topical antibiotic such as silver sulfadiazine or mafenide acetate to a thickness of 1-2 mm. If an antibiotic cream is not available, sterile petrolatum will be useful. Modified Dakins solution (sodium hypochlorite) was used in World War I and in Iranian casualties for irrigation and as an antiseptic.

Multiple or large areas of vesication suggest the need for hospitalization and whirlpool bath irrigation.

Systemic analgesics should be used liberally, particularly before manipulation of the patient or irrigation of the burn areas. Systemic antipruritics such as trimeprazine should be tried if needed. Monitoring of fluids and electrolytes is important in any sick patient, but it must be recognized that fluid loss is not of the magnitude seen with thermal burns. Clinicians accustomed to treating patients with thermal burns must resist the temptation to overhydrate a mustard casualty with a similar amount of burned body surface.

Eyes. Conjunctival irritation from a low Ct will respond to any of a number of available ophthalmic solutions after the eyes are thoroughly irrigated. Regular application of homatropine (or

Adapted and reprinted with permission from the United States Army Medical Research Institute of Chemical and Defense–Chemical Casualty Care Division; 1999

other anticholinergic drug) ophthalmic ointment will reduce or prevent future synechiae formation. A topical antibiotic applied several times a day will reduce the incidence and severity of infection. Vaseline or a similar substance should be applied to the edges of the lids regularly to prevent them from sticking together. This prevents adhesions and later scarring during healing and also permits drainage of any underlying infection or pus. Topical analgesics may be useful initially if blepharospasm is too severe to permit an adequate examination, but topical analgesics should otherwise be avoided and systemic analgesics should be given for eye pain. Topical steroids are not of proven value, but their use during the first day or two might reduce inflammation. Further use should be relegated to an ophthalmologist. Sunglasses may reduce discomfort from photophobia.

The patient should be constantly reassured that complete healing and restoration of vision will be the outcome.

Pulmonary. Upper airway symptoms (sore throat, nonproductive cough, and hoarseness) may respond to steam inhalation and cough suppressants. Although a productive cough and dyspnea accompanied by fever and leukocytosis occurring 12 to 24 hours after exposure may suggest a bacterial process to the clinician, he must resist the urge to use antibiotics for this process, which in fact is a sterile bronchitis or pneumonitis. Infection often occurs on about the third day. Its presence is signaled by an increased fever, an increase in the pulmonary infiltrate by x-ray, and an increase in sputum production and a change in sputum character to purulent. Appropriate antibiotic therapy should await confirmation of the clinical impression by positive sputum studies (Gram stain and culture).

Intubation should be performed early before laryngeal spasm or edema make it difficult or impossible. Intubation permits better ventilation and facilitates suction of the necrotic and inflammatory debris. Oxygen may be needed, and early use of PEEP or CPAP may be of benefit. If there is a suggestion of pseudomembrane formation, bronchoscopy should be done to permit suctioning of the necrotic debris by direct vision.

Bronchodilators may be of benefit for bronchospasm. If they fail, steroids may be tried. There is little evidence that the routine use of steroids is beneficial. The need for continuous use of assisted or controlled ventilation suggests a poor prognosis.

Death often occurs between the fifth and tenth day after exposure because of pulmonary insufficiency and infection complicated by a compromised immune response from agent-induced bone marrow damage.

Gastrointestinal. Atropine (0.4–0.6 mg, i.m. or i.v.), another anticholinergic drug or antiemetic, should control the early nausea and vomiting. Prolonged vomiting or voluminous diarrhea beginning days after exposure suggests direct involvement of the GI tract by severe systemic poisoning, a poor prognostic sign.

Bone marrow. Sterilization of the gut by nonabsorbable antibiotics should be considered to reduce the possibility of sepsis from enteric organisms. Cellular replacement (bone marrow transplants or transfusions) may be successful, as intact mustard does not persist beyond the few minutes following absorption and would not damage the new cells.

General. A patient severely ill from mustard poisoning requires the general supportive care provided for any severely ill patient, as well as the specific care given to a burn patient. Liberal use of systemic analgesics and antipruritics, as needed, maintenance of fluid and electrolyte balance, and other supportive measures are necessary. Parenteral food supplements including vitamins may also be helpful.

Other. Sulfur donors such as sodium thiosulfate decreased systemic effects and elevated the LD_{50} when given before exposure or within 20 minutes after exposure in experimental animals. Activated charcoal given orally to casualties was of no value. Hemodialysis was not only ineffective, but was actually harmful in several casualties. The rapid biotransformation of the mustard molecule suggests that none of these measures would be beneficial hours or days after exposure.

TRIAGE

Most mustard casualties will be triaged as **delayed**. Those with skin lesions covering several percent to 50% of the BSA will require further medical care but do not need immediate life-saving assistance. (In contrast, patients with thermal burns covering 20 to 70% of their BSA are considered immediate because of their fluid requirements.) Those with mild to moderate pulmonary effects will also eventually require further care, but are not in the immediate category for triage. Eye injuries from other causes require immediate care, but by the time the mustard eye lesion develops, there is no possibility of reducing the injury. These casualties are also in the delayed category.

Patients with skin lesions covering a small percent of BSA (under 5%), when the lesions are not in vital areas (a burn on the face might prevent mask donning), are triaged as **minimal**. Clinical judgement should dictate whether these patients should be evacuated for care or whether they can return to duty. The tactical situation will also be a factor in the decision. Patients with minor eye injuries to include irritation and reddening can be treated and returned to duty. Those with slight upper respiratory complaints of a hacking cough and an irritated throat which developed 12 hours or longer after exposure might be given symptomatic therapy and returned to duty.

The only mustard casualties who might be triaged as **immediate** are those with moderately severe to severe pulmonary signs and symptoms. Two factors should temper this decision. (1) Casualties who develop severe pulmonary effects within four to six hours of exposure will probably not survive despite maximal medical care, and it might be better to expend limited medical resources elsewhere. (2) If evacuation to a maximal medical care facility is required, the casualty may survive the lengthy trip, but during the delay his lesion may progress to an irreversible stage.

A mustard casualty who has severe pulmonary effects that developed within four to six hours of exposure should be triaged as **expectant**. A casualty who has over 50% BSA burns from mustard liquid might also be categorized as **expectant**, but this decision would depend on available medical resources at the far rear echelons of medical care. (The LD_{50} for liquid mustard is about 7 grams, or between one and one and a half teaspoons of liquid. This amount will cover about 25% BSA, so an individual with a

Adapted and reprinted with permission from the United States Army Medical Research Institute of Chemical and Defense–Chemical Casualty Care Division; 1999

50% BSA burn could possibly have two LD_{50}s on his skin. This person might be saved, but at great expenditure of medical resources.)

LONG-TERM EFFECTS

Repeated symptomatic exposures to mustard over a period of years (as in manufacturing workers) seem to be well established as a causal factor in an increased incidence of upper airway cancer. However, the association between a single exposure to mustard and airway cancer is not well established. A single, severe exposure to mustard may have contributed to other airway problems, such as chronic bronchitis, based on World War I data. A new complication seen in Iranian casualties from the Iran-Iraq War in the 1980s was late-onset tracheobronchial stenosis, which presumably would have been seen in World War I casualties had antibiotic therapy been available to allow those who died from secondary bacterial pneumonia to survive.

Several eye diseases, such as chronic conjunctivitis and delayed keratitis, may follow a single, severe exposure of the eye to mustard. Skin scarring and pigment changes may follow a severe skin lesion from mustard; cancer sometimes develops in scarred skin.

Mustard is classed as a mutagen and carcinogen based on laboratory studies. However, there are no data to implicate mustard as a reproductive toxin in man, and there is no evidence that mustard is a causative factor in nonairway, non-skin cancer in man.

LEWISITE, L

OVERVIEW

Lewisite is a vesicant that damages the eyes, skin, and airways by direct contact. After absorption, it causes an increase in capillary permeability to produce hypovolemia, shock, and organ damage. Exposure to Lewisite causes immediate pain or irritation, although lesions require hours to become full-blown. Management of a Lewisite casualty is similar to management of a mustard casualty, although a specific antidote, British-Anti-Lewisite (BAL, dimercaprol), will alleviate some effects.

PHYSICOCHEMICAL CHARACTERISTICS

Lewisite is an oily, colorless liquid with the odor of geraniums. It is more volatile than mustard.

MECHANISM OF TOXICITY

Lewisite is readily absorbed from the skin, eyes, and respiratory tract, as well as by ingestion and via wounds. It is systemically distributed to almost all organs and tissues of the body where it participates in a variety of chemical reactions. It is eventually eliminated primarily as reaction products in the urine.

TOXICITY

Lewisite causes nasal irritation at a Ct of about 8 mg-min/m³, and its odor is noted at a Ct of about 20 mg-min/m³. Lewisite causes vesication and death from inhalation at the same Ct as mustard. Liquid Lewisite causes vesication at about 14 mcg, and the LD50 of liquid Lewisite applied to the skin is about 2.8 grams.

TOXICODYNAMICS (MECHANISM OF ACTION)

Although Lewisite contains trivalent arsenic and combines with thiol groups in many enzymes, its exact mechanism of biological activity is unknown.

CLINICAL EFFECTS

Organ Systems. Unlike mustard, Lewisite vapor or liquid causes immediate pain or irritation. A person with a droplet of Lewisite on his skin will note the burning and will immediately take steps to try and remove it. The vapor is so irritating that a person will seek to mask or leave the contaminated area if possible. Because this warning causes the person exposed to take immediate steps to decontaminate, the Lewisite lesion will probably not be as severe as the lesion from mustard, as exposure to mustard is often undetected and decontamination is not done.

There are almost no data on humans exposed to Lewisite. The following information is based on animal investigations.

Skin. Within about five minutes after contact, liquid Lewisite will produce a grayish area of dead epithelium. Erythema and blister formation follow more rapidly than in a similar lesion from mustard, although the full lesion does not develop for 12 to 18 hours. The lesion has more tissue necrosis and tissue sloughing than does a mustard lesion.

Eyes. Lewisite causes pain and blepharospasm on contact. Edema of the conjunctiva and lids follows, and the eyes may be swollen shut within an hour. Iritis and corneal damage may follow if the dose is high. Liquid Lewisite causes severe eye damage within minutes of contact.

Respiratory. The extreme irritancy of Lewisite to the nasal area and upper airways causes the person to mask or exit the area. Scanty data indicate that Lewisite causes the same airway signs and symptoms as does mustard. The airway mucosa is the primary target, and damage progresses down the airways in a dose-dependent manner. Pseudomembrane formation is prominent. Pulmonary edema, which occurs rarely and usually only to a minimal degree after mustard exposure, may complicate exposure to Lewisite.

Other. Available data suggest that Lewisite causes an increase in permeability of systemic capillaries with resulting intravascular fluid loss, hypovolemia, shock, and organ congestion. This may lead to hepatic or renal necrosis with more prominent GI effects (including vomiting and diarrhea) than after mustard.

Physical findings. The findings are similar to those caused by mustard. As noted, the tissue damage at the site of the skin lesion may be more severe.

TIME COURSE OF EFFECTS

Pain and irritation from either liquid or vapor Lewisite are immediate. Early tissue destruction is more obvious than after mustard, but the lesion is not full-blown for 12 hours or longer.

DIFFERENTIAL DIAGNOSIS

Although differences have been reported between the skin

Adapted and reprinted with permission from the United States Army Medical Research Institute of Chemical and Defense–Chemical Casualty Care Division; 1999

lesions from mustard and Lewisite (less surrounding erythema and more tissue destruction characterize Lewisite blisters), these are of little diagnostic assistance in a single patient. The history of immediate pain on contact is absent after mustard exposure and present after Lewisite or phosgene oxime exposures.

Other substances cause erythema and blisters, and often the history of exposure is the most helpful tool in diagnosis.

LABORATORY FINDINGS

There is no specific diagnostic test for Lewisite. Leukocytosis, fever, and other signs of tissue destruction will occur.

MEDICAL MANAGEMENT

Early decontamination is the only way of preventing or lessening Lewisite damage. Since this must be accomplished within minutes after exposure, this is self-aid rather than medical management.

The guidelines for the management of a mustard casualty will be useful. Lewisite does not cause damage to hematopoietic organs as mustard does; however, fluid loss from the capillaries necessitates careful attention to fluid balance.

British-Anti-Lewisite (BAL, dimercaprol) was developed as an antidote for Lewisite and is used in medicine as a chelating agent for heavy metals. There is evidence that BAL in oil, given intramuscularly, will reduce the systemic effects of Lewisite. However, BAL itself causes some toxicity, and the user should read the package insert carefully. British-Anti-Lewisite skin and ophthalmic ointment decreases the severity of skin and eye lesions when applied immediately after early decontamination; however, neither is currently manufactured.

TRIAGE

Casualties should be triaged using the guidelines for triage of mustard patients.

PHOSGENE OXIME CX

OVERVIEW

Phosgene oxime (CX) is an urticant or nettle agent that causes a corrosive type of skin and tissue lesion. It is not a true vesicant since it does not cause blisters. The vapor is extremely irritating, and both the vapor and liquid cause almost immediate tissue damage upon contact. There is very scanty information available on CX.

PHYSICOCHEMICAL CHARACTERISTICS

Phosgene oxime is a solid at temperatures below 95°F, but the vapor pressure of the solid is high enough to produce symptoms. Traces of many metals cause it to decompose; however, it corrodes most metals.

MECHANISM OF TOXICITY

The toxicokinetics of CX are not known in detail. Penetration

of exposed surfaces is rapid, and systemic distribution to most organs and tissues, including the GI tract, is probably important.

TOXICITY

The estimated LCt_{50} by inhalation is 1500–2000 mg·min/m^3. The LD_{50} for skin exposure has been estimated as 25 mg/kg.

TOXICODYNAMICS (MECHANISM OF ACTION)

The mechanism by which CX causes biological effects is unknown.

CLINICAL EFFECTS

Skin. Phosgene oxime liquid or vapor causes pain on contact, which is followed in turn by blanching with an erythematous ring in 30 seconds, a wheal in 30 minutes, and necrosis later. The extreme pain may persist for days.

Eyes. Phosgene oxime is extremely painful to the eyes. The damage is probably similar to that caused by Lewisite.

Pulmonary. Phosgene oxime is very irritating to the upper airways. This agent causes pulmonary edema after inhalation and after skin application.

Other. Some animal data suggest that CX may cause hemorrhagic inflammatory changes in the GI tract.

TIME COURSE OF EFFECTS

Phosgene oxime causes immediate pain and irritation to all exposed skin and mucous membranes. The time course of damage to other tissue probably parallels that of damage to the skin.

DIFFERENTIAL DIAGNOSIS

Other causes of urticaria and skin necrosis must be considered. Common urticants do not cause the extreme pain that CX does.

LABORATORY FINDINGS

There are no distinctive laboratory findings.

MEDICAL MANAGEMENT

Management is supportive. The skin lesion should be managed in the same way that a necrotic ulcerated lesion from another cause would be managed.

TRIAGE

Because of the continuing pain, most casualties should be placed in the delayed category and evacuated.

NERVE AGENTS GA, GB, GD, GF, VX

OVERVIEW

Nerve agents are the most toxic of the known chemical agents. They are hazards in their liquid and vapor states and can cause death within minutes after exposure. Nerve agents inhibit

---

Adapted and reprinted with permission from the United States Army Medical Research Institute of Chemical and Defense–Chemical Casualty Care Division; 1999

acetylcholinesterase in tissue, and their effects are caused by the resulting excess acetylcholine.

PHYSICAL CHARACTERISTICS

Nerve agents are liquids under temperate conditions. When dispersed, the more volatile ones constitute both a vapor and a liquid hazard. Others are less volatile and represent primarily a liquid hazard. The "G-agents" are more volatile than VX. Sarin (GB) is the most volatile, but it evaporates less readily than water. GF is the least volatile of the G-agents.

Nerve agents can be dispersed from missiles, rockets, bombs, howitzer shells, spray tanks, land mines, and other large munitions.

MECHANISM OF TOXICITY

Nerve agents are organophosphorous cholinesterase inhibitors. They inhibit the butyrylcholinesterase in the plasma, acetylcholinesterase on the red cell, and acetylcholinesterase at cholinergic receptor sites in tissue. The three enzymes are not the same; even the two acetylcholinesterases have slightly different properties, although both have a high affinity for acetylcholine. The blood enzymes provide an estimate of the tissue enzyme activity. After acute exposure to a nerve agent, the erythrocyte enzyme activity most closely reflects the activity of the tissue enzyme, but during recovery the plasma enzyme activity more closely parallels tissue enzyme activity.

After a nerve agent inhibits the tissue enzyme, the enzyme cannot hydrolyze acetylcholine, the neurotransmitter, at cholinergic receptor sites. Acetylcholine accumulates and continues to stimulate the affected organ. The clinical effects from nerve agent exposure are caused by excess acetylcholine.

The attachment of the agent to the enzyme is permanent (unless removed by therapy). Erythrocyte enzyme activity returns at the rate of erythrocyte turnover, about 1% per day. Tissue and plasma enzyme activities return with synthesis of new enzymes. The rate of return of the tissue and plasma enzymes is not the same, nor is the rate the same for all tissue enzymes. However, the agent can be removed from the enzyme and the enzyme "reactivated" by several types of compounds, the most useful of which are the oximes. If the agent-enzyme complex has not "aged," oximes are useful therapeutically. Aging is a biochemical process by which the agent-enzyme complex becomes refractory to oxime reactivation of the enzyme. For most nerve agents, the aging time is longer than the time within which acute casualties will be seen. However, the aging time of the GD-enzyme complex is about two minutes, and the usefulness of oximes in GD poisoning is greatly decreased after this period.

Organs with cholinergic receptor sites include the smooth muscles, skeletal muscles, central nervous system (CNS), and most exocrine glands. In addition, cranial efferents and ganglionic afferents are cholinergic nerves.

Muscarine will stimulate some of the cholinergic sites, and these are known as muscarinic sites. Organs with these sites include the smooth muscles and glands. Nicotine will stimulate other cholinergic sites, known as nicotinic sites, which are those in skeletal muscle and ganglia. The CNS contains both types of receptors, but the pharmacology in the CNS is more complex and less well understood. Atropine and similar compounds block the effects of excess acetylcholine more effectively at muscarinic sites than at nicotinic sites.

Some commonly used pesticides (for example, the organophosphate (OP) Malathion and the carbamate Sevin) and some common therapeutic drugs (the carbamates pyridostigmine [Mestinon] and physostigmine [Antilirium]) also inhibit acetylcholinesterase and can be considered "nerve agents." However, while the OP pesticides cause the same biological effects as nerve agents, there are some important differences in the duration of biological activity and response to therapy.

CLINICAL EFFECTS

The initial effects of exposure to a nerve agent depend on the dose and route of exposure. The initial effects from a sublethal amount of agent by vapor exposure are different than the initial effects from a similar amount of liquid agent on the skin.

Toxicities. The estimated amounts to cause certain effects in man are shown in Tables I and II. In Table I, L indicates lethal, I indicates incapacitating (severe), and M indicates miosis. The large amounts of tabun (GA) and GB required to produce effects after skin application reflect the volatility of these agents. They evaporate rather than penetrate the skin. However, if these agents are occluded and prevented from evaporating, they penetrate the skin very well.

Sarin (GB), the agent studied most thoroughly in man, will cause miosis, rhinorrhea, and a feeling of tightness in the throat or chest at a Ct of 3 to 5 mg·min/m^3.

Effects. Exposure to a small amount of nerve agent vapor causes effects in the eyes, nose, and airways. These effects are from local contact of the vapor with the organ and do not indicate systemic absorption of the agent. In this circumstance, the erythrocyte-ChE may be normal or depressed. A small amount of liquid agent on the skin causes systemic effects initially in the gastrointestinal (GI) tract. Lethal amounts of vapor or liquid cause a rapid cascade of events culminating within a minute or two with loss of consciousness and convulsive activity, followed by apnea and muscular flaccidity within several more minutes.

Eye. Miosis is a characteristic sign of exposure to nerve agent vapor. It occurs as a result of direct contact of vapor with the eye. Liquid agent on the skin will not cause miosis if the amount of liquid is small. A moderate amount of liquid may or may not cause miosis. A lethal or near-lethal amount of agent usually causes miosis. A droplet of liquid in or near the eye will also cause miosis. Miosis will begin within seconds or minutes after the onset of exposure to agent vapor, but it may not be complete for many minutes if the vapor concentration is low. Miosis is bilateral in an unprotected individual, but occasionally may be unilateral in a masked person with a leak in his mask eyepiece.

Miosis is often accompanied by complaints of pain, dim vision, blurred vision, conjunctival injection, nausea, and occasionally, vomiting. The pain may be sharp or dull, in or around the eyeball, but more often is a dull ache in the frontal part of the head. Dim vision is due in part to the small pupil, and cholinergic mechanisms in the visual pathways also contribute. The complaint of blurred vision is less easily explained, as objective testing usually

Adapted and reprinted with permission from the United States Army Medical Research Institute of Chemical and Defense–Chemical Casualty Care Division; 1999

TABLE I: *Vapor Toxicity (mg-min/m³)*

Agent	LCt$_{50}$	ICt$_{50}$	MCt$_{50}$
GA	400	300	2-3
GB	100	75	3
GD	70	Unknown	<1
GF	Unknown	Unknown	<1
VX	50	35	0.04

TABLE II: *LD$_{50}$ on Skin*

Agent	Amount
GA	1000 mg
GB	1700 mg
GD	50 mg
GF	30 mg
VX	10 mg

indicates an improvement in visual acuity because of the "pin-hole" effect. Conjunctival injection may be mild or severe, and occasionally subconjunctival hemorrhage is present. Nausea (and sometimes vomiting) is part of a generalized complaint of not feeling well. Topical homatropine or atropine in the eye can relieve miosis, pain, dim vision, and nausea.

Nose. Rhinorrhea may be the first indication of nerve agent vapor exposure. Its severity is dose dependent.

Airways. Nerve agent vapor causes bronchoconstriction and increased secretions of the glands in the airways in a dose-related manner. The exposed person may feel a slight tightness in his chest after a small amount of agent and may be in severe distress after a large amount of agent. Cessation of respiration occurs within minutes after the onset of effects from exposure to a large amount of nerve agent. This apnea is probably mediated through the CNS, although peripheral factors (skeletal muscle weakness, e.g., the intercostal muscles, and bronchoconstriction) may contribute.

Gastrointestinal (GI) tract. After they are absorbed, nerve agents cause an increase in the motility of the GI tract and an increase in secretions by the glands in the wall of the GI tract. Nausea and vomiting are early signs of liquid exposure on the skin. Diarrhea may occur with large amounts of agent.

Glands. Nerve agent vapor causes increases in secretions from the glands it contacts, such as the lacrimal, nasal, salivary, and bronchial glands. Localized sweating around the site of liquid agent on the skin is common, and generalized sweating after a large liquid or vapor exposure is common. Increased secretions of the glands of the GI tract occur after systemic absorption of the agent by either route.

Skeletal muscle. The first effect of nerve agents on skeletal muscle is stimulation producing muscular fasciculations and twitching. After a large amount of agent, fatigue and weakness of muscles are rapidly followed by muscular flaccidity.

Fasciculations are sometimes seen early at the site of a droplet of liquid agent on the skin, and generalized fasciculations are common after a large exposure. These may remain long after most of the other acute signs decrease.

Central nervous system (CNS). The acute CNS signs of exposure to a large amount of nerve agent are loss of consciousness, seizure activity, and apnea. These begin within a minute after exposure to a large amount of agent vapor and may be preceded by an asymptomatic period of 1 to 30 minutes after contact of liquid with the skin.

After exposure to smaller amounts of nerve agents, CNS effects vary and are nonspecific. They may include forgetfulness, an inability to concentrate fully, insomnia, bad dreams, irritability, impaired judgement, and depression. They do not include frank confusion and misperceptions (i.e., hallucinations). These may occur in the absence of physical signs or other symptoms of exposure. After a severe exposure, these symptoms occur upon recovery from the acute severe effects. In either case, they may persist for as long as four to six weeks.

Cardiovascular. The heart rate may be decreased because of stimulation by the vagus nerve, but it is often increased because of other factors such as fright, hypoxia, and the influence of adrenergic stimulation secondary to ganglionic stimulation. Thus, the heart rate may be high, low, or in the normal range. Bradyarrhythmias such as first-, second-, or third-degree heart block may occur. The blood pressure may be elevated from adrenergic factors, but is generally normal until the terminal decline.

PHYSICAL FINDINGS

Physical findings depend on the amount and route of exposure. After exposure to small to moderate amounts of vapor, there are usually miosis and conjunctival injection, rhinorrhea, and pulmonary signs, although the latter may be absent even in the face of mild to moderate pulmonary complaints. In addition to these signs, an exposure to a high Ct may precipitate copious secretions from the nose and mouth, generalized muscular fasciculations, twitching or seizure activity, loss of consciousness, and apnea. Cyanosis, hypotension, and bradycardia may be present just before death.

Exposure to a small droplet of liquid on the skin may produce few physical findings. Sweating, blanching, and occasionally, fasciculations, at the site may be present soon after exposure, but may no longer be present at the onset of GI effects. After a large exposure, the signs are the same as after vapor exposure.

Adapted and reprinted with permission from the United States Army Medical Research Institute of Chemical and Defense–Chemical Casualty Care Division; 1999

Miosis is a useful sign of exposure to vapor but does not occur after a liquid exposure unless the amount of exposure is large or the exposure is in or close to the eye.

TIME COURSE OF EFFECTS

Effects from nerve agent vapor begin within seconds to several minutes after exposure. Loss of consciousness and onset of seizure activity have occurred within a minute of exposure to a high Ct. After exposure to a very low Ct, miosis and other effects may not begin for several minutes, and miosis may not be complete for 15 to 30 minutes after removal from the vapor. There is no latent period or delay in onset from vapor exposure. Effects may continue to progress for a period of time, but maximal effects usually occur within minutes after exposure stops.

A large amount of liquid on the skin causes effects within minutes. Commonly there is an asymptomatic period of 1 to 30 minutes, and then the sudden onset of an overwhelming cascade of events, including loss of consciousness, seizure activity, apnea, and muscular flaccidity. After small amounts of liquid agent on the skin, the onset of effects has been delayed for as long as 18 hours after contact. These effects are initially gastrointestinal and are usually not life threatening. Generally, the longer the interval, the less severe are the effects.

DIFFERENTIAL DIAGNOSIS

The effects caused by a mild vapor exposure, namely rhinorrhea and tightness in the chest, may easily be confused with an upper respiratory malady or an allergy. Miosis, if present, will help to distinguish these, but the eyes must be examined in very dim light to detect this. Similarly, GI symptoms from another illness may be confused with those from nerve agent effects, and in this instance there will be no useful physical signs. History of possible exposure will be helpful, and laboratory evidence (decreased RBC-ChE activity), if available, will be useful to distinguish the two.

The diagnosis is easier in the severely intoxicated patient. The combination of miosis, copious secretions, and generalized muscular fasciculations in a gasping, cyanotic, and convulsing patient is characteristic.

LABORATORY FINDINGS

Nerve agents inhibit the cholinesterase activity of the blood components, and estimation of this activity is useful in detecting exposure to these agents. The erythrocyte enzyme activity is more sensitive to acute nerve agent exposure than is the plasma enzyme activity.

The amount of inhibition of this enzyme activity does not correlate well with the severity of local effects from mild to moderate vapor exposure. The enzyme activity may be from 0 to 100% of the individual's normal activity in the face of miosis, rhinorrhea, and/or airway symptoms. Normal or nearly normal erythrocyte acetylcholinesterase activity may be present with moderate effects in these organs. At the other extreme, the enzyme may be inhibited by 60 to 70% when miosis or rhinorrhea is the only sign of exposure. Severe systemic effects generally indicate inhibition of the erythrocyte acetylcholinesterase by 70 to 80% or greater.

Other laboratory findings will relate to complications. For example, acidosis may occur after prolonged hypoxia.

MEDICAL MANAGEMENT

Management of a casualty with nerve agent intoxication consists of decontamination, ventilation, administration of the antidotes, and supportive therapy. The condition of the patient dictates the need for each of these and the order in which they are done.

Decontamination is described elsewhere in this manual. Skin decontamination is not necessary after exposure to vapor alone, but clothing should be removed because it may contain "trapped" vapor.

The need for **ventilation** will be obvious, and the means of ventilation will depend on available equipment. Airway resistance is high (50-70 cm of water) because of bronchoconstriction and secretions, and initial ventilation is difficult. The resistance decreases after atropine administration, after which ventilation will be easier. The copious secretions that may be thickened by atropine also impede ventilatory efforts and require frequent suctioning. In reported cases of severe nerve agent exposure, ventilation has been required from 0.5 to 3 hours.

Three drugs are used to treat nerve agent exposure, and another is used as pretreatment for potential nerve agent exposure. The three therapeutic drugs are atropine, pralidoxime chloride, and diazepam. The use of the pretreatment drug pyridostigmine bromide is discussed later in this chapter.

Atropine is a cholinergic blocking or anticholinergic compound. It is extremely effective in blocking the effects of excess acetylcholine at peripheral muscarinic sites. Under experimental conditions, very large amounts may block some cholinergic effects at nicotinic sites, but these antinicotinic effects are not evident even at high clinical doses. When small amounts (2 mg) are given to normal individuals without nerve agent intoxication, atropine causes mydriasis, a decrease in secretions (including a decrease in sweating), mild sedation, a decrease in GI motility, and tachycardia. The amount in three MARK I Kits may cause adverse effects on military performance in a normal person. In people not exposed to nerve agents, amounts of 10 mg or higher may cause delirium. Potentially, the most hazardous effect of inadvertent use of atropine (2 mg, i.m.) in a young person not exposed to a cholinesterase inhibiting compound in a warm or hot atmosphere is inhibition of sweating, which may lead to heat injury. In the military, atropine is packaged in autoinjectors, each containing 2 mg.

Pralidoxime chloride (Protopam chloride, 2-PAMCl) is an oxime. Oximes attach to the nerve agent that is inhibiting the cholinesterase and break the agent-enzyme bond to restore the normal activity of the enzyme. Clinically, this is noticeable in those organs with nicotinic receptors. Abnormal activity in skeletal muscle decreases and normal strength returns. The effects of an oxime are not apparent in organs with muscarinic receptors; oximes do not cause a decrease in secretions, for example. They also are less useful after aging occurs, but with the exception of GD (soman) intoxicated individuals, casualties will be treated before significant aging occurs. Pralidoxime chloride (600 mg) is in an autoinjector for self-use along with the atropine injector.

Adapted and reprinted with permission from the United States Army Medical Research Institute of Chemical and Defense–Chemical Casualty Care Division; 1999

These atropine and pralidoxime chloride autoinjectors are packaged together in a MARK I Kit. Each soldier is issued three MARK I Kits.

Diazepam is an anticonvulsant drug used to decrease convulsive activity and reduce the brain damage caused by prolonged seizure activity. Without the use of pyridostigmine pretreatment, experimental animals died quickly after superlethal doses of nerve agents despite conventional therapy. With pyridostigmine pretreatment (followed by conventional therapy), animals survived superlethal doses of soman but had prolonged periods of seizure activity before recovery. They later had performance decrements and anatomic lesions in their brains. The administration of diazepam with other standard therapy to soman-poisoned animals pretreated with pyridostigmine reduced the seizure activity and its sequelae. Current military doctrine is to administer diazepam with other therapy (three MARK I Kits) at the onset of severe effects from a nerve agent, whether or not seizure activity is among those effects. Each soldier carries one autoinjector containing 10 mg of diazepam for his buddy to administer to him (if he could self-administer it, he would not need it). **Diazepam should be administered with the three MARK I Kits when the casualty's condition warrants the use of three kits at the same time.** Medical personnel can administer more diazepam to a casualty if necessary. The medical corpsman carries extra diazepam injectors and is authorized to administer two additional injectors at ten-minute intervals to a convulsing casualty.

The doctrine for **self-aid** for nerve agent intoxication states that if an individual has effects from the agent, he/she should self-administer one MARK I Kit. If there is no improvement in ten minutes, he/she should seek out a buddy to assist in the evaluation of his/her condition before further MARK I Kits are given. If a buddy finds an individual severely intoxicated (e.g., gasping respirations, twitching, etc.) so that the individual cannot self-administer a MARK I Kit, the buddy should administer three MARK I Kits and diazepam immediately. The discussion below is advice for medical assistance.

The appropriate number of MARK I Kits to administer initially to a casualty from nerve agent vapor depends on the severity of the effects. Systemic atropine will not reverse miosis (unless administered in very large amounts), and miosis alone is not an indication for a MARK I Kit. If the eye or head pain and nausea associated with the miosis are severe, topical application of atropine (or homatropine) in the eye will bring relief. Topical atropine should not be used without good reason (severe pain), because it causes blurred vision for a day or longer. A casualty with miosis and rhinorrhea should be given one MARK I Kit only if the rhinorrhea is severe and troublesome (he cannot keep his mask on because of fluid). A casualty with mild to moderate dyspnea should be given one or two MARK I Kits, depending on the severity of his distress and the time between exposure and therapy. Some of the respiratory distress from a mild exposure will spontaneously decrease within 15 to 30 minutes after termination of exposure, so if the casualty is not severely uncomfortable, only one MARK I Kit should be used initially. Atropine is quite effective, and care should be taken not to give too much in a casualty who does not need it.

A severe casualty from nerve agent vapor has miosis, copious secretions from the nose and mouth, severe difficulty breathing or apnea, possibly some degree of cyanosis, muscular fasciculations, and twitching or convulsive activity, and is unconscious. He should be given three MARK I Kits and diazepam immediately. Ventilation will be needed and should be done via an endotracheal airway if possible. Suctioning of the excessive airway secretions will be necessary to enhance air exchange and will make ventilatory efforts easier. Atropine, 2 mg, should be repeated at three to five-minute intervals and should be titrated to a reduction of secretions and to reduction of ventilatory resistance. When the intravenous preparation is available, the preferred route of atropine administration is via the intravenous route, but this route should be avoided until hypoxia is corrected, because intravenously administered atropine in hypoxic animals has produced ventricular fibrillation. In a hypotensive patient or a patient with poor veins, atropine might be given intratracheally, either via the endotracheal tube or directly into the trachea, for more rapid absorption via the peribronchial vessels.

The medical care provider might err in giving too much atropine to a mild to moderate casualty. More importantly, the care provider might err by giving too little atropine to a severe casualty. In a severe casualty, atropine should be pushed at frequent intervals until secretions are dry (or nearly dry) and until ventilation can be accomplished with ease. In reported cases this has required 10 to 20 mg of atropine within the first several hours. A conscious, less-severely exposed casualty should receive atropine until he is breathing comfortably, and he will be able to communicate this. Dry secretions need not be an endpoint in mild to moderate casualties.

The casualty with skin exposure to liquid is more difficult to evaluate and manage than is a vapor exposure casualty. Agent on the surface of the skin can be decontaminated, but agent absorbed into the skin cannot be removed. The initial effects from absorbed liquid agent can start two to three hours after thorough decontamination of agent droplets on the skin. A casualty from liquid exposure on the skin may continue to worsen because of continued absorption of the agent from the skin depot.

The first effects of a liquid droplet on the skin are sweating with or without blanching, and occasionally, muscular fasciculations at the site. Gastrointestinal effects (nausea, vomiting, and sometimes diarrhea) are the first systemic effects, and these may start from 0.5 to 18 hours after contact with the agent. If these effects occur within the first several hours after exposure, they may portend more severe effects, and initial therapy should be two MARK I Kits. If effects begin later, initial therapy should be one MARK I Kit.

A large amount of liquid agent on the skin will cause effects 1 to 30 minutes after contact, whether or not decontamination was done. Nevertheless, early decontamination may lessen the magnitude of the effects. After a 1 to 30-minute latent or asymptomatic period, the casualty will suddenly lose consciousness and begin seizure activity. The condition of the casualty and management are the same as described for a severe casualty from vapor exposure.

Adapted and reprinted with permission from the United States Army Medical Research Institute of Chemical and Defense–Chemical Casualty Care Division; 1999

Further care of the severe casualty consists of atropine administration to minimize secretions and ventilation until spontaneous respiration resumes. Oxime administration should be repeated at hourly intervals for two or three additional doses. The preferred method of administration of the oxime is by intravenous drip of 1 gram over 20 to 30 minutes (more rapid administration will cause hypertension), but 3 additional oxime autoinjectors (total dose of 1.8 grams) may be given if the intravenous route cannot be used. The need for ventilation may continue for 0.5 to 3 hours. Unless prolonged hypoxia or other complications have occurred, the casualty will eventually begin having spontaneous muscular activity and make sporadic attempts to breathe. Muscles will become stronger and breathing more regular, and the casualty will have intermittent episodes of conscious behavior. Within an hour or two, he will be breathing, moving, and conscious, although he will be weak and intermittently obtunded.

PRETREATMENT

In late 1990, the United States military fielded pyridostigmine bromide as a pretreatment for nerve agent exposure. Each individual received a blister pack containing twenty-one 30-mg tablets. The dose regimen is one 30-mg tablet every eight hours. When to start and stop dosing is a division or corps' command decision and is made with the advice of the intelligence, chemical, and medical staffs. To use or to stop the pretreatment is not a local decision, nor is it an individual decision.

When given before soman exposure and when that exposure is followed by the standard MARK I therapy, the use of pretreatment will increase the LD$_{50}$ several fold over the LD$_{50}$ obtained without the use of the pretreatment. When soman is the nerve agent, the use of pyridostigmine increases survival. When the agent is GB or VX, survival after standard MARK I therapy is essentially the same whether or not pyridostigmine pretreatment is used, i.e., pyridostigmine use provides no benefit in GB or VX poisoning. Current data are not adequate to evaluate the effectiveness of pyridostigmine pretreatment for GA or GF exposure.

Pyridostigmine is not an antidote, and it should not be taken after soman exposure. Its use will not decrease the effects of soman. It is ineffective unless standard MARK I therapy is also used in the appropriate manner.

One consequence of the greater survival from the use of pyridostigmine is prolonged seizure activity and subsequent brain damage in the survivors. The early administration of diazepam will decrease these effects.

About 50 years ago, it was noted that carbamates bind to the active site of cholinesterase in a similar manner to the binding of organophosphorus cholinesterase inhibitors to cholinesterase. Additionally, while the carbamate was attached to the active site, an organophosphorus compound could not attach to the enzyme. The carbamate-enzyme binding, or carbamylation, lasts only for hours, rather than for the lifetime of the enzyme as the organophosphorus compound attachment does. While the enzyme is carbamylated, the active site is protected from attack by other compounds such as organophosphorous cholinesterase inhibitors, including nerve agents. After several hours, the carbamate leaves

TABLE III: NERVE AGENTS EFFECTS. *Vapor Exposure*

Mild
- Eyes: miosis, dim vision, headache
- Nose: rhinorrhea
- Mouth: salivation
- Lungs: dyspnea ("tightness in the chest")
- Time of onset: seconds to minutes after exposure

Severe
All of the above, plus
- Severe breathing difficulty or cessation of respiration
- Generalized muscular twitching, weakness, or paralysis
- Convulsions
- Loss of consciousness
- Loss of bladder, bowel control
- Time of onset: seconds to minutes after exposure

TABLE IV: NERVE AGENTS EFFECTS. *Liquid on Skin*

Mild/moderate
- Muscle twitching at site of exposure
- Sweating at site of exposure
- Nausea, vomiting
- Feeling of weakness
- Time of onset: 10 minutes to 18 hours after exposure

Severe
All of the above, plus
- Severe breathing difficulty or cessation of breathing
- Generalized muscular twitching, weakness, or paralysis
- Convulsions
- Loss of consciousness
- Loss of bladder and bowel control
- Time of onset: minutes to an hour after exposure

Adapted and reprinted with permission from the United States Army Medical Research Institute of Chemical and Defense–Chemical Casualty Care Division; 1999

the enzyme (that is, decarbamylation occurs), and the enzyme becomes completely functional again. Thus, the carbamate provides temporary protection for the enzyme against nerve agent attack.

Over the past several decades, many carbamates have been investigated for their effectiveness in animals and their safety in man. Pyridostigmine was chosen and underwent extensive testing in humans. Investigations indicated that it did not interfere with the performance of military tasks and caused no adverse physiological disturbances. The incidence of side effects from the drug during these studies was reported as fewer than 5%.

Tens of thousands of United States troops took pyridostigmine during the recent Gulf War Conflict. The incidence of side effects (primarily gastrointestinal and urinary) was over 50%, but only a few percent of the troops sought medical help because of the severity of these effects. The drug was discontinued in less than 1% of cases.

TRIAGE

A severe nerve agent casualty who is unconscious, convulsing or post-ictal, breathing with difficulty or apneic, and possibly flaccid will survive with appropriate, immediate therapy (including ventilation) if he still has an intact circulation. He should be triaged as **immediate** if that therapy can be provided. If a blood pressure cannot be obtained, he should be considered **expectant**.

The casualty with severe symptoms who is spontaneously breathing, has not lost consciousness, and has not seized has an excellent chance of survival with a minimal amount of therapeutic effort. He should be categorized as **immediate** and given three MARK I Kits and diazepam. He may worsen if his exposure was to liquid, and atropine administration should be repeated at frequent intervals. If he loses consciousness, seizes, and becomes apneic, he will be retriaged, and his further care will depend on available resources.

Casualties who are walking and talking will usually be triaged as **minimal**. If a casualty can walk and talk, he is breathing and his circulation is intact. He would not appear to need immediate, life-saving care. This does not preclude self-administration or medic-administration of further antidotes for symptoms, and these should be given as necessary.

A casualty recovering from a severe exposure who has received large amounts of antidotes and has been ventilated will be triaged as **delayed**, because he is in need of further medical observation or care.

LONG-TERM EFFECTS

Minor electroencephalographic changes were noted more than a year after nerve agent exposure when averaged EEGs in a group of people who had been exposed to a nerve agent were compared to a control group. Changes could not be identified in individuals. Neuropsychiatric changes have been noted in individuals for weeks to months after exposure to insecticides.

Polyneuropathy, reported after OP insecticide poisoning, has not been reported in humans exposed to nerve agents and has been produced in animals only at doses of nerve agents so high that survival would be unlikely. The Intermediate Syndrome has not been reported in humans after nerve agent exposure, nor has it been produced in animals by nerve agent administration. Muscular necrosis has been produced in animals after high dose nerve agent exposure but reverses within weeks; it has not been reported in humans.

Adapted and reprinted with permission from the United States Army Medical Research Institute of Chemical and Defense–Chemical Casualty Care Division; 1999

SECTION **THREE**

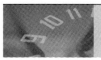

Reference Resources on Biological and Chemical Terrorism

INTRODUCTION

Preparedness for biological and chemical terrorism is a process that must be an ongoing priority. Experience will guide preparedness activities, but biological and chemical terrorism agents are associated with a great deal of uncertainty. Few people have had the experience of managing anthrax or smallpox. A limited number of individuals have experience in the treatment of exposure to nerve gas or mustard. Few health-system pharmacists or other health professionals have the experience with biological and chemical terrorism agents that is needed to develop preparedness plans. The literature can help to bridge the gap between uncertainty and the development of preparedness plans that meet the needs of your community and institution.

The section that follows presents a survey of the contemporary literature. It is not an exhaustive reference list, but it is representative of the key papers, books, and Internet resources that are available on the topic of biological and chemical terrorism. Exploring the reference lists of key papers and the hotlinks on Internet sites can provide the health-system pharmacist with the literature that is necessary to tailor a preparedness plan for his or her institution. The day of the next biological or chemical terrorism incident is not the time to search the literature and establish a reference library for the health-system pharmacy. Anticipate that more biological and chemical terrorism events will occur and build a reference library that will support staff and institutional needs. Ultimately, preparedness planning will improve the level of pharmaceutical care that is provided to the victims of biological and chemical terrorism.

REFERENCES

BIOLOGICAL AGENTS

Anon. Recognition of illness associated with the intentional release of a biologic event. *JAMA* 2001;286:2088-2090.

Anon. Suspected brucellosis case prompts investigation of possible bioterrorism-related activity—New Hampshire and Massachusetts, 1999. *MMWR* 2000;49:509-512.

Danzig R, Berkowsky PB. Why should we be concerned about biological warfare? *JAMA* 1997;278:431-432.

Darling RG, Catlett CL, Huebner KD, et al. Threats in bioterrorism I: CDC category A agents. *Emerg Med Clin N Am* 2002;20:273-309.

Franz DR, Jahrling PB, Friedlander AM, et al. Clinical recognition and management of patients exposed to biological warfare agents. *JAMA* 1997;278:300-411.

Greenfield RA, Brown BR, Hutchins JB, et al. Microbiological, biological, and chemical weapons of warfare and terrorism. *Am J Med Sci* 2002;323:326-340.

Hayes DP, Marrese M. Chemical-biological warfare: Medical logistics and defense. *Mil Med* 1991;156:321-327.

Henretig FM, Cieslak TJ, Kortepeter MG, et al. Medical management of a suspected victim of bioterrorism: An algorithmic approach to the undifferentiated patient. *Emerg Med Clin N Am* 2002;20:351-364.

Holloway HC, Norwood AE, Fullerton CS, et al. The threat of biological weapons: Prophylaxis and mitigation of psychological consequences. *JAMA* 1997;278:425-427.

Kolavic SA, Kimura A, Simons SL, et al. An outbreak of Shigella dysenteriae type 2 among laboratory workers due to intentional food contamination. *JAMA* 1997;278:396-398.

Kortepeter MG, Parker GW. Potential biological weapons threats. *Emerging Infect Dis* 1999;5:523-527.

McGovern TW, Christopher GW, Eitzen EM. Cutaneous manifestations of biological warfare and related threat agents. *Arch Dermatol* 1999;135:311-322.

Moran GJ. Threats in bioterrorism II: CDC category B and C agents. *Emerg Med Clin N Am* 2002;20:311-330.

Pavlin Ja, Gilchrist MJR, Osweiler GD, et al. Diagnostic analyses of biological agent-caused syndromes: Laboratory and technical assistance. *Emerg Med Clin N Am* 2002;20:331-350.

White SR, Henretig FM, Dukes RG. Medical management of vulnerable populations and co-morbid conditions of victims of bioterrorism. *Emerg Med Clin N Am* 2002;20:365-392.

Anthrax

Anon. Recognition of illness associated with the intentional release of a biologic agent. *MMWR* 2001;50:893-897.

Barakat LA, Quentzel HL, Jernigan JA, et al. Fatal inhalational anthrax in a 94-year-old Connecticut woman. *JAMA* 2002;287;863-868.

Bartlett JG. Applying lessons learned from anthrax case history to other scenarios. *Emerging Infect Dis* 1999;5:561-565.

Borio L, Frank D, Venkat M, et al. Death due to bioterrorism-related inhalational anthrax. *JAMA* 2002;287:2554-2559.

Borio LO, Inglesby T, Peters CJ, et al. Hemorrhagic fever viruses as biological weapons: Medical and public health management. *JAMA* 2002;2391-2405.

Bush LM, Abrams BH, Beall A, et al. Index case of fatal inhalational anthrax due to bioterrorism in the United States. *N Engl J Med* 2001;345:1607-1610.

Cieslak TJ, Eitzen EM. Clinical and epidemiologic principles of anthrax. *Emerging Infect Dis* 1999;5:552-560.

Freedman A, Olubunmi A, Chang MW, et al. Cutaneous anthrax associated with microangiopathic hemolytic anemia and coagulopathy in a 7-month-old infant. *JAMA* 2002;287:869-874.

Friedlander AM. Anthrax. In: Sidell FR, Takafuji ET, Franz DR, eds. *Textbook of military medicine: Medical aspects of chemical and biological warfare.* Washington, DC: Office of the Surgeon General, 1997:467-475.

Inglesby TV, O'Toole T, Henderson DA, et al. Anthrax as a biological weapon, 2002: Updated recommendations for management. *JAMA* 2002;287:2236-2252.

Kiratisin P, Fukuda CD, Wong A, et al. Large-scale screening of nasal swabs for Bacillus anthracis: Descriptive summary and discussion of the National Institutes of Health's Experience. *J Clin Microbiol* 2002;40:3012-3016.

Mayer TA, Bersoff-Matcha S, Murphy C, et al. Clinical presentation of inhalational anthrax following bioterrorism exposure: Report of 2 surviving patients. *JAMA* 2001;286:2549-2553.

REFERENCES

Mina B, Dym JP, Kuepper F, et al. Fatal inhalational anthrax with unknown source of exposure in a 61-year-old woman in New York City. *JAMA* 2002;287:858-862.

Pile JC, Malone JD, Eitzen EM, et al. Anthrax as a potential biological warfare agent. *Arch Intern Med* 1998;158:429-434.

Plotkin SA, Brachman PS, Utell M, et al. An epidemic of inhalation anthrax, the first of the twentieth century. *Am J Med* 1960;29:992-1001.

Smallpox

Barbera J, Macintyre A, Gostin L, et al. Large-scale quarantine following biological terrorism in the United States: Scientific examination, logistic and legal limits, and possible consequences. *JAMA* 2001;286:2711-2717.

Bardi J. Aftermath of a hypothetical smallpox disaster. *Emerging Infect Dis* 1999;5:547-551.

Boylston AW. Clinical investigation of smallpox in 1767. *N Engl J Med* 2002;346:1326-1328.

Breman JG, Henderson DA. Current concepts: Diagnosis and management of smallpox. *N Engl J Med* 2002;346:1300-1308.

Dworetzky M. Smallpox, October 1945. *N Engl J Med* 2002;346:1329.

Frey SE, Couch RB, Tacket CO, et al. Clinical responses to undiluted and diluted smallpox vaccine. *N Engl J Med* 2002;346:1265-1274.

Frey SE, Newman FK, Cruz J, et al. Dose-related effects of smallpox vaccine. *N Engl J Med* 2002;346:1275-1280.

Gani R, Leach S. Transmission potential of smallpox in contemporary populations. *Nature* 2001;414:748-751.

Henderson DA, Fenner F. Recent events and observations pertaining to smallpox virus destruction in 2002. *Clin Infect Dis* 2001;33:1057-1059.

Henderson DA, Inglesby TV, Bartlett JG, et al. Smallpox as a biological weapon: Medical and public health management. *JAMA* 1999;281:2127-2137.

Henderson DA. Smallpox: Clinical and epidemiologic features. *Emerging Infect Dis* 1999;5:537-539.

Inglesby TV, Dennis DT, Henderson DA, et al. Plague as a biological weapon: Medical and public health management. *JAMA* 2000;283:2281-2290.

Meltzer MI, Damon I, LeDuc JW, et al. Modeling potential responses to smallpox as a bioterrorist weapon. *Emerging Infect Dis* 2001;7:959-969.

O'Toole T. Smallpox: An attack scenario. *Emerging Infect Dis* 1999;5:540-546.

Plague

Inglesby TV, Dennis DT, Henderson DA, et al. Plague as a biological weapon. *JAMA* 2000;283:2281-2290.

Tularemia

Dennis DT, Inglesby TV, Henderson DA, et al. Tularemia as a biological weapon. *JAMA* 2001;285:2763-2773.

Botulism

Arnon SS, Schechter R, Inglesby TV, et al. Botulinum toxin as a biological weapon: Medical and public health management. *JAMA* 2001;285:1059-1070.

Hemorrhagic Viral Fevers

Borio LO, Inglesby T, Peters CJ, et al. Hemorrhagic fever viruses as biological weapons: Medical and public health management. *JAMA* 2002;2391-2405.

Vaccines

Albert MR, Ostheimer KG, Breman JG. The last smallpox epidemic in Boston and the vaccination controversy, 1901-1903. *N Engl J Med* 2001;344:375-379.

Benitez JG, Swanson-Biearman B, Krenzelok EP. Nystagmus secondary to fomepizole administration in a pediatric patient. *J Toxicol Clin Toxicol* 2000;38:795-798.

Bicknell WJ. The case for voluntary smallpox vaccination. *N Engl J Med* 2002;346:1323-1325.

Fauci AS. Smallpox vaccination policy—the need for dialogue. *N Engl J Med* 2002;346:1319-1320.

Frey SE, Couch RB, Tacket CO, et al. Clinical responses to undiluted and diluted smallpox vaccine. *N Engl J Med* 2002;346:1265-1274.

Frey SE, Newman FK, Cruz J, et al. Dose-related effects of smallpox vaccine. *N Engl J Med* 2002;346:1275-1280.

Friedlander AM, Pittman PR, Parker GW. Anthax vaccine: Evidence for safety and efficacy against inhalational anthrax. *JAMA* 1999;282:2104-2106.

Glass IA, Schoch-Spana M. Bioterrorism and the people. How to vaccine a city against panic. *Clin Infect Dis* 2002;34:217-223.

Kaplan EH, Craft DL, Wein LM. Emergency response to a smallpox attack: The case for mass vaccination. *Proc Natl Acad Sci USA* 2002;99:10935-10940.

REFERENCES

LeDuc JW, Jahrling PB. Strengthening national preparedness for smallpox: An update. Emerging Infect Dis 2001;7(1): http://www.medscape.com/viewarticle/414345 (accessed May 31, 2002).

Nierengarten MB, Lutwick LI. Developing new tularemia vaccines. Medscape Infect Dis 2002;4(1): http://www.medscape.com/viewarticle/431539 (accessed April 23, 2002).

Rosenthal SR, Merchlinsky M, Kleppinger C, et al. Developing new smallpox vaccines. *Emerging Infect Dis* 2001;7:920-926.

Russell PK. Vaccines in civilian defense against bioterrorism. *Emerging Infect Dis* 1999;5:531-533.

Strom BL, Barlow WE, Blazer DG, et al. The anthrax vaccine: Is it safe? Does it work? Institute of Medicine. http://www.iom.edu/iom/iomhome.nsf/WFiles/Anthrax-8-pager1FINAL/$file/Anthrax-8-pager1FINAL.pdf (accessed September 12, 2002).

Wiesen AR, Littell CT. Relationship between prepregnancy anthrax vaccination and pregnancy and birth outcomes among US Army women. *JAMA* 2002;287:1556-1560.

Zoon KC. Vaccines, pharmaceutical products and bioterrorism: Challenges for the US Food and Drug Administration. *Emerging Infect Dis* 1999;5:534-539.

CHEMICAL AGENTS

Aasted A, Dane E, Wilf HC. Mustard gas: Clinical, toxicological and mutagenic aspects based on modern experience. *Ann Plast Surg* 1987;19:330-333.

Amitai Y, Almog S, Singer R, et al. Atropine poisoning in children during the Persian Gulf crisis. *JAMA* 1992;268:630-632.

Borak J. Diller WF. Phosgene exposure: Mechanisms of injury and treatment strategies. *J Occup Environ Med* 2000;43:110-119.

Brennan RJ, Waeckerle JF, Sharp TW, et al. Chemical warfare agents: Emergency medical and emergency public health issues. *Ann Emerg Med* 1999;34:191-204.

Diller WF. Medical phosgene problems and their possible solution. *J Occup Med* 1978;20:189-193.

Evison D, Hinsley D, Rice P. Chemical weapons. *Br Med J* 2002;324:332-335.

Greenfield RA, Brown BR, Hutchins JB, et al. Microbiological, biological, and chemical weapons of warfare and terrorism. *Am J Med Sci* 2002;323:326-340.

Hayes DP, Marrese M. Chemical-biological warfare: Medical logistics and defense. *Mil Med* 1991;156:3231-3327.

Hu H, Fine J, Epstein P, et al. Tear gas-harassing agent of toxic chemical weapon. *JAMA* 1989;262:660-663.

Kadivar H, Adams SC. Treatment of chemical and biological warfare injuries: Insights derived from the 1984 Iraqi attack on Majnoon Island. *Mil Med* 1991;156:171-177.

Mccafferty RR, Lennarson PJ. Common chemical threats. *Neurosurg Focus* 2002;12(3): http://www.medscape.com/viewarticle/431312 (accessed May 13, 2002).

Morita H, Yanagisaw N, Nakajima T, et al. Sarin poisoning in Matsumoto Japan. *Lancet* 1995;346:290-293.

Nakajima T, Sato S, Morita H, et al. Sarin poisoning of a rescue team in Matsumoto sarin incident in Japan. *Occup Environ Med* 1997;54:697-701.

Nazaki H, Hari S, Shinonzawa Y, et al. Secondary exposure in medical staff to sarin vapor in the emergency room. *Intensive Care Med* 1995;21:1032-1035.

Ruhl C, Park SJ, Danisa O, et al. A serious sulfur mustard burn from an artillery shell. *J Emerg Med* 1994;12:159-166.

Sidell FR, Borak J. Agents of chemical warfare: Sulfur mustard. *Ann Emerg Med* 1992;21:303-308.

Sidell FR, Borak J. Chemical warfare agents: II. Nerve agents. *Ann Emerg Med* 1992;21:865-871.

Sidell FR. Chemical agent terrorism. *Ann Emerg Med* 1996;28:223-224.

Sidell FR. Chemical agent terrorism. http://www.nbc-med.org/SiteContent/MedRef/OnlineRef/Other/chagter.html (accessed February 14, 2002).

Sidell FR. What to do in case of an unthinkable chemical warfare attack or accident. *Postgrad Med* 1990;88:70-84.

Smith KJ, Hurst CG, Moeller RB, et al. Sulfur mustard: Its continuing threat as a chemical warfare agent, the cutaneous lesions induced, progress in understanding its mechanism of action, its long-term health effects and new developments for protection and therapy. *J Am Acad Dermatol* 1995;32:765-776.

Smith PR. Terrorism awareness: Weapons of mass destruction: Part I, chemical agents. Internet J Rescue Disaster Med 2000: http://www.ispub.com/journals/IJRDM/Vol2N1/terror1-a.html (accessed February 14, 2002).

REFERENCES

PREPAREDNESS PLANNING

Anon. Preparing for terrorism: Tools for evaluating the Metropolitan Medical Response System Program (2002). National Academy Press. http://www.nap.edu/books/0309084288/html (accessed August 21, 2002).

Bandyopadhyay K. The role of business impact analysis and testing in disaster recovery planning by health maintenance organizations. *Hosp Topics* 2001;79:16-22.

Bernardo LM, Kapsar P. Disaster preparedness at the University of Pittsburgh School of Nursing: Application of Haddon's 10 countermeasures to assess and plan. *Disaster Manage Response* 2002;1:18-20.

Burgess JL, Kirk M, Borron SW, et al. Emergency department hazardous materials protocol for contaminated patients. *Ann Emerg Med* 1999;34:205-212.

Burkle FM. Mass casualty management of a large-scale bioterrorist event: An epidemiological approach that shapes triage decisions. *Emerg Med Clin N Am* 2002;20:409-436.

California Department of Health Services. California hospital bioterrorism response planning guide. 2001.

Center for Civilian Biodefense Studies. Recommended actions for medicine and public health in the aftermath of anthrax attacks of 2001. http://www.hopkins-biodefense.org/interim.html (accessed August 18, 2002).

Clark D, Daniell WE, Treser CD. Hospital preparedness for victims of chemical and biological terrorism. *Am J Public Health* 2001;91:710-716.

Cutlip K. Strengthening the system: Joint Commission standards and building on what we know. *Hosp Topics* 2002;80:24-28.

Fee E, Brown TM. Preemptive biopreparedness: Can we learn anything from history? *Am J Public Health* 2001;91;721-726.

Flowers LK, Mothershead JL, Blackwell TH. Bioterrorism preparedness II: The community and emergency medical services systems. *Emerg Med Clin N Am* 2002;20:457-476.

Geiger HJ. Terrorism, biological weapons and bonanzas: Assessing the real threat to public health. *Am J Public Health* 2001;91:708-709.

Gerberding JL, Hughes JM, Koplan JP. Bioterrorism preparedness and response: Clinicians and public health agencies as essential partners. *JAMA* 2002;287:898-900.

Gostin LO, Sapsin JW, Teret SP, et al. The Model State Emergency Health Powers Act: Planning for and response to bioterrorism and naturally occurring infectious diseases. *JAMA* 2002;288:622-628.

Helget V, Smith PW. Bioterrorism preparedness: A survey of Nebraska health care institutions. *Am J Infect Control* 2002;30:46-48.

Henretig F. Biological and chemical terrorism defense: A view from the "front lines" of public health. *Am J Public Health* 2001;91:718-720.

Holloway HC, Norwood AE, Fullerton CS, et al. The threat of biological weapons: Prophylaxis and mitigation of psychological and social consequences. *JAMA* 1997;278:425-427.

Infectious Disease Society of America. IDSA and bioterrorism preparedness. http://www.idsociety.org/PA/PS&P/BT_Preparedness_10-2-01.htm (accessed August 18, 2002).

Inglesby TV, O'Toole T, Henderson DA. Preventing the use of biological weapons: Improving response should prevention fail. *Clin Infect Dis* 2000;30:926-929.

Joint Commission. Backup communications needed during disaster. http://www.jcrinc.com/subscribers/perspectives.asp?durki=2525 (accessed August 18, 2002).

Joint Commission. Developing practical emergency: Preparing staff to respond to crisis. http://www.jcrinc.com/subscribers/perspectives.asp?durki=2520&site=10&return=1122 (accessed August 18, 2002).

Joint Commission. Managing people and resources: Transportation, security and volunteers. http://www.jcrinc.com/subscribers/perspectives.asp?durki=2523 (accessed August 18, 2002).

Joint Commission. Nuclear, biological and chemical: Checklist for bioterrorism preparedness. http://www.jcrinc.com/subscribers/perspectives.asp?durki=2527 (accessed August 18, 2002).

Joint Commission. Plan your response for common risks. http://www.jcrinc.com/subscribers/perspectives.asp?durki=2521&site=10&return=1122 (accessed August 18, 2002).

Joint Commission. Preparing your organization for any emergency. http://www.jcrinc.com/subscribers/perspectives.asp?durki=2517&site=10&return=1122 (accessed August 18, 2002).

REFERENCES

Joint Commission. Using JCAHO standards as a starting point: A comprehensive approach to emergency management. http://www.jcrinc.com/subscribers/perspectives. asp?durki=2541&site=10&return=1122 (accessed August 18, 2002).

Joint Commission. When code yellow is no longer a drill. http://www.jcrinc.com/subscribers/perspectives.asp?durki =2524 (accessed August 18, 2002).

Jones J, Terndrup TE, Franz DR, et al. Future challenges in preparing for and responding to bioterrorism events. *Emerg Clin N Am* 2002;20:501-524.

Keim M, Kaufmann AF. Principles for emergency response to bioterrorism. *Ann Emerg Med* 1999;34:177-182.

Khan AS, Ashford DA. Ready or not-preparedness for bioterrorism. *N Engl J Med* 2001;345:287-289.

Khan AS, Sage MJ. Biological and chemical terrorism: Strategic plan for preparedness and response. *MMWR* 2000;49(RR04):1-14.

Kvetan V. Critical care medicine, terrorism and disasters: Are we ready? *Crit Care Med* 1999;27:873-874.

Mair JS, Sapsin J, Teret S. The Model State Emergency Health Powers Act and beyond. Biodefense Quarterly 2002;3(4): http/www.hopkins-biodefense.org/pages/ news/quarter.html (accessed August 12, 2002).

Mothershead JL, Tonat K, Koenig KL. Bioterrorism preparedness III: State and federal programs and response. *Emerg Med Clin N Am* 2002;20:477-500.

Okumura T, Suzuki K, Fukuda A, et al. The Tokyo subway sarin attack: Disaster Management, part 1. *Acad Emerg Med* 1998;5:613-617.

Okumura T, Suzuki K, Fukuda A, et al. The Tokyo subway sarin attack: Disaster Management, part 2. *Acad Emerg Med* 1998;5:618-624.

Okumura T, Suzuki K, Fukuda A, et al. The Tokyo subway sarin attack: Disaster Management, part 3. *Acad Emerg Med* 1998;5:625-628.

Pesik N, Keim ME, Iserson KV. Terrorism and the ethics of emergency medical care. *Ann Emerg Med* 2001;37:642-646.

Relman DA, Olson JE. Bioterrorism preparedness: What practitioners need to know. *Infect Med* 2001;18:497-515.

Richards CF, Burstein JL, Waeckerle JF, et al. Emergency physicians and biological terrorism. *Ann Emerg Med* 1999;34:183-190.

Schultz CH, Mothershead JL, Field M. Bioterrorism preparedness I: The emergency department and hospital. *Emerg Med Clin N Am* 2002;20:437-455.

Shapira Y, Bar Y, Beerkenstadt H, et al. Outline of hospital organization for a chemical warfare attack. *Isr J Med Sci* 1991;27:616-622.

Sharp TW, Brennan RJ, Keim M, et al. Medical preparedness for a terrorist incident involving chemical or biological agents during the 1996 Atlanta Olympic Games. *Ann Emerg Med* 1998;32:214-223.

Sidell VW, Cohen HW, Gould RM. Good intentions and the road to bioterrorism preparedness. *Am J Public Health* 2001;91:716-719.

Simon JD. Biological terrorism: Preparing to meet the threat. *JAMA* 1997;278:428-430.

Stephens E. EMS and terrorism. *e Medicine J* 2001;2(9): http://www.emedicine.com/emerg/topic 712.htm (accessed February 2, 2002).

Stopford BM. Responding to the threat of bioterrorism: Practical resources and references, and the importance of preparation. *J Emerg Nurs* 2001;27:471-475.

Treat KN, Williams JM, Furbee PM, et al. Hospital preparedness for weapons of mass destruction incidents: An initial assessment. *Ann Emerg Med* 2001;38:562-565.

Tucker JB. National health and medical services response to incidents of chemical and biological terrorism. *JAMA* 1997;278;362-368.

Tur-Kaspa I, Lev EI, Hendler I, et al. Preparing hospitals for toxicological mass casualties events. *Crit Care Med* 1999;27:1004-1008.

Voelker R. Bioweapons preparedness chief discusses priorities in world of 21st century biology. *JAMA* 2002;287:573-575.

Waeckerle JF. Domestic preparedness for events involving weapons of mass destruction. *JAMA* 2000;283:252-254.

POSTEVENT LEARNING

Bardi J. Aftermath of a hypothetical smallpox disaster. *Emerging Infect Dis* 1999;5:547-551.

Bartlett JG. Applying lessons learned from anthrax case history to other scenarios. *Emerging Infect Dis* 1999;5:561-563.

REFERENCES

Benedek DM, Holloway HC, Becker SM. Emergency mental health management in bioterrorism events. *Emerg Med Clin N Am* 2002;20:393-407.

Fine A, Layton M. Lessons from the West Nile viral encephalitis outbreak in New York City, 1999: Implications for bioterrorism preparedness. *Clin Infect Dis* 2001;32:277-282.

Inglesby TV, Grossman R, O'Toole T. A plague on your city: Observations from TOPOFF. *Clin Infect Dis* 2001;32:436-445.

Inglesby TV. Anthrax: A possible case history. *Emerging Infect Dis* 1999;5:556-560.

Long AE. Crisis and recovery: Lessons in readiness on bioterrorism's front lines. *Healthplan* 2002;434:20-24.

Mitchell AM, Sakraida TJ, Kameg K. Overview of post-traumatic stress. *Disaster Manage Response* 2002;1:10-14.

Schoch-Spana M. Implications of pandemic influenza for bioterrorism response. *Clin Infect Dis* 2000;31:1409-1413.

Schuster MA, Stein BD, Jaycox LH. A national survey of stress reactions after the September 11, 2001, terrorist attacks. *N Engl J Med* 2001;345:1507-1512.

Silver RC, Holman A, McIntosh DN, et al. Nationwide longitudinal study of psychological responses to September 11. *JAMA* 2002;288:1235-1244.

SURVEILLANCE/COMMUNICATIONS

Barthell EN, Cordell WN, Moorhead JC, et al. The frontlines of medicine project: A proposal for the standardized communication of emergency department data for public health uses including syndromic surveillance for biological and chemical terrorism. *Ann Emerg Med* 2002;39:422-429.

Castrodale L, Beller M, Jenkerson SA, et al. Using e-mail to investigate outbreaks. *West J Med* 2002;176:181-183.

Garshnek V, Burkle FM. Telecommunications systems in support of disaster medicine. *Ann Emerg Med* 1999;34:213-218.

Mrvos R, Krenzelok EP. Poison Center Surveillance for bio-chem terrorism. *J Toxicol Clin Toxicol* 2002;40:638.

Shapiro RL, Hatheway C, Becher J, et al. Botulism and emergency response: A public health strategy for a global challenge. *JAMA* 1997;278:433-435.

Talan DA, Moran GJ, Mower MR, et al. *EMERGE*ncy ID NET: An emergency department-based emerging infections sentinel network. *Ann Emerg Med* 1998;32:703-711.

Zeng X, Wagner MM, Mrvos R, et al. Certified specialists in poison information as investigators of epidemics. *J Toxicol Clin Toxicol* 2002;40:639.

BOOKS

Alibek K, Handelman S. *Biohazard: The chilling true story of the largest covert biological weapons program in the world, told from the inside by the man who ran it.* New York: Random House, 1999.

Anon. *Chem-bio: frequently asked questions: guide to better understanding chem-bio.* Alexandria, VA: Tempest Publishing, 1998.

Bartlett JG. *Bioterrorism and public health: An Internet resource guide.* Montvale, NJ: Thomson Medical Economics, 2002.

Croddy E, Perez-Armandariz C, Hart J. *Chemical and biological warfare: A common-sense guide for the concerned citizen.* New York: Copernicus, 2002.

Dando M, Pearson GS, Kriz B, North Atlantic Treaty Organization. Scientific Affairs Division. *Scientific and technical means of distinguishing between natural and other outbreaks of disease.* Dordrech, The Netherlands; Boston: Kluwer Academic Publishers, 2001.

Eberhart-Phillips J. *Outbreak alert: responding to the increasing threat of infectious diseases.* Oakland, CA: New Harbinger Publications, 2000.

Eitzen E, Pavlin J, Cieslak T, Christopher G, Culpepper R, eds. *Medical management of biological casualties handbook,* 4th ed. Fort Detrick, MD: US Army Medical Research Institute of Infectious Diseases, 2001.

Ellison DH. *Handbook of chemical and biological warfare agents.* Boca Raton: CRC Press, 2000.

Frist WH. *When every moment counts: What you need to know about bioterrorism from the Senate's only doctor.* Lanham, MD: Rowman & Littlefield Publishers, 2002.

Guillemin J. *Anthrax: The investigation of a deadly outbreak.* Berkeley: University of California Press, 1999.

Hilborne LH, Marshall GN, Spektor DM, Rettig RA, Golomb BA, Augerson WS, Cecchine G; U.S. Department of Defense, Office of the Secretary of Defense; and National Defense Research Institute (U.S.). *A review of the scientific literature as it pertains to Gulf War illnesses.* Santa Monica, CA: Rand, 1998.

REFERENCES

Institute of Medicine. *Biological threats and bioterrorism: Assessing the science and response capabilities—workshop summary.* Washington, DC: National Academy Press, 2002.

Marrs TC, Maynard RL, Sidell FR. *Chemical warfare agents: toxicology and treatment.* Chichester, NY: Wiley, 1996.

McEvoy GK, ed. *AHFS DI bioterrorism resource manual.* Bethesda, MD: American Society of Health-System Pharmacists, 2002.

Sidell FR, Takafuji ET, Franz DR, eds. *Textbook of military medicine: Medical aspects of chemical and biological warfare.* Washington, DC: Office of the Surgeon General, 1997.

Sidell, FR, Patrick WC, Dashiell TR. *Jane's chem-bio handbook.* Alexandria, VA: Jane's Information Group, 2000.

Sifton, DW. *PDR® guide to biological and chemical warfare response.* Montvale, NJ: Thomson/Physicians' Desk Reference, 2002.

Somani SM, Romano JA. *Chemical warfare agents: Toxicity at low levels.* Boca Raton: CRC Press, 2001.

Tucker JB. *Toxic terror: Assessing terrorist use of chemical and biological weapons.* Cambridge, MA: MIT Press, 2000.

U.S. Army Medical Research Institute of Chemical Defense, Chemical Casualty Care Division. *Medical management of chemical casualties handbook,* 3rd ed. Aberdeen Proving Ground–Edgewood Area, MD, 1998.

World Health Organization. *Public health response to biological and chemical weapons—WHO guidance.* Geneva, 2001.

INTERNET RESOURCES

American Academy of Family Physicians. Btresponse.org. http://www.btresponse.org/ (accessed September 17, 2002).

American Association of Health-System Pharmacists. Emergency Preparedness-Counterterrorism Resource Center. http://www.ashp.org/public/proad/emergency/em_prep.html (accessed August 19, 2002).

American College of Physicians—American Society of Internal Medicine. *Bioterrorism resources.* http://www.acponline.org/bioterro/ (accessed September 17, 2002).

American Hospital Association. *Chemical and bioterrorism preparedness checklist.* http://www.aha.org/Emergency/Content/MaAtChecklistB1003.doc (accessed on August 21, 2002).

American Medical Association. *Disaster preparedness and medical response.* http://www.ama-assn.org/ama/pub/category/6206.html (accessed September 17, 2002).

American Pharmaceutical Association Pharmacist Response Center. http://www.aphanet.org/pharmcare/ResponseCenter.htm (accessed September 17, 2002).

Anthrax Vaccine Immunization Program. http://www.anthrax.osd.mil/ (accessed September 17, 2002).

Association for Professionals in Infection Control and Epidemiology, Inc. *Bioterrorism resources.* http://www.apic.org/bioterror/ (accessed August 18, 2002).

Centers for Disease Control. *Public health preparedness and emergency response.* http://www.bt.cdc.gov/Agent/Agentlist.asp (accessed September 17, 2002).

Chemical and Biological Defense Information Analysis Center. http://www.cbiac.apgea.army.mil/ (accessed September 17, 2002).

Emergency Response and Research Institute, Inc. Emergency.com. http://www.emergency.com/ (accessed September 17, 2002).

Federal Emergency Management Agency. http://www.fema.gov/rris/reflib.htm (accessed September 17, 2002).

Health Sciences & Human Services Library. *Terrorism resources for the health care community.* http://www.hshsl.umaryland.edu/resources/terrorism.html (accessed August 21, 2002).

John Hopkins University, Center for Civilian Biodefense Strategies. http://www.hopkins-biodefense.org/ (accessed August 21, 2002).

Mayo Clinic.com. *Biological, chemical weapons: Arm yourself with information.* http://www.mayoclinic.com/invoke.cfm?id=MH00027 (accessed August 19, 2002).

McGraw-Hill: Access Medicine. *Bioterrorism watch.* http://www.harrisononline.com/amed/public/amed_news/news_article/281.htm. (accessed August 21, 2002).

Medical NBC Online Information Server. http://www.nbc-med.org/SiteContent/main.asp (accessed August 21, 2002).

REFERENCES

Monterey Institute of International Studies. *Chemical and biological weapons resource page.* http://www.cns.miis.edu/research/cbw/cbterror.htm (accessed September 17, 2002).

National Association of County and City Health Officials. *Bioterrorism and emergency response program.* http://www.naccho.org/project63.cfm (accessed September 17, 2002).

National Center for Complementary and Alternative Medicine. *Bioterrorism and CAM: What the public needs to know.* http://nccam.nih.gov/health/alerts/bioterrorism/ (accessed August 19, 2002).

National Library of Medicine–Medline Plus. *Disaster and emergency preparedness.* http://www.nlm.nih.gov/medlineplus/disastersandemergencypreparedness.html (accessed September 17, 2002).

San Francisco Department of Public Health. *Educational resources for bioterrorism preparedness.* http://www.healthysf.org/pharmacy/education/ (accessed August 21, 2002).

The National Academies. *Responding first to bioterrorism.* http://bob.nap.edu/shelves/first/ (accessed August 21, 2002).

The New England Journal of Medicine. *Smallpox and smallpox vaccination.* http://nejm.org/earlyrelease/index.asp (accessed August 21, 2002).

United States Army Research Institute of Chemical Defense. http://chemdef.apgea.army.mil/ (accessed September 17, 2002).

UPMC Health System. *Coping with terrorism.* http://www.coping.upmc.com (accessed September 17, 2002).

U.S. Army Soldier and Biological and Chemical Command. http://www.sbccom.army.mil/ (accessed September 17, 2002).

U.S. Food and Drug Administration. *Bioterrorism.* http://www.fda.gov/oc/opacom/hottopics/bioterrorism.html (accessed September 17, 2002).

USAMRIID. *Medical management of biological casualties handbook.* http://www.usamriid.army.mil/education/bluebook.html (accessed September 17, 2002).

World Health Organization. *Communicable disease surveillance and response.* http://www.who.int/emc/index.html (accessed September 17, 2002).

SECTION **FOUR**

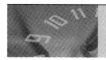 Hospital Pharmacy Preparedness

INTRODUCTION

There is a general consensus that America's hospitals may be the weakest link in the preparedness for biological and chemical terrorism. Many hospitals have not considered the need to work cooperatively with local, state, and federal anti-terrorism planners, nor are they prepared to respond to the needs of several hundred patients who may appear in the aftermath of a terrorist event. These oversights illustrate the need for health care professionals, including all pharmacists across the continuum of pharmaceutical care, to develop terrorism preparedness response plans to address the immediate questions that may arise as the consequence of a biological or chemical terrorism incident. Such questions include whether there is/are:

- Ample bed space?
- Sufficient staff?
- Adequate decontamination facilities?
- Protective clothing for health care providers?
- Sufficient medications, including antidotes and antibiotics?
- Adequate medical supplies (e.g., dressings, ventilators)?
- A plan to treat the family members of hospital staff?
- Adequate security?
- Triage and treatment guidelines?
- An established chain of command?
- Open communication channels within the hospital and with local officials?

- Redundant communication technology (e.g., radios, cell phones, fax machines)?
- Staff who understand biological and chemical terrorism agents?
- Places where patients can be quarantined?
- A designated temporary morgue?
- Fact sheets for patients?
- Access to interpreters (especially in highly populated urban areas)?

In the wake of the terrorism events of the last decade, hospitals have been challenged and face even more significant challenges as the threat of terrorism continues to grow. This was exemplified by the surge of over 5,500 patients who presented to Tokyo hospitals after the release of sarin gas in the subway system: the hospitals were unprepared, and the surge capacity of the hospitals was overwhelmed.[1] Even superb preparedness would be tested under this type of circumstance. However, the potential for mass casualties is very real, and every hospital and health care facility must be prepared to deal with challenges that exceed its capabilities. Proactive preparedness will allow for optimal reaction when a terrorism event occurs and the number of patients threatens to overwhelm a hospital's capabilities. Rapid and appropriate response to a terrorism event will limit morbidity and mortality and reduce the event's economic impact on the community, institution, and pharmacy.

Every hospital must develop a terrorism preparedness plan that addresses a number of issues, including the questions posed above. The overall hospital preparedness strategy must include a plan from every department that encompasses issues common to the hospital plan and specific to each department in support of the hospital and the patients it will manage. While every department has an important role to play in the success of a hospital plan, the pharmacy plan is critical to the successful implementation of a hospital's biological and chemical terrorism preparedness plan. However, hospitals and pharmacy

departments are but one component of the emergency response to a biological or chemical terrorism event. It is critical for the hospital to integrate its emergency preparedness plans with those of local, state, and federal authorities and other health care entities to prevent unnecessary duplication of effort and expense and, most important, to insure that patients will receive optimal care.

The importance of the pharmacy and pharmacists in terrorism preparedness was recognized by the American Society of Health-System Pharmacists (ASHP) Executive Session on Emergency Preparedness and the Pharmaceutical Supply Chain:[2]

> Responsibility for responding to homeland terrorist attacks and other emergencies begins at the local level and is grounded in collaboration between private and public sectors. Effective response also requires the cooperation of individual health care professionals at the local level. Among those professionals whose participation is vital are pharmacists. . . .

The ASHP position statement emphasizes local initiatives, cooperation, and the vital role of the pharmacist. Cooperation during the response to a terrorism event is essential. However, cooperation may be difficult to achieve without preparedness planning. It is critical that the pharmacy be a leader within its own institution. Equally important is preparedness planning with entities outside the institution. At a minimum, the pharmacy leadership must know about local, regional, state, and national terrorism preparedness. Traditionally, pharmacists have had little participation in planning preparedness activities external to their own institution.[3] The preferred course of action is to become better prepared, especially by participating in local and regional preparedness. This level of participation will insure that the pharmacy leadership is aware of both state and national preparedness and response capabilities and responsibilities. Involvement in institutional, local, and regional preparedness planning will formalize relationships and facilitate collegial cooperation.

The day of a disaster should not be the first time that individuals who are essential to patient care meet and exchange business cards. Developing professional relationships prior to a terrorist event is key to the successful mitigation of the crisis.

Pharmacist participation in local and regional planning is a mutually beneficial experience. Pharmacists will learn new roles and become more cognizant of the threats posed by biological and chemical terrorism. Colleagues across all aspects of emergency planning and response will realize that pharmacists possess a complex skill set and should be thought of as pharmaceutical care professionals, not merely the purveyors of physical responsibilities such as storing and dispensing medications.

Preparedness: A Tiered Response

Local response will be the key to reducing the morbidity and mortality associated with a biological or chemical terrorist event. The federal government will not be in a position to render support in the immediate postevent period. Thousands of victims may overwhelm a region's health care system. The potential magnitude of the problem is incomprehensible. The impact of a wide-scale biological or chemical terrorism incident may make the response to other disasters seem small by comparison. Pharmacists may be responsible for caring for the needs of hundreds of patients for 24 to 48 hours until federal resources can be mobilized. This reinforces the importance of having well-conceived pharmacy, hospital, and local/regional preparedness plans. However, understanding the hierarchy of preparedness is critical to disaster planning.

Federal Initiatives

The U.S. Office of Emergency Preparedness (OEP) directs the National Disaster Medical System (NDMS), which operates as a partnership between several federal agencies (see Table 4.1) and state and local government.[3] The National Strategy for Homeland Security was developed by the president in early 2002 and includes the current Office of Homeland Security and legislation for the proposed Department of Homeland Security, which will coordinate the terrorism mitigation efforts of the federal government and its many organizations, departments, and divisions.

Table 4.1 Federal Agency Partners in the NDMS

- Department of Health and Human Services
  - Centers for Disease Control (CDC)
  - National Pharmaceutical Stockpile Program (NPSP)
- Department of Veterans Affairs
- Department of Defense
- Federal Emergency Management Agency

National Pharmaceutical Stockpile Program

Each federal agency has specific responsibilities in responding to biological or chemical terrorism. For example, the Centers for Disease Control (CDC), a division within the Department of Health and Human Services, is charged with the administration of the National Pharmaceutical Stockpile Program (NPS). The mission of the NPS is to insure the availability of lifesaving pharmaceuticals, antidotes, and other medical supplies and equipment necessary to counter the effects of biological and chemical agents. The caches of medical supplies are located strategically at multiple sites in the United States and capable of being deployed promptly and delivered to the site of a biological or chemical terrorism incident (or other equivalent major disaster) in all U.S. states and territories within 12 to 24 hours after being summoned by a predesignated official (often the state governor).[3, 4, 5]

A team of CDC advisors designated as the Technical Advisory Response Unit (TARU) will accompany each deployment of the NPS for the purpose of advising local authorities on receiving, distributing, dispensing, replenishing, and recovering unused assets of the NPS. However, the TARU team is purely advisory, and the NPS assets will be transferred to local and state government officials once the NPS arrives at the airport nearest the disaster.

The NPS is positioned throughout the country in environmentally controlled and secure warehouses and stored in shipping containers, referred to as "push packages," that will be dispatched according to need. State and territorial government officials will predesignate nonhospital medication distribution sites (e.g., gymnasiums, convention centers, schools) and have preestablished local teams to distribute NPS contents. Health care facilities are not preferred distribution sites due to their need to provide direct patient care and their physical inability to provide assistance to hundreds, if not thousands, of individuals who may need prophylactic antibiotics instead of emergent care.

Each push package contains 50 tons of material that is designed to meet the needs of a mass casualty incident and includes containers of bulk antibiotics for asymptomatic individuals, medical and surgical supplies (e.g., parenteral fluids, airway supplies, dressings), chemical terrorism medications (e.g., atropine, pralidoxime), vaccines (e.g., for smallpox), and convenient unit-of-use oral antibiotics for prophylaxis against bacterial terrorist agents (e.g., anthrax, plague, tularemia). To assist in the dispensing and distribution of medications, each push pack contains medication packaging machines, tablet-counting machines, and extremely accurate volumetric hand-held devices that will allow manual "scooping" and dispensing of medications from bulk supplies.

However, the delay from the recognition of a terrorist incident to the acquisition of the NPS may exceed 24 hours and necessitates the need for local preparedness. It is not the purpose of the NPS to serve as a distribution resource to restock pharmacy medication inventories. Therefore, it is essential that there is good local planning between and among all health-system pharmacies (e.g., clinic, community, and hospital pharmacies) and drug distributors to insure that optimal supplies of desired pharmaceuticals are available in response to the enhanced demands that a biological or chemical terrorism event may pose. Many pharmacists are under the false impression that they need to stock only minimal quantities of antidotes and antibiotics because of rapid access to the NPS.

National Pharmacists Response Team

The Department of Health and Human Services, in conjunction with the Joint Commission of Pharmacy Practitioners, is working on the establishment of the National Pharmacists Response Team (NPRT).[6] When active, the NPRT will consist of 10 regionally based teams of 200 pharmacists, pharmacy students, and pharmacy technicians that when activated would be called upon to assist with vaccinations and/or distribution of medications. Pharmacists are invited to join, and participation is contingent upon the successful completion of continuing education. Deployed individuals would be:

- Paid as federal civil service employees
- Reimbursed for all expenses
- Protected from medical–legal liability
- Activated for no more than two weeks

While the NPRT is an example of how a pharmacist can become involved nationally and learn a great deal about how to assist in the local and institutional response to a biological or chemical terrorist event, directors of health-system pharmacies may want to restrict the number of staff members who can participate in the NPRT, since their deployment may leave staffing gaps that may compromise a pharmacy's operation.

Local Initiatives

Every municipality in the United States is vulnerable to biological and chemical terrorism. A rural Wisconsin high school basketball game may bring hundreds of individuals into a gymnasium—an ideal venue for a terrorist event. A Monday night NFL football game will be attended by tens of thousands of people and attract a national television audience—another perfect opportunity to affect large numbers of individuals and begin a cascade of fear and terrorism nationally without warning. A Broadway musical convenes hundreds of people and provides another opportunity for terrorists to use biological and chemical agents. Each community, large or small, is vulnerable and every town, city, hospital, health-system pharmacy, and local/regional government must have a terrorism preparedness plan.

Approximately half of the 200 largest metropolitan regions of the United States participate in the federally developed Metropolitan Medical Response System (MMRS).[7] The MMRS is neither a federal agency nor an entity. MMRS is a program that is administered by the OEP to assist communities in the development of a coordinated first-response strategy to any type of terrorism event. The OEP provides grant support to communities that meet established guidelines and performance standards. New agencies are not developed; instead MMRS coordination builds on the existing network of local, county, and state agencies to prepare for a mass casualty event. MMRS coordinates emergency response systems such as ambulances and hospitals, organizes morticians to establish temporary morgues, secures coordination with poison center services, and so forth.

An important function of the MMRS is to develop and implement a plan for securing and storing pharmaceuticals that would be used to treat a portion of the affected population, in addition to those being treated in local hospitals, prior to the arrival of the NPS. Since pharmacists have not been traditional participants in emergency planning, many MMRS bodies have not included a pharmacist on their local pharmaceutical cache committee. However, the input of the pharmacist as a pharmaceutical care specialist is critical to proper decision making with regard to product selection, stability issues, storage concerns, proper dispensing, and responsible fiscal considerations.

Preexisting relationships between pharmacists and drug distribution firms can be taken advantage of to secure the optimal cache for a given community. For example, instead of having a cache located in several sites within a community (waiting for an incident to occur), the cache could be purchased via MMRS and rotated continuously throughout the stock of a regional pharmacy wholesaler to eliminate the inordinate expenses associated with expired medications (e.g., ciprofloxacin).[8] MMRS participation is an excellent way for the pharmacist to become involved in local disaster preparedness planning, to reinvigorate his or her role as a provider of public health, and to have others recognize the inherent value of the pharmacist as a purveyor of pharmaceutical care.

The pharmacist may also become involved in local emergency preparedness planning through participation on the Local Emergency Planning Committee (LEPC). LEPCs are usually a function of county government and local emergency response systems. An easy way to find your LEPC is via the following Website: http://www.lepcinfoexchange.com/lepclists.html#contacts. It is the responsibility of the LEPC to develop an emergency plan to respond to chemical emergencies, such as a hazardous materials spill. The LEPC consists of individuals who represent law enforcement, civil defense, firefighters, first responders, local transportation agencies, hospitals, news media, the local poison information center, community groups, and industry.[9] Based on their education, pharmacists are qualified uniquely to provide valuable expertise to the local LEPC with regard to the toxicity of chemicals and the treatment of overexposure to chemicals.[10] Many LEPC members are MMRS participants or are in some way involved in the planning for and response to biological and chemical terrorism. Therefore, the LEPC provides the pharmacist with another opportunity to learn, share information, and prepare for disasters, some of which may be acts of terrorism.

Developing relationships with local government and law enforcement and public health officials will also allow pharmacists to become aware of syndromic surveillance activities. Intelligence shared with the pharmacy about emerging disease patterns or sentinel events may provide early warning signs that activation of the pharmacy's biological and chemical terrorism preparedness plan is imminent. Advance notice or anticipation of a pending crisis is to the pharmacist's benefit.

Development of a Pharmacy Biological and Chemical Terrorism Preparedness Plan

The contemporary medical literature contains hundreds of papers that describe emergency preparedness for general disasters, hazardous materials incidents, and nuclear, biological, and chemical terrorism. The pharmacy literature has a limited number of papers that address the topic of disaster preparedness and more specifically terrorism preparedness.[2, 3, 10–33] Most of the key pharmacy-related papers have been published in the *American Journal of Health-System Pharmacy (AJHP)* and are reproduced in their entirety in this book. The *AJHP* papers provide an excellent foundation for the development of a comprehensive biological and chemical terrorism pharmacy preparedness plan. While biological and chemical terrorism have unique features, the principles associated with general disaster preparedness planning can be applied to the preparation for a biological or chemical terrorism incident. Therefore, biological and chemical terrorism preparedness could be one aspect of a pharmacy's general disaster plan. This approach may temper the daunting task of developing yet another disaster plan.

Traditional disasters such as hurricanes, tornadoes, hazardous materials incidents, plane crashes, and anticipated technology crises (e.g., Y2K) may be used as models to develop terrorism preparedness plans.[10, 28, 29] A number of authors have proposed templates for developing a preparedness plan. Augustine recommended the following approach:[34]

- Avoid the crisis
- Prepare to manage the crisis
- Contain the crisis
- Resolve the crisis
- Profit from the crisis

Pearson and colleagues, in their paper entitled "Managing the Unthinkable," indicated that each disaster has five phases:[35]

- Signal detection
- Preparation
- Damage containment
- Recovery
- Learning

Johnston and Stepanovich identified four criteria associated with a crisis and how they relate to pharmacy practice.[11] They stated that disasters have low probability, high impact, ambiguity, and the necessity to resolve the problem expeditiously. Three key features were identified as critical to the crisis management process:

- Planning: What to do; how to avoid, prevent or lessen the crisis
- Acting: What to do in the midst of a crisis
- Learning: What to do afterwards to enhance crisis management

Preparation, action, and learning are common to all three approaches to crisis management. However, learning from experience stimulates improvement of both the planning and acting phases and is an important aspect of every disaster plan that should not be minimized or overlooked.

Planning

With regard to biological and chemical terrorism, planning should begin with an understanding of what to anticipate. An attempt to address every possible biological and chemical terrorism agent and contingency would doom any plan for pharmacy preparedness immediately. Each hospital, in conjunction with local and federal government recommendations, should focus its attention on identifying a limited number of agents and dedicating precious financial resources to the agents that pose the highest risk and greatest probability. Proximity to commercial targets such as oil refineries and chemical plants or to military biological and chemical storage or research facilities may dictate special needs. The plan should be coordinated closely with departments such as emergency medicine, infectious disease, nursing, and intensive care so that mutual needs and expectations can be matched. Unlike natural disasters (e.g., floods, hurricanes) or mass destruction and casualty incidents (e.g., an airliner crash), which generally have a distinct beginning and end,[16] terrorism incidents, especially biological ones, may take days to manifest themselves and weeks to resolve, as is the case with anthrax.[36] Therefore, every aspect of pharmaceutical care must be considered in the plan. Biological and chemical terrorism incidents represent unconventional disasters that have not been addressed in typical health-system pharmacy disaster plans. Since these are atypical disasters, pharmacists are encouraged to think beyond traditional planning strategies and consider the unthinkable in the development of a terrorism preparedness plan. Examples of issues that should be considered in the terrorism preparedness plan include:

- Staffing
- Formulary exceptions
- Refills
- Dispensing limitations
- Use of child-resistant containers
- Labeling
- Documentation
- Prescriber approval and validation
- Patient counseling
- Provisions for patients who do not have their maintenance medications
- Communication with staff, within the institution, with external colleagues, and with local government and public health officials
- Financial implications
- Adequate supplies of critical medications (e.g., antidotes, antibiotics)
- Provisions to provide staff with prophylactic medications for themselves and their families
- Emergency dispensing policy
- Patient records
- Staff education, initial and continuing
- Understanding communicable diseases
- Security
- Legal implications
- Anticipation of technology failure
- Staff counseling
- Fact sheets for patients on biological and chemical terrorism agents
- Medication procurement
- Mutual aid agreements with other pharmacies
- Integration with the hospital and community plans

A question that arises often during the planning process relates to having adequate stores of medications to address the adverse effects of a biological or chemical terrorism incident. One way to determine need is to know the emergency capability of your institution. Consult with the emergency department to establish the maximum number of patients that it can manage. The response capability will depend on the type of agent that was used. Biological terrorism is more insidious than chemical terrorism, and patient volume may increase over several days rather than precipitously; whereas chemical terrorism is generally associated with the rapid development of symptoms and a surge of patients within minutes to hours after their exposure. Considering these factors may help to establish an approximate quantity of antibiotics or antidotes, such as atropine or pralidoxime, that you may need to stock.

For example, the initial dose of atropine sulfate to treat a patient suffering from acute sarin (anticholinesterase nerve agent) exposure may be 2–6 mg IV, with repeated doses of 2–4 mg every 30 to 60 minutes depending on the severity of the patient's exposure. The dose and administration intervals of subsequent atropine doses should be titrated to patient need. Some patients may require smaller or larger doses more frequently or at longer intervals, and others may not require additional atropine administration. It may be judicious to assume that some patients may need treatment for 2 to 3 days until the situation is stabilized and the NPS has arrived.

If the local emergency medical response system is prepared for terrorism that involves nerve agents, a loading dose and perhaps maintenance doses of atropine will have been administered in the field prior to patient arrival at a hospital or emergency clinic. However, this contingency should not be assumed, and adequate supplies of atropine should be stocked.

In the event that biological terrorism with a bacterial agent occurs, a good plan should include a protocol for dispensing prophylactic antibiotics to both the hospital staff and their immediate families. The implementation of prophylactic antibiotic administration should be consistent with the recommendations of local public health officials and not decided arbitrarily by pharmacy personnel or other hospital staff. However, if antibiotic prophylaxis is indicated, an internal plan to provide the staff with the assurance that they and their families are safe from the threat of illness from a biological agent such as anthrax may reduce their hesitance to work during the crisis.

Larger communities may have a local pharmaceutical cache that is capable of meeting the emergent pharmaceutical needs for a thousand or more individuals. However, the pharmacy preparedness plan, especially for smaller communities with only one or two hospitals, should consider the pharmaceutical needs of community political leaders, law enforcement officials, fire service personnel, hospital volunteers, and others integral to the operation of the community in the overall pharmacy preparedness plan.

Consider developing a "pharmacist response team" for your pharmacy. Within the community there may be retired pharmacists and pharmacists from across the continuum of pharmaceutical care who could be invaluable in the time of crisis.[15] Consider establishing a proactive formal relationship with these pharmacists that would allow them to be of assistance if the pharmacy terrorism preparedness plan is activated. This is in contrast to the utilization of pharmacists who volunteer as a civic duty in response to a disaster. While there may be potential roles for volunteers after a biological or chemical incident is stabilized, their presence during an immediate crisis may interfere with the efficient operation of a pharmacy. In communities where there are schools of pharmacy, pharmacy students and faculty may provide an additional human resource. Pharmacists employed by industry are yet another source of professionals. All of these pharmacists need to have formal training with regard to the operation of your pharmacy, be credentialed by your institution, and be trained on a continuous basis about biological and chemical terrorism. Therefore, commitment to this approach must be proactive and ongoing for it to be successful in response to a biological or chemical terrorist incident.

Health-system pharmacy security issues should be addressed in the preparedness plan. Pharmacies are especially vulnerable to both internal and external security compromise since they possess lifesaving antidotes and antibiotics. For example, the panic that may arise following an actual or alleged anthrax terrorism incident may place the pharmacy in a position that is vulnerable to individuals who are seeking unlawful access to antibiotics such as doxycycline or ciprofloxacin. Armed robbery and after-hours break-ins are distinct possibilities. Security plans should include securing the pharmacy's physical confines and having security personnel available to guard the pharmacy. Internal security plans should include preventing the theft of medications by hospital and pharmacy staff. Satellite pharmacy security must also be considered in the plan.

It is anticipated that a pharmacy staff will respond willingly when conventional natural disasters mandate enhanced staffing. Natural disasters generally have a finite end and present little or no risk to pharmacy staff and their families. The issue of terrorism, especially biological terrorism, presents an unknown challenge with regard to emergency staffing. The risk of being exposed to patients with a life-threatening contagious disease such as smallpox or plague must be considered personally by each staff member, and the potential risk to staff members' families may preclude some staff from working. Will parents place their professional commitments above the safety and security of their families? The pharmacy preparedness plan must include provisions for assuring pharmacy staff that they will be safe and that their families will not be at risk. A proactive agreement with medical staff experts (e.g., infectious disease experts, clinical toxicologists) and mental health counselors to counsel pharmacy staff may be a useful strategy.

Biological and chemical terrorism incidents have been rare. It is unlikely that most health care professionals and health-system pharmacies will personally experience such an incident. However, the impact on morbidity, mortality, and general panic is so significant that no health-system pharmacy can afford to be unprepared. The emphasis should be on *overplanning* to insure that every potential contingency is addressed.

Planning efforts should not overlook the efforts of others. This book includes papers that deal directly with the anthrax crisis of 2001 and provide excellent models upon which to build.[21, 22] Other models describe disaster plans and response following natural disasters and human-induced disasters that can be applied to the development of a pharmacy terrorism plan.[10, 28, 29]

Action

In all likelihood, public health or law enforcement officials will alert your institution that a biological or chemical terrorism incident has occurred. It is also plausible that you will hear about the incident via the news media before you receive formal notification. It is advisable to begin to implement the preliminary aspects of your pharmacy preparedness plan as soon as there is reasonable confirmation of an incident. Begin to assess your current staffing and anticipate your staffing needs in the event that the hospital preparedness plan is activated. Have a sufficient number of copies of your plan for distribution to the staff, and begin to prioritize staff allocation according to basic operational needs and the needs associated with addressing the sequelae of the terrorism event. The preparedness plan should have identified the chain of command and who is in charge of the pharmacy plan. It is important that:[11]

- A crisis management team be formed
- A clear chain of command be established
- A single individual be in charge
- One spokesperson be identified
- Decision makers be predetermined so that action is not delayed
- The pharmacy leadership maintain high visibility during the response to the crisis

Teamwork within the pharmacy is critical to the successful implementation of the pharmacy preparedness plan. Each staff member must understand the entire plan and his or her specific responsibilities. An individual should be designated as the team leader (e.g., director, assistant director, supervisor—someone with organizational knowledge and skills and decision-making authority within the organizational structure) for disaster or terrorism preparedness.

This individual should be responsible for working with other hospital departments, outside agencies, pharmaceutical distributors, and others essential to the development and implementation of a pharmacy preparedness plan. As the department expert on biological and chemical terrorism, the pharmacy preparedness team leader may be the most appropriate individual to conduct initial and continuing education for the pharmacy staff. The time and financial resources to develop a pharmacy preparedness plan are not inconsequential. It may be necessary to delegate some of the team leader's pharmacy responsibilities to other department members. After the plan has been developed, it will require several hours per month of the team leader's time to participate in activities related to ongoing preparedness, such as meetings and educational programs. Unfortunately, there is no universal federal, state, or community funding to compensate the pharmacy for this preparedness activity. For the present, it will continue to be an unreimbursable, but absolutely necessary, function of the pharmacy department.

The demands of providing extensive pharmaceutical care in a biological or chemical terrorism incident will challenge pharmacy staffing. A mutual aid agreement with other hospital departments, especially nonclinical departments, for assistance to provide personnel to help support the pharmacy (e.g., security, medication delivery, order submissions, supply procurement) is advised. Conversely, it is conceivable that pharmacists and pharmacy technicians may have to respond to needs within the institution but totally outside the realm of their normal responsibilities.[23, 28] For example, pharmacy staff may be directed to assist with patient decontamination, triage, or even security. Therefore, all members of the pharmacy staff should be familiar with the entire hospital biological and chemical terrorism preparedness plan. The pharmacy plan should address maximal effectiveness with minimal staff.

A disaster is not the time to determine if the pharmacy biological and chemical terrorism preparedness plan is viable and to identify its limitations. Full-scale drills should be conducted internally and in conjunction with the institution and local agencies to insure that the plan will meet the needs of those who must be served through the delivery of pharmaceutical care. Repetition, through frequent simulated exercises, will help staff understand and remember their responsibilities and identify and minimize the plan's limitations. The pharmacy plan must recognize the importance of continuous learning and incorporate it as a key aspect of the plan.

Learning

While retrospective learning may be the third aspect of a pharmacy's biological and chemical terrorism preparedness plan, learning is actually the first aspect of a proactive plan. To plan effectively, the problem must first be identified. The following questions should be asked with reference to both biological and chemical agents:

- What diseases, toxins, or chemicals are the most likely terrorism agents?
- What are the typical routes or venues of exposure?
- What is the onset of illness following the exposure?
- What is the clinical presentation of the illness?
- Is the illness communicable?
- How long will the illness persist?
- What are the preferred and alternative treatments?

Understanding the agents that may pose a threat will allow the pharmacy to plan accordingly. This book includes basic information on some of the most likely biological and chemical terrorism agents. The time to learn is prior to the development of a plan and on a continuous basis to facilitate implementation of the terrorism preparedness plan. Since the occurrence of the sarin gas release in the Tokyo subway in 1995 and the biological terrorism (anthrax) events during the fall of 2001, a plethora of Websites, texts, videotapes, and medical literature contributions have made learning about biological and chemical terrorism less of a mystery. Although these educational opportunities are accessed easily, the lack of personal initiative and the lengthening temporal separation between the incidents and today have resulted in a degree of complacency about biological and chemical terrorism. Pharmacists and support staff must be active participants in the educational process. Hospital and pharmacy administration must provide financial and logistical support to insure that optimal initial and continuing education occur. It must be emphasized to a hesitant and resistant staff that training and preparedness are critical.[15]

Learning should be systematic because there are a large number of potential biological and chemical agents to consider. For example, categorizing agents is a valuable exercise since treatment of a bacterial exposure differs considerably from that of exposure to a viral agent. Dividing chemicals into groups, such as nerve agents and vesicants, simplifies treatment since the similar therapies may pertain to nearly every agent within each of these two chemical groups.

Once the specific poisons or disease processes have been identified, the use of a template approach to teaching, such as the RaPiD-T Program, will standardize the learning and thinking process during education programs and encourage uniformity in case the principles need to be applied during an actual terrorism response.[37] The RaPiD-T approach addresses four specific components: R stands for recognition, P for protection, D for decontamination, and T for triage and treatment.

A simulated or actual terrorist event provides a valuable opportunity to learn from the crisis. An objective debriefing exercise provides important feedback about the successes, limitations, and failures associated with the activation of a pharmacy terrorism preparedness plan. The information should be used to enhance the plan, and this exercise should be performed continuously—the pharmacy terrorism preparedness plan will be of no value if it is shelved and merely serves as a trophy for the next Joint Commission review.

Each pharmacy should have a comprehensive literature file that includes key publications that relate to the terrorism plan. This book provides a basis for the development of the pharmacy terrorism-literature file. Additionally, the pharmacy should insure that the regional poison information center telephone number (nationwide toll-free access to the nearest center: 1-800-222-1222) is posted prominently throughout the facility.[20, 35] The poison information center will be able to provide the pharmacy with specific information about biological or chemical terrorism agents, as well as contemporary treatment information.

Financial Considerations

The response to a terrorism event will be very costly to the institution that manages the victims. However, the preparation for an event may be even more expensive. Decontamination and personal protective equipment must be purchased to treat the victims and protect the health care management team. Antibiotics such as ciprofloxacin and antidotes like pralidoxime are expensive and sometimes difficult to secure in adequate quantities. Ventilation patterns within the institution may need to be reengineered to prevent the contamination of the entire building from an infectious agent like smallpox or noxious chemicals. Countless hours will be spent developing plans, training staff, and networking with local and regional public health and law enforcement officials. Since terrorism events are rare, expertise may be obtained only through constant reinforcement and simulated drills. These activities are no longer optional and require an inordinate investment by every institution and health-system pharmacy in the United States.

The Nunn-Lugar legislation appropriated funds to provide training and equipment. However, most of the funds were invested in local government equipment and programs, with little of the funding channeled directly to hospitals. Additional bioterrorism funds were allocated by the federal government in 2002 and directed to state governments. As with the Nunn-Lugar funds, little of the 2002 federal money will be available directly to institutions or health-system pharmacies to offset their preparedness activities. Developing mutual aid agreements with other health-system pharmacies and active participation in local preparedness endeavors may help to reduce expenses and identify grant funds to assist terrorism preparedness planning. Preparedness activities can be justified from both a humane and financial perspective.[38]

Summary

A biological and chemical terrorism preparedness plan is essential for each and every pharmacy. The grave consequences associated with terrorism mandate proactive development of such a plan to minimize the morbidity and mortality, as well as the negative financial impact of such a disaster on an institution. The focus of the pharmacy plan should be to plan, train, recover, and learn. Execution of each aspect is critical to the success of this important endeavor.

REFERENCES

1. Tetsu O, Takasu N, Ishimatsu S, et al. Report on 640 victims of the Tokyo subway sarin attack. *Ann Emerg Med* 1996;28:129-135.

2. Anon. Summary. Executive session on emergency preparedness and the pharmaceutical supply chain: November 9, 2001. http://www.ashp.org/public/proad/emergency/exec_summary2001.html (accessed September 4, 2002).

3. Anon. Summary of the second executive session on emergency preparedness and the pharmaceutical supply chain. *Am J Health-Syst Pharm* 2002;59:1057-1065.

4. Anon. National Pharmaceutical Stockpile aids homeland health security. *Am J Health-Syst Pharm* 2001;58:2112, 2115.

5. Centers for Disease Control. National Pharmaceutical Stockpile Program. http://www.cdc.gov/nceh/nps/default.htm (accessed September 11, 2002).

6. Anon. National Pharmacists Response Team—Be Prepared to Respond! http://www.aphanet.org/pharmcare/nationalpharmacistsresponseteam.htm (accessed September 10, 2002).

7. Mothershead JL, Tonat K, Koenig KL. Bioterrorism preparedness III: State and federal programs and response. *Emerg Med Clin N Am* 2002;20:477-500.

8. Mrvos R, Piposzar D, Stein T, et al. Regional pharmaceuticals for biological and chemical terrorism. *J Toxicol Clin Toxicol* 2001;39:538.

9. Anon. What are LEPCs? http://www.rtknet.org/lepc/webpage/info.html (accessed September 6, 2002).

10. Levy DB, Barone JA, Raia JJ, et al. Pharmacist participation in the management of incidents involving hazardous materials. *Am J Hosp Pharm* 1987;44:549-556.

11. Johnston WP, Stepanovich PL. Managing in a crisis: Planning, acting and learning. *Am J Health-Syst Pharm* 2001;58:1245-1249.

12. Anon. ASHP Statement on the role of health-system pharmacists in counterterrorism. http://www.ashp.org/public/proad/emergency/statement.html (accessed August 19, 2002).

13. Burda AM, Sigg T. Pharmacy preparedness for incidents involving weapons of mass destruction. *Am J Health-Syst Pharm* 2001;58:2274-2284.

14. Terriff CM, Tee AM. Citywide pharmaceutical preparation for bioterrorism. *Am J Health-Syst Pharm* 2001;58:233-237.

15. Teeter DS. Bioterrorism preparedness: Answers for the health-system pharmacist. *Am J Health-Syst Pharm* 2002;59:928-930.

16. Poe BM. Expanding disaster preparedness to include bioterrorism. *Am J Health-Syst Pharm* 2002;59:926-927.

17. Grabenstein JD. Public and patient concerns in catastrophic circumstances. *Am J Health-Syst Pharm* 2002;59:923-925.

18. Downs KE. Training requirements and opportunities in planning responses to bioterrorism. *Am J Health-Syst Pharm* 2002;59:1331-1332.

19. Montello MJ, Ames T. Therapeutic selection during an emergency response. *Am J Health-Syst Pharm* 1999;56:236-240.

20. Crouch BI. Role of poison control centers in disaster response planning. *Am J Health-Syst Pharm* 2002;59:1159-1163.

21. Haffer AST, Rogers JR, Montello MJ, et al. 2001 anthrax crisis in Washington, DC: Clinic for persons exposed to contaminated mail. *Am J Health-Syst Pharm* 2002;59:1189-1192.

22. Montello MJ, Ostroff C, Frank EC, et al. 2001 anthrax crisis in Washington, DC: Pharmacists' role in screening patients and selecting prophylaxis. *Am J Health-Syst Pharm* 2002;59:1193-1199.

23. Moore TD. Administrative approach to disaster preparedness in the pharmacy. *Am J Hosp Pharm* 1979;36:1137-1341.

24. Bradgon RL, Gousse GC, Piwarzyk P, et al. Regional disaster planning for hospital pharmacies. *Am J Hosp Pharm* 1982;39:1913-1915.

25. Ames TW, Montello MJ. Role of pharmacists on disaster response teams. *Am J Health-Syst Pharm* 1999;56:716, 718.

REFERENCES

26. Babb J, Downs K. Fighting back: Pharmacists' roles in the federal response to the September 11 attacks. *J Am Pharm Assoc* 2001;41:834-837.

27. Grabenstein JD. The pharmacist's response to biological and chemical terrorism: Developing a preparedness plan. *Hosp Pharm* 1998;33:1423-1431.

28. Carda E, Harcum J, Olthoff C. Mass casualty: A hospital pharmacist's call to action. *Hosp Pharm* 1989;24:697-699.

29. Cramer RL, Weeks KG. Pharmacy disaster emergency: The Huntsville tornado. *Hosp Pharm* 1990;25:523-526.

30. Anon. Extraordinary infections: A focus on bioterrorism. *J Am Pharm Assoc* 2000;40:S36-S37.

31. McKinney WP, Bia FJ, Stewart C, et al. Bioterrorism: An update for clinicians, pharmacists and emergency management planners. *Emerg Med Consensus Rep* November 1, 2001:1-12.

32. Teeter DS, Robbins W. US Pharmacist. http://www.uspharmacist.com/NewLook/DisplayArticle.cfm?item_num=887 (accessed August 21, 2002).

33. Gaudette R, Schnitzer J, George E, et al. Lessons learned from the September 11th World Trade Center disaster: Pharmacy preparedness and participation in an international medical and surgical response team. *Pharmacotherapy* 2002;22:271-281.

34. Augustine NR. Managing the crisis you tried to prevent. *Harv Bus Rev* 1995;73:147-158.

35. Pearson CM, Clair JA, Misra SK, et al. Managing the unthinkable. *Organ Dyn* 1997;26:51-64.

36. Inglesby, TV, Henderson, DA, Bartlett, JG, et al. Anthrax as a biological weapon: Medical and public health management. *JAMA* 1999; 281:1735-1745.

37. Krenzelok EP, Allswede MP, Mrvos R. The poison center role in biological and chemical terrorism. *Vet Human Toxicol* 2000;42:297-300.

38. Kaufmann AF, Meltzer MI, Schmid GP. The economic impact of a bioterrorist attack: Are prevention and post-attack intervention programs justifiable? *Emerging Infect Dis* 1997;3:83-94.

SUGGESTED READINGS

Ames TW, Montello MJ. Role of pharmacists on disaster response teams. *Am J Health-Syst Pharm* 1999;56:716-717.

Bragdon RL, Gousse GC, Piwarzyk P, et al. Regional disaster planning for hospital pharmacies. *Am J Hosp Pharm* 1982;39:1913-1915.

Crouch BI. Role of poison control centers in disaster response planning. *Am J Health-Syst Pharm* 2002;59:1159-1163.

Downs KE. Training and opportunities in planning responses to bioterrorism. *Am J Health-Syst Pharm* 2002;59:1331-1332.

Flowers LK, Mothershead JL, Blackwell TH. Bioterrorism preparedness II: The community and emergency medical services systems. *Emerg Med Clin N Am* 2002;20:457-476.

Grabenstein JD. Public and patient concerns in catastrophic circumstances. *Am J Health-Syst Pharm* 2002;59:923-925.

Krenzelok EP, Allswede MP, Mrvos R. The poison center role in biological and chemical terrorism. *Vet Human Toxicol* 2000;42:297-300.

Moore TJ. Administrative approach to disaster preparedness in the pharmacy. *Am J Hosp Pharm* 1979;36:1337-1341.

Mothershead JL, Tonat K, Koenig KL. Bioterrorism preparedness III: State and federal programs and response. *Emerg Med Clin N Am* 2002;20:437-455.

Schultz CH, Mothershead JL, Field M. Bioterrorism preparedness I: The emergency department and hospital. *Emerg Med Clin N Am* 2002;20:437-455.

READINGS

Summary of the executive session on emergency preparedness and the pharmaceutical supply chain

BETHESDA, MARYLAND
NOVEMBER 9, 2001

Am J Health-Syst Pharm. 2002; 59:247-53

Responsibility for responding to homeland terrorist attacks and other emergencies begins at the local level and is grounded in collaboration between the private and public sectors. The federal government is ready, at a state's bidding, to assist communities quickly and in powerful ways—supplying pharmaceuticals, trained personnel, equipment, and other resources. Effective response also requires the cooperation of individual health care professionals at the local level. Among those professionals whose participation is vital are pharmacists, who possess science-based knowledge and clinical acumen and are also widely accessible. The September 11th attacks in New York City and Washington, D.C., and the subsequent bioterrorist threat posed by anthrax challenged our nation's medical disaster-response system in unparalleled ways. Although the system rose to the occasion, there is ample room for improvement.

These are among the key points that emerged from an executive session on emergency preparedness and the pharmaceutical supply chain that was convened by the American Society of Health-System Pharmacists (ASHP) in Bethesda, Maryland, on November 9, 2001. The session brought together more than 35 representatives from federal public health and preparedness offices, pharmaceutical manufacturers, wholesalers, group purchasing organizations, academic health-science centers, community hospitals, and health organizations. The objectives of the session were to

1. Conduct an open, honest, noncompetitive review of the readiness of the pharmaceutical supply chain (and related decision-support and drug information mechanisms) related to projected demands on the system in the face of homeland terrorism, while considering all aspects of the supply chain, from procuring raw materials for use in manufacturing to the delivery of finished products and information to patients;
2. Identify significant vulnerabilities in the pharmaceutical supply chain and steps that should be considered to remedy those vulnerabilities;
3. Identify means to communicate the session's deliberations—particularly any vulnerabilities that are noted—to appropriate public and private offices.

This document summarizes the discussions that took place at the executive session. It gives an overview of the federal emergency response system, summarizes participants' remarks concerning the strengths and vulnerabilities of the nation's medical emergency-response system, and offers recommendations for improving this system. The opinions expressed at the meeting were candid and forthright. Given the diversity of the participants' backgrounds, a consensus on all issues was not expected. Nonetheless, as discussions proceeded, a shared resolve to work collaboratively and in new ways to meet the challenges posed by the threat of homeland terrorism was strikingly clear.

Federal emergency response system

Three participants in the executive session, representing the Office of Public Health and Science, Department of Health and Human Services (DHHS), Office of Emergency Preparedness, and the National Pharmaceutical Stockpile (NPS) program of the Centers for Disease Control and Prevention (CDC), described the systems, resources, and personnel involved in the nation's federal emergency response system. These presentations created a common context for the day's discussions and informed participants of the roles of these programs in handling the events of September 11th and thereafter.

An understanding of federal resources and how to access them is

Reprinted with permission from ASHP: *Am J Health-Syst Pharm*; February 1, 2002, Vol 59

essential for persons involved in disaster-response activities at any level. The three spokespersons emphasized that federal intervention in homeland terrorist attacks, as in hurricanes, fires, epidemics, and other crises, occurs only at the behest of a state governor, who has determined that local resources are not sufficient to deal with the problem. The system is a "bottom-up" operation, and all communities must have first-response capabilities. Once summoned, the federal government works with local public health authorities; its job is not to take charge of the situation. In a crisis, the federal government is in a position to supply the critical resources that are not available in the local community.

Requests for assistance from the states are submitted to the Federal Emergency Management Agency (FEMA). FEMA, termed the "switch point" in the nation's response system, has 14 "emergency support functions," covering such areas as firefighting, health and medical services, communications, and transportation. More than 25 federal agencies, including DHHS, have a designated responsibility to implement these support functions. After receiving a request for assistance, FEMA contacts the appropriate agencies, which will then work with the state to determine what resources are needed. FEMA then issues a task order so the response can be initiated. Disaster responses can be activated within minutes of receiving a request for assistance.

The Office of Emergency Preparedness (OEP) is the lead federal agency for providing emergency health and medical services. OEP directs the National Disaster Medical System (NDMS), which operates as a partnership between DHHS, the Department of Veterans Affairs (DVA), the Department of Defense, FEMA, and state and local governments. Major resources available through NDMS include hospital beds, phar-

maceutical supplies, personnel, and equipment.

Hospital beds. DHHS has contracts with civilian hospitals to identify beds that may be used in emergency situations. The core of the hospital-bed supply is DVA, which has 7500–9000 beds that can be made available. Military aircraft are available to transport patients to hospitals in other cities, if necessary.

Pharmaceutical supplies. Emergency pharmaceuticals and other products that cannot be supplied at the local level are available to local public health departments through NPS, which was created in 1999. (The Federal Emergency Response Plan does not have to be activated to request assistance from NPS.) One key component of this program, which is managed by CDC, are "push packages," which are stored in secure locations across the United States and can be delivered within 12 hours of the federal decision to deploy the supplies. The push packages contain pharmaceuticals, i.v. supplies, airway supplies, emergency medications, bandages, and wound dressings. Among the medications included are ciprofloxacin, doxycycline, gentamicin, dopamine, albuterol, lorazepam, morphine, atropine, diazepam, and pralidoxime. The quantities of antibacterials supplied are substantial; for example, one push package contains enough antibiotics to treat 50,000 persons for anthrax for 60 days. The quantities of other emergency medications are smaller. Most of the drug products are not in unit dose form and must be repackaged onsite. The push packages include counting machines, volumetric devices, packaging and labeling machines, and written patient and provider information. A CDC technical advisory team accompanies each push package that is deployed. The push packages are transported by aircraft and tractor-trailers. CDC has permission from the Federal Aviation Administration (FAA) to transport push packages on

aircraft if regular commercial air travel has been suspended.

These push packages are designed to augment local supplies and meet general emergency needs; they are described as containing "a little bit of everything." If a locality knows in advance what specific pharmaceuticals it needs, it may request aid from the vendor-managed inventory (VMI) component of NPS. VMI is a "cushion" that can be accessed rapidly in times of crisis. Emergency supplies of ciprofloxacin, for example, were made available from VMI in the wake of the recent anthrax exposures. After the delivery of a push package, supplies from VMI are delivered within 24 to 36 hours of being requested. VMI may also serve as an initial tailored response to an event involving a known agent, in which case pharmaceuticals can be delivered within 12 hours of a federal decision to deploy supplies.

Local communities must store sufficient pharmaceuticals and related supplies to respond to an attack and sustain victims for 24 hours or longer until federal assistance arrives.

Medical assistance teams. OEP directs the deployment of Disaster Medical Assistance Teams (DMATs), which are groups of medical personnel and logistic staff trained to provide emergency medical care. Principally a local resource, DMATs can be activated and deployed at other sites when needed. There are 98 DMATs stationed throughout the country. Each is sponsored by a local organization, such as a hospital or public health department. DMATs are equipped to sustain themselves for up to 72 hours after deployment. There are three specialized forms of DMATs: Disaster Mortuary Operational Response Teams (DMORTs), Veterinary Medical Assistance Teams (VMATs), and National Medical Response Teams.

Metropolitan Medical Response System. Another component of OEP's national disaster program is

Reprinted with permission from ASHP: *Am J Health-Syst Pharm*; February 1, 2002, Vol 59

the Metropolitan Medical Response System (MMRS). MMRS operates under contracts between DHHS and cities. It is a process or tool that OEP uses to bring together disparate agencies in the public and private sectors that share responsibility for emergency preparedness and response. Each project is led by a steering committee that includes representatives of local police and fire departments, hospitals, professional organizations, community and state agencies, and federal partners. Each MMRS site must produce 12 documents outlining its plan for responding to local emergencies in a coordinated manner. The plans must cover the spectrum of disaster-response functions, ranging from the acquisition of local caches of pharmaceuticals and equipment to the development of protocols for postevent surveillance.

MMRSs are key to a community's first-response strategy. Ninety-seven MMRSs have been funded, and 23 others are slated for funding within the next year. One goal of MMRS is to enable cities to learn from each other. For this reason, a summary of lessons learned and best practices will be published and made available on MMRS's Web site.

Strengths of the pharmaceutical supply chain

As participants began to tackle the session's first objective—the readiness of the current pharmaceutical supply chain—the many strengths of the current system emerged.

Faced with a crisis of any dimension, hospital pharmacy managers routinely solve problems by calling their drug distributors or other hospitals. Distributors, in turn, have developed their own disaster-preparedness programs. They have internal electronic networks and are accustomed to responding quickly to unanticipated demands. Through the efforts of the Food and Drug Administration (FDA), health-professional organizations, and individual pharma-

cists, who monitor prescription and nonprescription drug sales patterns, drug supplies are monitored on an ongoing basis. Distributors have implemented systems to limit, when necessary, the amount of drug products supplied to certain customers and divert supplies to the areas in most critical need. They stated that they can generally respond to unanticipated requests within three or four hours. Given these practices, one participant noted that his industry finds the word "stockpile" a misnomer. "We don't use the word," he said. Instead, his firm thinks in terms of "inventory" and has a plan to ensure that drugs are made available to the places in the most need.

By and large, this system worked well in the days and weeks following September 11. For example, the November 1, 2001, issue of the *American Journal of Health-System Pharmacy* (AJHP) cites examples of how hospitals, wholesalers, and distributors, supported by ground transport companies and local police escorts, collaborated to deliver supplies to New York City and Washington, D.C. Faced with several "logistic nightmares," *AJHP* reported, the organizations "rallied to get supplies to hospitals." For example, there was a critical need for human albumin, used to stabilize patients in shock. Within hours, a supply sufficient for 25,000 patients was on its way to the attacked sites. The product was shipped on a chartered FedEx Boeing 747 freight jetliner. "Lifeguard" flight approvals from FAA during the week of September 11 made it possible to transport products and rescue supplies to areas of need. Later, when the anthrax threats emerged, Bayer Corporation, which produces Cipro (ciprofloxacin), began a "24/7" production schedule; it also had a factory in Germany ready to begin production of the drug.

The system, participants concluded, deals with crises on a routine basis and generally handles them well.

As one discussant said, "Our business is to keep the day-to-day supply chain going. Fires, storms, and similar crises are routine. We have programs to survey our inventories and quickly move stuff to where it is needed. Regardless if you're our customer or not, you'll get it. . . . Each crisis is different. We learn from them, and we communicate. Flexibility is key."

Emergency personnel also rose to the occasion on September 11 and thereafter. DMATs and DMORTs were deployed in New York City and Washington, D.C. One participant in the discussions gave "high grades" to CDC for the delivery of products and to the actions of support personnel in New Jersey. Health care professionals were on the scene from the beginning. Pharmacists, physicians, and other health care professionals worked side-by-side. Patients' medical histories were taken before drugs were distributed. Team members provided counseling and followed the patients through the entire process.

Vulnerabilities in the system

Despite the success stories, participants agreed that the events of September 11th served as a "wake-up call." Individual components of these systems often worked well; nonetheless, the whole was not greater than the sum of its parts. An overall coordinated plan was missing. "We don't have a network," said one participant, "we respond in an unorganized organized way." Or, to quote another participant, "There are a lot of good folks doing good things. The problem is that they're not always on the same page."

There is a need not only to "bind the public and private sectors" more effectively but also to improve coordination within and among the agencies and organizations charged with disaster-response responsibilities. Absent an overall plan, some essential piece of the complicated drug supply chain will prove to be the weakest link. For example, a shortage

Reprinted with permission from ASHP: *Am J Health-Syst Pharm*; February 1, 2002, Vol 59

of dispensing containers hampered the otherwise well-structured drug distribution activity in New Jersey in response to anthrax exposure. The continuing problem of drug product shortages suggests that some aspects of the supply chain are fragile.

The discussions revealed that one fundamental weakness in the current system is a failure to appreciate the full context and complexity of the medication use process. As one participant stated, drug products are not "jellybean commodities." Their manufacture, distribution, and safe use depends on coordinated interactions among a variety of players. Locating a sufficient supply of a product, while sometimes difficult in itself, is far from enough. There must be a system to ensure that the product is packaged and labeled and accompanied by written product information. Personnel must be available to take patients' medical histories, counsel them, and answer questions. Appropriate follow-though measures must be established.

Another major vulnerability of the pharmaceutical supply chain is a lack of communication. This may be attributed in part to the historical lack of interaction between the public and private sectors of the U.S. health care system. This vulnerability is heightened by the current status of the nation's public health infrastructure, which has, according to many accounts, deteriorated in recent decades. Forging a strong bond between these two sectors is essential for emergency response, but it is at present, in one participant's words, an "unnatural marriage." The lack of communication and coordination continues at many levels—between individual professional disciplines, such as pharmacy and medicine, between agencies and organizations, and between cities and states. Overcoming "parochial barriers" is essential.

Also missing is a system by which health-professional volunteers can be drawn into the system when needed. Concerns for professional liability and state board regulations were seen as significant barriers to ensuring that pharmacists, physicians, and other providers can be mobilized to serve in areas of need.

Lack of pharmacist involvement is a particular vulnerability in the current system. Pharmacists have not participated in most emergency-preparedness planning processes. They have not assumed a community leadership role in this area. This is unfortunate because pharmacists have a "pragmatic and science-based knowledge" that is invaluable. Their accessibility in hospitals and the community is an additional benefit.

A final vulnerability of the pharmaceutical supply chain is a lack of education and awareness, which extends to all persons directly and indirectly involved in disaster response. Overcoming this barrier requires a multifaceted approach. The media need to be educated to ensure that the general public receives accurate information. Physicians need drug-use guidelines and an awareness of the resources available to them. Health professionals need to know how to volunteer in disaster-response and disaster-planning processes. Federal agencies need information from the frontline to tailor programs and services more effectively. The need for a unified, credible voice at the federal level—which might be provided by, for example, the United States Surgeon General—has been evident in recent weeks. The absence of such a voice leads to inconsistent messages that may cause undue public alarm and an inappropriate use of resources.

Recommendations for improvement

Participants offered many suggestions for improving the nation's capability to respond to acts of homeland terrorism and other emergencies. Central to their recommendations was the need to dramatically strengthen the country's public health system. Investments in the country's beleaguered public health system would have tremendous payoffs, not only in enhancing responses in times of a crisis but also in improving the overall health status of the U.S. population. There is enormous potential for pharmacist involvement in this effort; the current situation, said one participant, offers the opportunity to "reinvigorate the profession's public health roots."

Discussions about overcoming these perceived vulnerabilities also focused on the following points, which were identified for further consideration and analysis (the group did not attempt to reach a consensus on these matters): collaboration, education and information sharing, federal responsibilities, and legislative and regulatory activities.

Collaboration

The federal government has created and established an effective infrastructure for emergency preparedness and response. To ensure maximum efficiency and eliminate redundancy, organizations and individuals should tap into this national system rather than undertake separate efforts. For example, health-professional organizations wishing to become involved in planning and response systems should contact their local MMRS. Most of the MMRSs are still working on their plans and offer many opportunities for pharmacist participation. Only if such a group does not exist in their areas should health professionals undertake a new effort, and if they do, their plans should be based on the MMRS collaborative model focused on the overall needs of the community.

Collaboration is a "push–pull" affair. Public health departments should reach out to health professionals in the private sector, including pharmacists. These departments rarely have pharmacists on staff.

The community pharmacist should be an integral part of disaster-

Reprinted with permission from ASHP: *Am J Health-Syst Pharm*; February 1, 2002, Vol 59

response efforts. For example, patients might receive a few days' supply of a medication at an emergency distribution center; a prescription could then be filled by a community pharmacist, who would assume responsibility for additional counseling and follow-up.

Distributors and wholesalers should consider being more forthcoming in sharing information with appropriate officials about where their products are stored. General information on storage locations is already known, but by sharing specific information with the appropriate federal authorities, responding to requests in times of emergency would be simpler and would not put anyone at a competitive disadvantage.

Education and information sharing

Information of many kinds, such as clinical guidelines for the use of medications or other issues and lists of frequently asked questions, should be developed and disseminated. The federal government could take a lead role in this; however, professional organizations could also develop the needed material and share it with the government. These documents should be available in print and electronic formats. Of particular value would be the following:

- A diagram showing the components of the disaster-response system and illustrating how the components can be accessed;
- Recommendations for the appropriate responses to attacks by specific bioweapons. Had such a document been available before the anthrax episode, it might have saved a great deal of confusion and frustration; and
- Emergency-response guides for state and local pharmaceutical and medical organizations.

National organizations such as ASHP, the American Medical Associa-

tion, and the American Hospital Association, which have strong state affiliate systems, should use these networks for information sharing.

Members of the pharmaceutical industry should take a more active role in educating the public, media, and health professionals. They can mobilize their sales forces and science liaisons to serve in educational roles.

Group purchasing organizations can facilitate communications with their constituents and provide educational programs.

Hospital drug information centers and poison control centers are natural allies and should be included in the resource and information-sharing process.

Federal responsibilities

The federal government should have a single designated authority—an individual with scientific credibility and the ability to connect with the public and media—to serve as a spokesperson for the health system.

FDA should take a more active role in identifying and resolving problems stemming from drug shortages. This is a matter of increasing concern with respect to the day-to-day drug supply, and it is critical in times of emergency.

OEP should provide more guidance to local communities regarding planning for, procuring, distributing, and controlling pharmaceuticals in a local cache. Information should be provided on how a local cache relates to NPS and vendor-managed inventories. The OEP effort to develop "best practices" guidelines should be expedited to the extent possible.

CDC should do more to inform local emergency-preparedness officials about NPS. Sites that receive push packages must be made aware in advance of the packages' contents, onsite services that will be needed to use them, and how to replenish them.

Legislative and regulatory activities

State boards of pharmacy and medicine should explore ways that make it easier for health professionals to provide crisis-response services in states other than those in which they are licensed. This is particularly important at a time when there is a shortage of pharmacists in the national workforce. A model for this already exists: for health professionals participating in federal disaster-response programs, credentialing and liability responsibilities are assumed by the U.S. government.

State legislatures will be seeking ways to increase emergency preparedness within their jurisdictions. Some states have already done this, and the provisions in state law cover diverse areas. For example, Colorado recently passed legislation that addresses quarantines. Health-professional organizations should provide information that will enable elected officials to make informed decisions as they draft and vote for new legislation.

One reason for hospitals' interest in stockpiling of pharmaceutical products is the concern for liability. This issue could be addressed in legislation.

Next steps

Participants agreed that the executive session had laid a solid foundation for future cooperative efforts. They expressed a desire to hold at least one additional large-group session and discussed the possibility of forming work groups around specific issues. The creation of a "listserv" (i.e., an electronic mailing list) was suggested. Group members concurred that the inclusion of persons with a variety of perspectives was essential to any deliberations and, in that vein, suggested that the group be expanded to include representatives from FEMA, appropriate agencies within the Department of Transportation, professional nursing organizations, and security agencies.

Reprinted with permission from ASHP: *Am J Health-Syst Pharm*; February 1, 2002, Vol 59

Conference participants, by affiliation

Government Offices

CAPT Charles Bruner
U.S. Coast Guard
Washington, D.C.

Tomas Daley
Chief, Pharmaceuticals Group
Directorate of Medical Materiel
Defense Supply Center
Philadelphia
Philadelphia, Pennsylvania

CAPT Kathleen Downs
Office of Emergency Preparedness
U.S. Department of Health and
Human Services
Rockville, Maryland

Susan E. Gorman, Pharm.D., DABAT
Senior Science Officer
National Pharmaceutical
Stockpile Program
Centers for Disease Control and
Prevention
Atlanta, Georgia

COL W. Mike Heath, M.S.
Pharmacy Consultant, U.S. Army
Office of the Army Surgeon General
Falls Church, Virginia

RADM Arthur Lawrence
Office of Public Health and Science
Acting Principal Deputy Assistant
Secretary for Health
Washington, D.C.

CAPT Thomas J. McGinnis
Deputy Associate Commissioner
Office of Policy, Planning & Legislation
Food and Drug Administration
Rockville, Maryland

COL Ardis J. Meier
Pharmacy Consultant to USAF
Surgeon General
Associate Chief, Biomedical Sciences
Corps for Pharmacy
Andrews Air Force Base,
Maryland

Jimmy R. Mitchell, M.P.H., M.S.
Director, Office of Pharmacy Affairs
Health Resources and Services
Administration
U.S. Department of Health and
Human Services
Bethesda, Maryland

John E. Ogden, M.S., FASHP
Chief Consultant for Pharmacy
Benefits Management
Department of Veterans Affairs
Washington, D.C.

CAPT Jerry Phillips
Associate Director
Medication Error Prevention
Office of Postmarketing Drug Risk
Assessment
Food and Drug Administration
Center for Drug Evaluation and
Research
Rockville, Maryland

CDR James Sabatinos
Office of Emergency Preparedness
U.S. Department of Health and
Human Services
Rockville, Maryland

RADM Richard S. Walling
Director, Office of the Americas &
Middle East ORIH
Rockville, Maryland

Drug Manufacturers

Dan Horn
Vice President
Distribution & Customer Service
Abbott Laboratories
Abbott Park, Illinois

Frank J. Malinoski, M.D., Ph.D.
Assistant Vice President
Global Medical Affairs
Wyeth-Ayerst Pharmaceuticals
St. Davids, Pennsylvania

W. B. Novotny
Director, Pharmaceutical Supply
Planning
Wyeth-Ayerst Laboratories
Frazer, Pennsylvania

Group Purchasing Organizations

Allen Dunehew
Vice President of Pharmacy
AmeriNet Inc.
St. Louis, Missouri

Mick Hunt, Jr., M.S., FASHP
Senior Director of Pharmacy
Novation
Irving, Texas

Weldon Johnson
Director of Contracting
Premier, Inc.
Oak Brook, Illinois

Wholesalers

Mark Hartman
Senior Vice President, Operations
and Planning
Cardinal Distribution
Dublin, Ohio

Dan Skalecki
Corporate Vice President, Health
Systems Grp.
AmeriSourceBergen
Carmel, Indiana

Ronald J. Streck
President and CEO
Healthcare Distribution
Management Assoc.
Reston, Virginia

James Trance
Vice President
Distribution Operations
McKesson Corporation
Rocky Hill, Connecticut

Community Pharmacy

Calvin J. Anthony
Executive Vice President
National Community Pharmacists
Association
Alexandria, Virginia

Bruce Roberts
Executive Vice President–Designate
National Community Pharmacists
Association
Alexandria, Virginia

Edward J. Staffa
Director
Pharmacy Practice &
Communications
National Association of Chain
Drug Stores
Alexandria, Virginia

Practitioners

Paul W. Abramowitz, Pharm.D., FASHP
Director of Pharmacy and Professor
Department of Pharmaceutical
Care
University of Iowa Hospitals and
Clinics
Iowa City, Iowa

David Chen, M.B.A.
Pharmacy Director
Shady Grove Adventist Hospital
Rockville, Maryland

Reprinted with permission from ASHP: *Am J Health-Syst Pharm*; February 1, 2002, Vol 59

Douglas J. Scheckelhoff, M.S., FASHP
 Children's National Medical Center
 Pharmacy Department
 Washington, D.C.

Other Associations

Steve Bende, Ph.D.
 Vice President
 Science, Professional &
  Regulatory Affairs
 The Generic Pharmaceutical Association
 Washington, D.C.
Barry Dickinson, Ph.D.
 Director, Science Policy
 American Medical Association
 Chicago, Illinois
Mitchel Rothholz
 Vice President
 Professional Practice
 American Pharmaceutical Association
 Washington, D.C.
Douglas R. Smith, Pharm.D.
 Senior Director, Pharmacy and
  Oncology

University HealthSystem
 Consortium
 Oak Brook, Illinois
R. Joseph Trauger
 Associate Director
 Congressional & Executive Branch
  Relations
 American Hospital Association
 Washington, D.C.

Other

David A. Zilz, B.S., M.S.
 Consultant to ASHP
 Iola, Wisconsin

American Society of Health-System Pharmacists

Henri R. Manasse, Jr., Ph.D., Sc.D.
 Executive Vice President and
  Chief Executive Officer
 American Society of Health-System
  Pharmacists
 Bethesda, Maryland

Charles E. Myers, M.S., M.B.A.
 Vice President
 Professional and Scientific Affairs
  Office
 American Society of Health-System
  Pharmacists
 Bethesda, Maryland
Steven L. Sheaffer, Pharm.D., FASHP
 President
 American Society of Health-System
  Pharmacists
 Associate Professor and Vice Chair for
  Experiential Learning
 University of the Sciences in Phila-
  delphia
 Philadelphia, Pennsylvania
William A. Zellmer, M.P.H.
 Deputy Executive Vice President
 American Society of Health-System
  Pharmacists
 Bethesda, Maryland

Reprinted with permission from ASHP: *Am J Health-Syst Pharm*; February 1, 2002, Vol 59

Summary of the second executive session on emergency preparedness and the pharmaceutical supply chain

BETHESDA, MARYLAND
MARCH 8, 2002

Am J Health-Syst Pharm. 2002; 59:1057-65

What can be done to prevent shortages of emergency drug products—not only during emergencies but also as part of ongoing preparedness? How can pharmacists' skills and knowledge be better tapped by local emergency-response systems? How can "best practices" developed by local emergency-response programs be shared?

These were among the questions confronting some 40 representatives from federal agencies, pharmaceutical manufacturers, drug wholesalers, group purchasing organizations, pharmacy and other health associations, and hospital and community pharmacies who convened on March 8, 2002, for the Second Executive Session on Emergency Preparedness and the Pharmaceutical Supply Chain. The meeting was hosted by the American Society of Health-System Pharmacists (ASHP).

Participants in the first executive session, held November 9, 2001, engaged in a wide-ranging discussion of issues related to emergency preparedness. Speakers at that meeting presented an overview of the federal emergency-response system and discussed its performance following the terrorist attacks of September 11. Within that context, group members identified the strengths and weaknesses of the pharmaceutical supply chain. ASHP published a summary of the November meeting in the *American Journal of Health-System Pharmacy*[1] and disseminated copies for participants' use in their own organizations and agencies.

The purpose of the second executive session was to continue the dialogue and to focus on three objectives:

1. Examine and recommend appropriate interfaces between community emergency offices, local supply networks, and health-system pharmacists to ensure the availability of appropriate medications and their safe and effective use during the initial and sustained phases of emergencies,

2. Review what has been learned from existing Metropolitan Medical Response System (MMRS) plans with respect to best medication-use practices that can be recommended to others, and

3. Propose solutions to gaps in emergency preparedness identified at the November 9, 2001, executive session and identify the next steps.

Meeting overview

The meeting agenda featured brief presentations, as well as opportunities for discussion. Participants received updated information on two federal initiatives discussed at the November session: the MMRS and the National Pharmaceutical Stockpile (NPS). The MMRS is a contract mechanism through which the U.S. Department of Health and Human Services' Office of Emergency Preparedness supports activities among public and private agencies to achieve an operational system at the local level to respond to a weapon of mass destruction incident. The NPS, which is managed by the Centers for Disease Control and Prevention (CDC), consists of large, strategically positioned caches of drugs and other agents ("push packages") that can be sent to disaster sites. As well as pre-existing agreements with wholesalers to utilize vendor managed inventory during a response.

Meeting participants were also introduced to relevant developments that were not explored at the November meeting. One presenter described a proposed electronic data information network for monitoring the manufacture, distribution, and dispensing of pharmaceutical products nationwide. Another speaker described a proposed Institute of Medicine (IOM) study of the pro-

Reprinted with permission from ASHP: *Am J Health-Syst Pharm*; June 1, 2002, Vol 59

duction and availability of vaccines and antiinfective agents.

During the discussions, participants were asked to propose solutions or "next steps" to overcoming the gaps in emergency preparedness identified at the November 9 executive session. These gaps were

- Insufficient coordination of plans at the local level,
- Lack of awareness of the contents of the NPS push packages,
- Lack of pharmacist participation in local emergency-response planning and implementation,
- Insufficient appreciation of the complexity of the medication-use process,
- Lack of awareness of where emergency medications are located in the postdistribution network,
- Lack of communication between the private and public sectors,
- Lack of a means for drawing on qualified pharmacists' expertise during emergencies,
- Insufficient pharmacist involvement in emergency planning, and
- Lack of education and awareness.

Federal emergency response initiatives

MMRS update. The purpose of the MMRS program is to encourage private- and public-sector cooperation at the local level and to ensure that major metropolitan areas of the country have an appropriate response capability. As the program grows, its leaders are intent on ensuring that communities learn from one another: "My job," said one speaker, "is to make shameless thefts of what works."

Recent developments in the MMRS program were described from the federal perspective. The MMRS program will be expanded to 122 cities that cover two thirds of the U.S. population. Increased human resources will accompany the influx of financial support.

Commissioned Corps of the U.S. Public Health Service. The Commis-

sioned Corps Readiness Force (CCRF) is being expanded. All active-duty Public Health Service (PHS) commissioned officers may be deployable in times of emergency.

National Vaccine Advisory Committee. The National Vaccine Advisory Committee and a new assistant secretary will focus on ensuring that the vaccine supply is adequate.

Medical Reserve Corps. The Secretary of the Department of Health and Human Services (DHHS) plans to establish the Medical Reserve Corps as a component of the United States Freedom Corps, under which local volunteers with expertise in various areas, backed by federal resources, will be organized for community service. Building local infrastructure is critical, because responsibility for first response to disasters resides at the community level.

Survey of MMRS best practices. A speaker representing the DHHS' Office of Emergency Preparedness described the results of an informal survey done to identify MMRS best practices at the local level. One purpose of the survey was to determine the extent of pharmacist involvement in MMRS program development. Of 25 respondents, over 80% indicated that they did have pharmacists involved in inventory management. The same number of respondents stated that pharmacists are involved in overall emergency response planning through subcommittee representation. Some of the MMRS jurisdictions developed several years ago did not include pharmacists in their emergency response planning because pharmacists are not traditionally known as "first responders" (i.e., police, firefighters, and emergency medical technicians). This lack of pharmacist involvement was underscored by another survey, performed by University HealthSystem Consortium. This survey, reporting 26 responses concerning MMRS plans in 23 cities, revealed that there were no pharmacists on MMRS steer-

ing committees; pharmacists were represented on subcommittees. The 2002 MMRS program contract requires participation of pharmacists on the steering committee.

MMRS practices vary and are customized for local needs and resources. The best plans and practices, however, share one characteristic: They build on the combined abilities of individuals, organizations, and agencies in the private and public sectors to create a program that fits local needs. Examples of site-specific best practices:

- Several jurisdictions for mass-immunization or prophylaxis campaigns have been developed. Including a plan initiated by the health department within 24 hours of the recognized event, in collaboration with the state pharmacy association. One program has developed a partnership with the local school of pharmacy in which 500-600 volunteers can be utilized to assist with immunizations and breakdown of the NPS. Another program has created a step-by-step biological response plan involving community pharmacies.
- A jurisdiction has developed an innovative method for the procurement and provision of pharmaceutical products. A computer-based system identifies over 70 wholesale drug distributors and over 500 community pharmacies throughout the region. This system is utilized to complete a monthly survey of chemical antidotes and antibiotic stockpiles.
- Several jurisdictions have created policies and procedures for inventory management that define factors as location, storage, security, stock rotation, and access. In fact, one program has developed a unique areawide system to categorize inventory on the basis of response-time availability.
- Several jurisdictions have established partnerships with pharmacy and medical schools to assist with emergency response.
- Several jurisdictions have established

Reprinted with permission from ASHP: *Am J Health-Syst Pharm*; June 1, 2002, Vol 59

arrangements with drug wholesalers for inventory management. One program has made arrangements with drug wholesalers that guarantee around-the-clock access to antibiotic stockpiles, delivery of biological response agents to sites where mass prophylaxis is needed, redistribution of needed products to targeted areas, and assistance in obtaining extra supplies in times of crisis.

- Many jurisdictions have established wide networks of pharmacists that can be tapped to assist in the response efforts. One program has developed a "telephone tree" by which pharmacists can be summoned to assist in repackaging and distributing NPS push packages.
- One well-developed jurisdiction includes the formation of a "strike team" with representation by approximately 100 pharmacists and technicians. All team members undergo orientation and training in the breakdown and distribution of stockpiled drugs. Team members are prepared to collect and analyze adverse-drug-reaction reports from any mass-prophylaxis campaigns. The team includes pharmacists with specialized training in such areas as pediatrics and geriatrics.
- A college of pharmacy, a poison and drug information center, a college of public health, and the local fire department have joined forces in an MMRS program to offer a seminar on bioterrorism and weapons of mass destruction. Continuing-education units were available to participants.

National Pharmaceutical Stockpile. Within the NPS program, the number of push packages has been increased from 8 to 12, and the vendor-managed inventory stock has been increased. The goal of the NPS is to deliver push packages to the disaster site within 12 hours. Commercial contractors transport products to the site. With vastly increased post-September 11 funding, the NPS will provide more assistance to the states.

A state participating in the program must submit a plan for how it will manage the push packages upon their arrival within its borders. NPS has developed a computer-based tool to help states develop their plans. A planning guide, which includes recommended pharmacist functions, is also available, and a videotape is in production.

The Office of the Inspector General is conducting an audit of state preparedness to receive the NPS materials; the outcome of this report will shape future NPS activities. Areas of planned activity include enabling the states to improve transport, facilitating more localized deployment of chemical agents, and making it easier to break down the push packages through the use of industrial packaging machines and unit-of-dispensing containers.

Emergency-preparedness activity in the private sector

Real-time electronic information. The desirability of a nationwide, real-time electronic network among all organizations in the public and private sectors that are involved in the manufacture, distribution, and dispensing of pharmaceutical products was a major topic at the November 2001 executive session. During the second session, a potential plan for such a system was outlined. The proposed Product Availability Inquiry and Response (PAIR) Network would take advantage of existing connectivity and interfaces among manufacturers, distributors, hospital and community pharmacies, and government and public health agencies at the federal, state, and local levels and link them via electronic data interchange (EDI).

Manufacturers would submit product information for entry into PAIR's item-level database. The system would be event triggered; the moment an emergency occurred, the relevant government agency could send a message through the system to

determine the availability of needed products—their quantities, their estimated delivery times, and any special instructions governing their use. Relevant providers would respond to this alert. The agency placing the request would determine the source from which the product would be procured, which could be the NPS, an MMRS or other cache, or any other source in the PAIR Network. The system, its designers believe, would serve as a "secure electronic pipeline for seeking, tracking, and accessing inventories on specific pharmaceutical products and for communicating special instructions concerning their use." Implementing the PAIR Network would begin with a needs analysis. Also required would be someone to manage the network.

Study of vaccines and antiinfective agents. Late in 2001, IOM convened a panel of experts from industry, academia, and practice to discuss IOM's role in ensuring the availability of vaccines and antiinfective agents. Participants concluded that any study by IOM should be grounded in an in-depth analysis of the economic forces that drive the pharmaceutical and biotechnology industries and that such a study should explore the incentives for the development of products that could be used, not only in attacks with bioterrorism agents but also for other purposes.

The study is expected to take 18 to 24 months. The economic analysis would be carried out by a firm with expertise in economic and systems analysis. IOM is currently looking for a study sponsor. A committee with 5 subcommittees or panels would explore the following areas: A vaccine and drug development subcommittee would examine economic, government, and social barriers to the development and maintenance of these agents and explore how the government and academia can join with industry to make needed products available. A panel on production

Reprinted with permission from ASHP: *Am J Health-Syst Pharm*; June 1, 2002, Vol 59

issues would study how the pharmaceutical industry could work more effectively with regulatory agencies. A third panel would analyze government policy on the use of antimicrobial agents. Another panel would study how to improve communication about the safe use of antiinfective agents. A fifth panel would explore vulnerabilities in the global drug distribution system.

Problems and answers

Participants used the list of gaps identified during the first executive session, as well as new ideas that arose during the second session, as a basis for discussion. The major problems identified and solutions suggested are described below.

Problem: Disasters and emergencies aside, drug shortages are a problem of growing significance nationwide. *Background.* Drug shortages are a matter of growing significance for pharmacists and the health care community. Reflecting members' concern, ASHP, in cooperation with the Drug Information Service of the University of Utah, publishes online Drug Product Shortage Bulletins.[2] The information in the bulletins is drawn from reports shared by ASHP members, the Food and Drug Administration (FDA), the University of Utah, pharmaceutical manufacturers, and other sources. The March 6 list, a typical example, contained more than 40 items.

Group members agreed that this is a serious problem and were intent on exploring ways to solve it. Approaches that focus on one particular product are often needed, but a broader approach is essential. "We need to come up with a way to focus on the *process* of the shortage and what can be done about it," said one participant.

Looking at process is important, because shortages arise for different reasons and are varied. Some are predictable; these include shortages that develop when the sole source of a medication decides to curtail production. Some shortages are absolute and have a nationwide impact; others affect only a certain geographic area. Shortages may develop because of hoarding. Some shortages emerge as a result of an FDA action resulting from a violation of good manufacturing practices (GMPs). Finally, some shortages involve products for which there is no alternative; in a much larger number of cases, acceptable alternatives are available.

Even when there are alternatives, drug shortages have a powerful effect. When one product is not available, prescribers turn to another, and then to another; the items in these categories, said one participant, tend to "domino." Eventually, several related items may end up on the shortage list. Switching products, moreover, has enormous implications for patient safety, staff training, and pharmacy logistics.

Solutions. Some participants suggested that shortages are not only a manufacturing issue; they are a public policy issue. They are also a knowledge issue. "In many cases, the word [on product availability] is not getting out," said one participant. Said another, "Once you have the information, you can analyze the shortage. You can tell what exists and why."

The information needed may eventually be available, online and in real time, through an EDI system like the PAIR Network. Other solutions that were proposed include the following:

- Ensure that all parties in the drug supply chain have a better understanding of production time lines. For example, when a company has met its sales target, it may temporarily shut down production of a product. Should an unanticipated need for that product develop, it may take several weeks to return production to normal.
- Consider negotiating with manufacturers who intend, for economic reasons, to stop producing items for which there are no or few alternatives.
- Through education and reassurance, discourage hoarding.
- Engage in "collaborative forecasting" for critical and unique products. Such forecasting could have been helpful in preventing or minimizing problems associated with protopam, which caused broad concern last year.
- Clarify FDA procedures related to curtailing manufacture of a product because of failure to comply with GMPs. Determine, if violations are minor, if there is a way to continue production of items for which there is no alternative without jeopardizing the public health.

Problem: There is too little sharing of information on pharmaceutical caches. *Background.* Awareness of the placement, contents, and availability of various caches of pharmaceuticals in the United States is key to overcoming shortages. Since 1999, the NPS has been a major cache for emergency use. The Department of Veterans Affairs (VA) is now developing caches of emergency drugs that will be placed in its medical centers. The Department of Defense and Office of Emergency Preparedness have supplies, as do MMRS cities. The ultimate "caches" are those under the control of community and hospital pharmacies, drug manufacturers, and wholesalers and suppliers. For a variety of reasons—chief among which are security concerns and a proprietary mindset—information on drug supplies and availability is not shared. Lack of information leads to uncertainty, unnecessary redundancies, and hoarding. It may create the impression of a shortage when none exists.

There is some sharing of information. For example, VA worked with CDC and the Office of Emergency Preparedness in developing its list of stored items. Individual MMRS jurisdictions, as illustrated in the best practices cited earlier, are sharing information; in addition, NPS makes

---

Reprinted with permission from ASHP: *Am J Health-Syst Pharm*; June 1, 2002, Vol 59

information on the contents of push packages available to MMRS jurisdictions. Openness and willingness to share, nonetheless, are too often the exception rather than the rule. "Does anyone know the total combined assets of all the caches?" asked one participant. Unfortunately, the question was rhetorical. Participants expressed divided opinions on the reluctance to share. One asserted that we have a "war mindset" that makes sharing information difficult, while another asserted that "we have no intention of being self-sufficient . . . we're not thinking of ourselves only."

Awareness of what is *not* in the caches is as important as knowing what is in them. For example, 15% of residents in a given community may be receiving hypertensive medication. An emergency-oriented cache could not be relied on to fill this need.

Solutions. To ensure optimum use of resources, people and organizations associated with the acquisition and maintenance of pharmaceutical supplies must be more willing to share information. This could be achieved in the following ways:

- Strengthen the mandate of the Federal Medical Materials Coordinating Group, which is charged with overseeing government caches.
- Encourage ASHP or another organization to work with DHHS and other federal agencies to bring the data together.
- In all discussions of resource sharing, acknowledge the role of human resources and the need to have personnel trained and deployed so that limited supplies can be used with the greatest safety and efficacy.
- Reexamine state public health laws; consider adding provisions that would enable governments to seize and redeploy inventories in times of emergency.
- Recognize that, in a major crisis, cities and states may not be able to rely on goodwill; legal mechanisms must be in place to facilitate resource sharing.

Problem: Activities surrounding the transport, unpacking, and use of materials in the NPS push packages need to be examined and improved. *Background.* Broader awareness of the content and estimated time of arrival of the NPS push packages is highly recommended, but that is only a beginning. Cities and states should also be able to plan for the transport, unpacking, and dispensing of pharmaceuticals. Health professionals need to be able to counsel patients and track them over time. Better plans are needed for integrating NPS deployment with existing onsite resources. Working out this integration must entail two-way discussions.

Solutions. The following suggestions were discussed with respect to optimum use of the push packages. Cost-effectiveness, as well as convenience, were driving forces behind these ideas.

- Encourage NPS to take a collaborative approach to policy development—one that takes advantage of local resources and responds to local needs.
- Establish connectivity with local wholesalers, which have established transportation systems in place, for secondary distribution of the push packages after their arrival at the crisis site. Wholesalers also have systems to track product distribution that might be valuable during emergencies.
- Think creatively; for example, refrigerator vans from local supermarkets could be used for transport.
- Expand dosage information, which is currently based on adult men.
- Instead of flagging expired products and returning them to their sources, consider retesting them. Redate products that remain potent and reintegrate them into the supply.
- Think creatively about logistics; for example, local sites may make arrangements with hotels to accommodate personnel.

Problem: Understanding of the medication-use process is inade-

quate. *Background.* Safe medication use involves more than dispensing a drug product to a patient. Failing to appreciate the many steps involved in safe medication use poses an even greater risk to patients during an emergency than it does under ordinary circumstances. First responders focus on getting medications to patients in acute need; they have little knowledge of, or time to consider, the other aspects of safe medication use: accurate diagnosis, laboratory tests, product packaging and labeling, counseling, dosage, drug interactions, tracking of distributed products, and patient follow-up.

Participants in the first executive session noted newspaper stories of ciprofloxacin being dispensed in resealable plastic bags in the wake of the anthrax contamination at a post office in Washington, D.C. They cited incidents in which patient counseling was insufficient or nonexistent. Such events did occur in the immediate aftermath of the terrorist events, but in a majority of cases, onsite health personnel moved quickly to correct them. Nonetheless, the experience underscores that a thorough understanding of the medication-use process is an essential component of an effective emergency response.

Solutions. The following answers to this problem were proposed:

- Mobilize pharmacists to take the lead in increasing understanding of the medication-use process. Participation of a pharmacist on the MMRS steering committees—now required—can expedite this.
- Develop and disseminate to each MMRS steering committee a statement that articulates the role of the pharmacist in the safe use of medications.
- Ensure that the MMRS plans cover such activities as patient diagnosis and testing, drug prescribing, dispensing, labeling, and packaging; tracking; patient counseling; and follow-up.
- Encourage MMRS pharmacists to assume responsibility for developing

Reprinted with permission from ASHP: *Am J Health-Syst Pharm*; June 1, 2002, Vol 59

medication-use documentation, including prescription-dispensing labels, site case report forms, medical supply order forms, patient-flow diagrams, and written health provider and patient information.

- Provide preservice, inservice, and continuing-education programs on safe medication use as a required part of the professional development of the staff of disaster-preparedness programs.
- Develop pharmacist-designed, pharmacist-led courses on various aspects of medication use for first responders.
- Invite distributors to be involved in planning at the local level.

Problem: Pharmacists are not sufficiently involved in disaster-response planning or in providing services at disaster sites. *Background.* Pharmacists, according to one federal spokesperson at the executive session, are uniquely qualified to participate in disaster-response efforts. "They are not just logisticians . . . pharmacists need to be involved in planning and in the ramp-up of disaster planning at the local level," he said. Such participation is far from optimal, as reflected by the survey of pharmacist participation in MMRS steering committees cited earlier in this report.

The encouraging news is that pharmacists are willing to get involved. More than 700 pharmacists responded to a call for volunteers included in a state board of pharmacy survey in Alabama; a Maryland survey produced similar results. Pharmacy organizations are attempting to spur action in this area. For example, ASHP communicates with its state societies on this issue and is creating a database that identifies pharmacists involved in disaster-response efforts. The Joint Commission of Pharmacy Practitioners (JCPP) has formed a work group that is exploring ways to reach out to and involve local pharmacists.

Solutions. Expanding pharmacist involvement will require concerted efforts at many levels. For example, planners could

- Consider making the new regulation mandating pharmacist participation on MMRS steering committees retroactive, so that all programs will have pharmacists in this key position.
- Urge pharmacists to be more proactive. Instead of waiting for an invitation, pharmacists should attend and take active roles in meetings.
- Encourage state chapters of pharmacy associations and state boards of pharmacy to expand their current efforts to inform pharmacists of the need for their collaboration and to suggest specific opportunities for such involvement.
- Create and disseminate a list of pharmacist consultants who can be tapped to provide advice to frontline providers and others. Some state pharmacy associations and schools of pharmacy have already created such lists for use in immunization programs; these could serve as a prototype for emergency-response lists.
- Include pharmacy students, pharmacy residents, and pharmacy technicians in outreach efforts.
- Encourage state boards of pharmacy to modify regulations so that pharmacists licensed in one state can practice in other states during emergencies.
- As long as pharmacist resources remain limited, make sure they are focused on areas where their impact can be greatest. One such area is instructing first responders in the appropriate handling of drug products.
- Take maximum advantage of pharmacists' numbers and accessibility to engage them in public education about the real and imagined risks of bioterrorism. Increased public understanding is key to preventing inappropriate emotional responses, such as those that followed the anthrax cases in October 2001.

Problem: Pharmacists need more training in disaster response. *Background.* Emergency preparedness is not a core topic in the pharmacy curriculum. Some schools have begun to incorporate this information into course work; however, much effort is needed to ensure that future, as well as current, practitioners are prepared to take leadership roles in disaster response.

Members of the CCRF are now required to complete online courses in disaster response. Pharmacists members of the National Disaster Medical System are strongly encouraged to complete the training. American Council on Pharmaceutical Education credit is granted to those who complete this course. A second course is being planned; this one will be conducted on-site and will model hands-on skills and feature topics such as setting up a mass-prophylaxis campaign. The Department of Defense has inquired about making the online course available to its pharmacists; however, funding for this is currently insufficient.

Pharmacy organizations like ASHP and the American Pharmaceutical Association are offering continuing-education programs at their educational meetings. A JCPP working group is collaborating with PHS to expand educational opportunities for pharmacists.

Solutions. Suggestions for expanding training opportunities included the following:

- Consider creating an ASHP specialty residency standard in disaster preparedness or adding requirements in this area to other ASHP residency accreditation standards.
- Urge state boards of pharmacy to mandate completion of course work in disaster preparedness for licensure and license renewal.
- Work with schools of pharmacy and associations such as the American Association of Colleges of Pharmacy to develop course materials for pharmacy students.
- Regularly offer continuing-education programs in emergency preparedness

Reprinted with permission from ASHP: *Am J Health-Syst Pharm*; June 1, 2002, Vol 59

at national and state pharmacy association meetings; publish articles in the pharmacy literature.

Problem: Communication at all levels is not as strong as it should be. One result is that best practices are not being shared. Instead of learning from one another, communities and organizations reinvent the wheel. *Background.* Many of the solutions to improving and expanding emergency-response capacity—particularly the acquisition of pharmaceutical supplies and the development of new educational programs—are expensive to implement and maintain. Improving communication can also be expensive, particularly if it involves new technology, such as EDI.

Better communication—perhaps the single most powerful means of improving emergency preparedness—can cost very little. It does, however, require a change in mindset. It also requires taking advantage of existing opportunities for information sharing and creating new ones. That sharing of information must take place among professions, organizations, and individuals and between the public and private sectors.

Solutions. Few would deny that improving communication is a laudable goal; it can also be nebulous. The following concrete ideas were suggested:

- Establish a central Web site and publicize its availability. Use this site to communicate information on all issues associated with disaster response. Even information on what donations are needed in a crisis could be put on the site.
- For MMRS, develop a centralized means of tracking, evaluating, and sharing best practices or prototypes.

- Find ways to communicate the importance of citizen involvement in public health. Preevent and postevent surveillance, for example, is an important public health activity. Innovative strategies should be used to encourage the citizen involvement in surveillance, as by placing kiosks in pharmacies or emergency rooms whereby patients could report their symptoms by ZIP code. Such systems would have many uses, such as tracking influenza outbreaks. Should a deadly threat posed by a pathogen be imminent, surveillance reports could provide an invaluable early-warning system.
- Encourage state regulatory boards to take part in promoting best practices.
- Convene pharmacy directors at the local and regional levels for information sharing; this is already taking place in New York.

Still more questions

Ensuring an adequate, accessible drug supply requires a high degree of collaboration between organizations and individuals in the public and private sectors at the local, state, and federal levels. Such collaboration is put to the test when disasters—floods, hurricanes, tornadoes, fires, or terrorist attacks—occur. The systems for pharmaceutical distribution and medication use will pass this test to the extent that they are grounded in a solid public health infrastructure.

The events of September 11 have led to positive actions on many fronts. None of these actions is more important than the commitment to reinvigorate the nation's public health infrastructure. Equally reassuring is that resources for emergency preparedness have increased, as has awareness of the need for emergency preparedness and the shared

responsibility for it. At the same time, hard questions remain. With finite resources and potentially infinite need, what is our national goal? Is it to protect everyone? If not, how should priorities be set? There is no public forum for the discussion of this fundamental question and little likelihood that it would be a popular topic for political debate.

Some resource-allocation questions will require more immediate answers. For example, what would happen if the federal government were no longer able to sustain its financial commitment to disaster response? When current caches are depleted or expired, how will they be replaced? Private organizations need resources, too. Working through their constituencies, these groups can take important roles in improving local emergency response. They do not, at present, benefit from the funding now being channeled into states and municipalities. Who will step forward to fund studies such as that proposed by IOM, the development of new technology such as the PAIR Network, or the design and conduct of needed educational programs?

Conclusion

As the meeting ended, participants expressed their willingness to serve as ambassadors by communicating the ideas generated to colleagues and others. They agreed that, given the size of the task, setting priorities will be essential.

References

1. Summary of the executive session on emergency preparedness and the pharmaceutical supply chain. *Am J Health-Syst Pharm.* 2002; 59:247-53.
2. American Society of Health-System Pharmacists. Drug product shortages management resources center. http://ashp.org/shortage (accessed 2002 Apr 18).

Conference participants, by affiliation

Government Offices

CDR Brian G. Kerr, M.S., M.B.A., MSC USN
  Deputy Chief, Pharmaceutical Division
  Defense Supply Center Philadelphia
  Philadelphia, Pennsylvania

CAPT Kathleen Downs, M.P.H.
  Medical Readiness Coordinator,
    Education Specialist
  Commissioned Corps Readiness Force
  Office of Emergency Preparedness
  U.S. Department of Health and
    Human Services
  Rockville, Maryland

Susan E. Gorman, Pharm.D., DABAT
  Senior Science Officer
  National Pharmaceutical Stockpile
    Program
  Centers for Disease Control and
    Prevention
  Atlanta, Georgia

CAPT Elizabeth A. Nolan, M.B.A., MSC USN
  Pharmacy Consultant/Specialty Leader
  Health Care Operations
  Bureau of Medicine and Surgery
  Washington, D.C.

COL W. Mike Heath, M.S.
  Pharmacy Consultant, U.S. Army
  Office of the Army Surgeon General
  Falls Church, Virginia

RADM Arthur Lawrence
  Acting Principal Deputy Assistant
    Secretary for Health
  Office of Public Health and Science
  Washington, D.C.

CAPT Thomas J. McGinnis
  Deputy Associate Commissioner
  Office of Policy, Planning & Legislation
  Food and Drug Administration
  Rockville, Maryland

Jimmy R. Mitchell, M.S., M.P.H.
  Director, Office of Pharmacy Affairs
  Health Resources and Services
    Administration
  U.S. Department of Health and
    Human Services
  Bethesda, Maryland

John E. Ogden, M.S., FASHP
  Chief Consultant for Pharmacy
    Benefits Management
  Department of Veterans Affairs
  Washington, D.C.

Wesley D. Robbins, Pharm.D.
  Associate Chief Consultant
  Emergency Pharmacy Services
  Department of Veterans Affairs
  Hines, Illinois

CAPT Jerry Phillips
  Associate Director for Medication
    Error Prevention
  Office of Drug Safety
  Food and Drug Administration
  Center for Drug Evaluation and
    Research
  Rockville, Maryland

CDR Matthew J. Tarosky, Pharm.D.
  U.S. Public Health Service
  Office of Emergency Preparedness
  Department of Health and Human
    Services
  Rockville, Maryland

Drug Manufacturers

Stephen D. Christian
  Director
  Logistics and Customer Service
  Abbott Laboratories
  Abbott Park, Illinois

Raymond W. Tiedemann
  Assistant Vice President
  Pricing, Forecasting, & Contracting
  Wyeth-Ayerst Pharmaceuticals
  St. Davids, Pennsylvania

Paul Minicozzi, Ph.D.
  Director, Scientific Affairs
  Wyeth-Ayerst Pharmaceuticals
  St. Davids, Pennsylvania

R. Duane Tackitt, M.S., FAPhA
  Director, Global Professional Affairs
  Wyeth Pharmaceuticals
  St. Davids, Pennsylvania

William B. Novotny
  Director, Pharmaceutical Supply
    Planning
  Wyeth Ayerst Laboratories
  Frazer, Pennsylvania

Michael A. Friedman, M.D.
  Senior Vice President, R&D
  Medical and Public Policy
  Pharmacia Corporation
  Peapack, New Jersey

Group Purchasing Organizations

Allen Dunehew, M.P.A.
  Vice President of Pharmacy
  AmeriNet Inc.
  St. Louis, Missouri

Wayne L. Russell, Pharm.D., FASHP
  Director of Pharmacy
  Novation, L.L.C.
  Irving, Texas

Weldon Johnson
  Director of Contracting/
    Environmental Purchasing
  Premier, Inc.
  Oak Brook, Illinois

Wholesalers

David Fister, M.B.A.
  Director, Quality and Government
    Contracts Compliance
  Cardinal Distribution
  Dublin, Ohio

Kent Rischar, B.S.
  Vice President, Government Accounts
  Health Systems Group
  AmerisourceBergen Corporation
  Chesterbrook, Pennsylvania

Ronald J. Streck
  President and CEO
  Healthcare Distribution Management
    Association
  Reston, Virginia

Sheri Fink
  Director, E-business Process
    Development
  Healthcare Distribution Management
    Association
  Reston, Virginia

Jeffrey L. Hill, Ph.D.
  President
  Healthcare Business Associates
  Research Triangle Park
  North Carolina

Reprinted with permission from ASHP: *Am J Health-Syst Pharm*; June 1, 2002, Vol 59

Community Pharmacy

Edward J. Staffa
   Director
   Pharmacy Practice & Communications
   National Association of Chain Drug
      Stores
   Alexandria, Virginia

Practitioners

David Chen, M.B.A.
   Pharmacy Director
   Shady Grove Adventist Hospital
   Rockville, Maryland

Joseph G. Barbaccia, Pharm.D.
   Director, Pharmacy Department
   Washington Hospital Center
   Washington, D.C.

Other Professional Associations and Organizations

Steve Bende, Ph.D.
   Vice President
   Science, Professional & Regulatory
      Affairs
   The Generic Pharmaceutical Association
   Washington, D.C.

Mitchel Rothholz
   Vice President, Professional Practice
   American Pharmaceutical Association
   Washington, D.C.

Douglas R. Smith, Pharm.D.
   Senior Director, Pharmacy and
      Oncology
   University HealthSystem Consortium
   Oak Brook, Illinois

Curtis Rooney
   Senior Associate Director & Counsel,
      Federal Affairs
   American Hospital Association
   Washington, D.C.

Richard A. Levinson
   Associate Executive Director
   American Public Health Association
   Washington, D.C.

Joseph Mislowack, M.S.
   Assistant Vice President, Pharmacy
      Services
   Greater NY Hospital Association
      Services, Inc.
   New York, New York

Rick Erdtmann, M.D., M.P.H.
   Senior Program Officer
   Medical Follow-Up Agency
   Washington, D.C.

Jane E. Henney, M.D.
   Scholar in Residence
   Association of Academic Health
      Centers
   Washington, D.C.

Lawrence H. Mokhiber, R.Ph.
   Executive Secretary
   New York Board of Pharmacy
   Albany, New York

Other

David A. Zilz, B.S., M.S.
   Consultant to ASHP, Past President
      and Treasurer
   Iola, Wisconsin

American Society of Health-System Pharmacists

Steven L. Sheaffer, Pharm.D., FASHP
   President
   American Society of Health-System
      Pharmacists
   Associate Professor and Vice Chair for
      Experiential Learning
   University of the Sciences in
      Philadelphia
   Philadelphia, Pennsylvania

Henri R. Manasse, Jr, Ph.D., Sc.D.
   Executive Vice President and Chief
      Executive Officer
   American Society of Health-System
      Pharmacists
   Bethesda, Maryland

William A. Zellmer, M.P.H.
   Deputy Executive Vice President
   American Society of Health-System
      Pharmacists
   Bethesda, Maryland

Charles E. Myers, M.S., M.B.A.
   Vice President
   Professional and Scientific Affairs
      Office
   American Society of Health-System
      Pharmacists
   Bethesda, Maryland

Brian M. Meyer
   Director, Government Affairs Division
   American Society of Health-System
      Pharmacists
   Bethesda, Maryland

Gary C. Stein, Ph.D.
   Director, Federal Regulatory Affairs
   Government Affairs Division
   American Society of Health-System
      Pharmacists
   Bethesda, Maryland

Kristina E. Lunner
   Director, State Legislative and
      Regulatory Affairs
   American Society of Health-System
      Pharmacists
   Bethesda, Maryland

Gerald K. McEvoy, Pharm.D.
   Assistant Vice President
   Publications and Drug Information
      Systems Office
   Editor, *AHFS Drug Information*
   American Society of Health-System
      Pharmacists
   Bethesda, Maryland

David R. Witmer, Pharm.D.
   Director, Professional Practice and
      Scientific Affairs Division
   American Society of Health-System
      Pharmacists
   Bethesda, Maryland

Douglas J. Scheckelhoff, M.S., FASHP
   Director, Division of Practice
      Leadership and Management
   American Society of Health-System
      Pharmacists
   Bethesda, Maryland

Joseph H. Deffenbaugh, M.P.H.
   Professional Practice Associate,
      Professional   Practice and Scientific
      Affairs Division
   American Society of Health-System
      Pharmacists
   Bethesda, Maryland

Jamilla-Ann V. Bethune, Pharm.D.
   Executive Resident
   Administration and Information
      Systems Technology
   American Society of Health-System
      Pharmacists
   Bethesda, Maryland

Writer

Linda Harteker
   Washington, D.C.

Reprinted with permission from ASHP: *Am J Health-Syst Pharm*; June 1, 2002, Vol 59

ASHP Statement on the Role of Health-System Pharmacists in Counterterrorism

Am J Health-Syst Pharm. 2002; 59:282-3

As the United States began to enhance counterterrorism measures in response to the homeland terrorist attacks of September 11, 2001, it became clear that hospital and health-system pharmacists have an essential role to play in those measures. The American Society of Health-System Pharmacists (ASHP) believes that hospital and health-system pharmacists must assertively exercise their responsibilities to counter terrorist acts, and the leaders of emergency planning at the federal, regional, state, and local levels must call on pharmacists to participate in the full range of issues related to pharmaceuticals.

General principles

1. On the basis of their education, training, experience, and legal responsibilities, pharmacists should have a key role in the planning and execution of (a) pharmaceutical distribution and control and (b) drug therapy management of patients in the event of a homeland terrorist attack with weapons of mass destruction (WMD), especially chemical, biological, and nuclear agents.
2. The expertise of the pharmacist must be sought in (a) selecting pharmaceuticals and related supplies for national and regional stockpiles and local emergency inventories in counterterrorism programs, (b) ensuring proper packaging, storage, handling, labeling, and dispensing of emergency supplies of pharmaceuticals, (c) ensuring appropriate deployment of emergency supplies of pharmaceuticals in the event of a terrorist attack, (d) developing guidelines for the diagnosis and treatment of victims of WMD, and (e) ensuring appropriate education and counseling of individuals who receive pharmaceuticals from an emergency supply after a terrorist attack.
3. Pharmacists must be in a position to advise public health officials on appropriate messages to convey to the public about the use of essential pharmaceuticals after terrorist attacks, giving consideration to issues such as adverse effects, contraindications, the effectiveness of alternative pharmaceuticals, and the potential development of drug-resistant infectious agents.
4. In the event of a terrorist attack, pharmacists should be called on to collaborate with physicians and other prescribers in the drug therapy management of individual victims.

Advice to hospital and health-system pharmacy directors

Every hospital and health-system pharmacy director (or designee) should

The ASHP Board of Directors welcomes comments on this document, which is subject to ratification by the ASHP House of Delegates at its next session in June 2002. The Board may make revisions, based on comments received, before the final vote by the House. Please send comments to the ASHP Executive Office, 7272 Wisconsin Avenue, Bethesda, MD 20814 (email address: evp@ashp.org) by March 15, 2002.

1. Become thoroughly informed of federal, regional, state, local, and institutional plans for emergency preparedness, especially those related to the distribution, control, and use of pharmaceuticals;
2. Ensure that the pharmaceutical components of the institution's emergency plans are coordinated with the overall local preparedness plans involving other institutions, community pharmacies, and wholesalers as well as coordinated with federal, regional, and state plans;
3. Ensure that the appropriate pharmaceuticals and related equipment and supplies are in stock at the institution, consistent with the overall local preparedness plan, which

Approved by the ASHP Board of Directors on November 27, 2001. Subject to ratification by the ASHP House of Delegates.

The bibliographic citation for this document is as follows: American Society of Health-System Pharmacists. ASHP Statement on the Role of Health-System Pharmacists in Counterterrorism. *Am J Health-Syst Pharm.* 2002; 59:282-3

Index terms: Administration; American Society of Health-System Pharmacists; Antidotes; Biological warfare; Chemical warfare; Disaster planning; Drugs; Emergency services; Guidelines; Nuclear warfare; Organizations; Patient information; Pharmacists, hospital; Pharmacists, institutional; Public health; Violence

Copyright © 2002, American Society of Health-System Pharmacists, Inc. All rights reserved. 1079-2082/02/0201-0282$06.00

should account for the interim between the occurrence of a terrorist attack and the receipt of federal or state assistance;

4. Ensure that information about the appropriate use of pharmaceuticals in response to a terrorist attack is available to the health professionals in the institution;

5. Ensure that the institution does not engage in stockpiling of pharmaceuticals without regard to local counterterrorism plans that are designed to meet the needs of the whole community; and

6. Ensure that pharmacy personnel are trained to implement the institution's emergency plans.

Advice to hospital and health-system pharmacists

Every hospital and health-system pharmacist should

1. Become well informed about the threats of chemical, biological, and nuclear terrorism, including potential agents that could be used in an attack and the related diagnostic and treatment issues;

2. Share with professional colleagues and patients evidence-based information on pharmaceuticals used to respond to terrorist attacks;

3. Act assertively to prevent and allay panic and irrational responses after acts of terrorism;

4. Strongly discourage individuals from developing personal stockpiles of pharmaceuticals for use in the event of chemical, biological, or nuclear terrorism;

5. Consider volunteering in advance of any terrorist attack to assist in (a) distributing emergency supplies of pharmaceuticals and (b) managing the

drug therapy of individual victims; and

6. Develop and maintain first-aid skills.

Advice to hospital and health-system administrators

Hospital and health-system administrators should

1. Ask the pharmacy director to participate in preparing the institution's emergency preparedness plan;

2. Consult with the pharmacy director to coordinate the institution's participation in the building of emergency pharmaceutical supplies for use in the community;

3. Refrain from building institutional stockpiles of pharmaceuticals that are not coordinated with the local plan;

4. Encourage local preparedness-planning officials to involve pharmacists in the full range of issues related to pharmaceuticals; and

5. Encourage and enable pharmacy personnel employed by the institution to volunteer for community service in the event of a terrorist attack.

Advice to emergency preparedness planners

Emergency preparedness planners at the federal, regional, state, and local levels should

1. Consult with qualified pharmacists in all areas in which the pharmacist's expertise is necessary to make workable plans;

2. Inform pharmacists, through national and state pharmacy organizations, of plans for deployment of emergency pharmaceutical supplies so that appropriate plans can be made at the local level; and

3. Consult with qualified pharmacists on messages that should be conveyed to

the public about the appropriate use of pharmaceuticals in the event of chemical, biological, or nuclear terrorism.

Advice to state societies of health-system pharmacists

State societies of health-system pharmacists should

1. Offer their assistance to state and local disaster-planning officials;

2. Advise their members of information unique to the state regarding pharmacists' participation in emergency preparedness planning and deployment efforts; and

3. Consider establishing a volunteer network of health-system pharmacists for deployment in the event of a terrorist attack.

Commitments made by ASHP

In support of the efforts of health-system pharmacists in counterterrorism, ASHP will

1. Maintain an electronic communications network of hospital pharmacy department directors that can be used to transmit urgent information related to counterterrorism;

2. Disseminate promptly to ASHP members important new information related to pharmacist involvement in counterterrorism;

3. Disseminate to ASHP members and others in the health-care community timely evidence-based information about pharmaceuticals used when responding to chemical, biological, or nuclear terrorism; and

4. Meet with government officials and others when necessary to clarify promptly important issues that affect the involvement of health-system pharmacists in counterterrorism.

Reprinted with permission from ASHP: *Am J Health-Syst Pharm*; February 1, 2002, Vol 59

Managing in a crisis: Planning, acting, and learning

WILLIAM P. JOHNSTON AND PAUL L. STEPANOVICH

Am J Health-Syst Pharm. 2001; 58:1245-9

As she drove into her neighborhood, Janice Parker felt the excitement beginning to grow. Although she had worked at her desk a few extra hours this Friday evening, her weekend off was about to begin. Just a few more hours of administrative on-call, and Saturday and Sunday would belong to her. She had only a moment to enjoy that thought before her pager buzzed. Calling from home, she learned that automated drug cabinets throughout the facility were "crashing" and that the pharmacy's computer system was down. Soon her car was pointed back toward the medical center. "The phone is ringing off the hook!" she had been told. Friday evening's reduced staff was probably overwhelmed by calls from nurses trying to obtain medications for the 8 p.m. administration time. Caught up in dealing with these phone calls, the staff was probably falling behind in processing new medication orders. That, in turn, would lead to more phone calls. Meanwhile, patients were not getting needed medications. Perhaps she should ask for more staff to meet her at the pharmacy. She could call for the controlled-substances pharmacists to come in to set up a backup dispensing system during the outage.

"I wonder how many nursing units are involved," she worried. "Is every unit without access to controlled drugs and floor stock? This could be bad! How should I respond? Should I go directly to the pharmacy, or should I go to the administrative wing, where the control panel for the drug cabinets is located? Perhaps I should go immediately to one of the nursing areas to gather information and smooth communication. I wonder what the pharmacy staff members on site are doing. Has anyone taken charge? Who's on duty tonight? Darn it! It's just one crisis after another! I spent last weekend getting the pharmacy ready for a hurricane that never showed up. This weekend I'm rushing back in because of some kind of technology failure!"

Most health-system pharmacy managers can identify with Janice. We often speak loosely of dealing with one crisis after another. In many cases, these "crises" are really minor aggravations that can be addressed with minimal expenditure of resources and with little risk to pharmacy operations or patient safety. However, we are always at risk of experiencing a true crisis, the type of situation that could test our management skills (or our luck). Hurricanes and floods, for example, have necessitated the implementation of disaster plans by many health-system pharmacies in recent years. The risks associated with technology failure were highlighted in 1999 with the approach of January 1, 2000, and a potential "Y2K" catastrophe. Having survived Y2K and other potential disasters, it is tempting to put crisis management activities on the back burner and become absorbed in more routine management activities. But perhaps crisis management should become one of those routine activities. And perhaps, with recent crises or threats in mind, we should ask just what constitutes a crisis and whether the pharmacy team can prepare to respond effectively to unexpected crises.

Where can we look for insights into the recognition and management of crises? Major crises are not new to the business community. Famous examples include the Tylenol-tampering incident, the Exxon Valdez oil spill, and the explosion of the Union Carbide chemical plant in

WILLIAM P. JOHNSTON, PH.D., is Staff Pharmacist, Department of Pharmacy Services, Medical University of South Carolina, Charleston. PAUL L. STEPANOVICH, PH.D., is Assistant Professor, Community and Environmental Health, Old Dominion University, Norfolk, VA.

Address correspondence to Dr. Stepanovich at Old Dominion University, 129 Spong Hall, Norfolk, VA 23529-0288 (pstepano@odu.edu).

Copyright © 2001, American Society of Health-System Pharmacists, Inc. All rights reserved. 1079-2082/01/0701-1245$06.00.

Bhopal, India. More recently, the news media have focused on Firestone's defective tires. A 1993 survey of Fortune 1000 companies identified crises actually faced by those companies.[1] The list included copyright infringement, rumors, executive kidnapping, extortion, bribery, computer breakdowns, product defects, environmental accidents, and sabotage. While kidnapping and bribery may seem improbable for the average pharmacy operation, it is clear that many businesses have found it necessary to prepare for a wide range of threats. In this article, we examine the business literature on the nature and management of crises and seek principles of crisis management that might offer guidance for health-system pharmacy managers.

The nature of crises. Early and well-publicized warnings allowed ample preparation time for Y2K. Even with hurricanes, whose paths cannot yet be precisely predicted, warning for regions at high risk is generally available hours or even days ahead. Most organizations already have policies and procedures in place for dealing with such natural disasters.[1] For many other types of crises, particularly human-induced ones, warnings may not be possible or at least may not be clear (until viewed in retrospect). Even so, it is crucial to prepare in advance for a variety of potential crises. What is a crisis, and what types of crises is a pharmacy vulnerable to?

Several definitions of crisis are found in the literature. Remarking on major corporate disasters, Mitroff et al.[2] ascribed causation to people, organizational structures, economics, and technology and noted the resulting devastation of organizations' finances and reputation. Greening and Johnson[3] described threat, surprise, and magnitude as attributes of crisis and discussed the need for a quick response and the implication of high costs if the event is not handled effectively. Of course, costs can be measured in dollars or in human comfort

and well-being. Pearson et al.[4] considered an event to be a crisis if it threatens the viability of the organizational unit, compromises health and safety, or threatens the public trust. A crisis is also, according to these authors, anything that "hyperextends" the organization, or stretches it beyond its capabilities. Stubbart[5] distinguished crises by their "wickedness"—their associated uncertainty, complexity, conflicts of interest, and emotional involvement. Stubbart pointed out that crises lack both a clear problem statement and an established set of criteria that might aid in selecting an effective solution from among numerous possibilities.

Pearson and Clair[6] incorporated a blend of aspects of crisis into their definition: "An organizational crisis is a low-probability, high-impact event that threatens the viability of the organization and is characterized by ambiguity of cause, effect, and means of resolution, as well as by a belief that decisions must be made swiftly." Since it brings together the perspectives of a number of authorities, the Pearson and Clair definition will serve as a foundation for our discussion. Four criteria (low probability, high impact, ambiguity, and pressure for a quick solution) appear to be applicable to health-system pharmacy. Situations that meet these criteria are clearly different from the average complications and challenges that arise from day to day.

Let us look at the example of technology failure experienced by Janice Parker's institution. The simultaneous failure of multiple, diversely located units of electronic equipment (e.g., computers and automated controlled-substance cabinets) is relatively unlikely in most pharmacy systems, assuming that this network of electronic devices has a history of reliable performance within the pharmacy. The Janice Parker example satisfies the second criterion also. Unanticipated technology failure presents the possibility of serious negative consequences of one type or another.

A major component or components of the distributive system have failed and could present harm to patients, as well as damage the confidence of patients, health professionals, and administrators in the system. The third criterion, ambiguity, also fits our example. Early in the developing crisis, Janice does not know what caused the automated drug cabinets to fail, which ones have failed so far, where the failed machines are located, and whether additional (perhaps all) machines will fail as the situation progresses. Nor does she know how long systems will be down. Meanwhile, stress is heightened as nurses, nurse administrators, hospital administrators, and others call in, anxious over lost access to vital medications. Certain only of uncertainty, Janice feels pressured to initiate, without delay, actions she believes will minimize damage and speed operations back to normal. She may have to act without a thorough analysis, which requires time and data.

For many managers, the example of failing hardware and software may be old hat. It does serve, however, to illustrate the nature of crises and the pressures often associated with crisis decision-making. Other possible pharmacy crises might include critical citations by accrediting or regulatory agencies, a series of catastrophic errors, medication tampering, computer hacking aimed at pharmacy systems, attacks by computer viruses, and work stoppages. With a handle on what constitutes a crisis, management can better identify the ones that present high risk to a given pharmacy operation and can formally prepare for them.

Managing crises. While the literature offers various definitions of crisis, there seems to be more agreement on what constitutes crisis management. Essentially, it is a systematic effort to avoid crises or to minimize the adverse effects of crises.[3] Crisis management implies a process that drives decision-making[4] and whose purpose is "to prepare an organiza-

Reprinted with permission from ASHP: *Am J Health-Syst Pharm*; July 1, 2001, Vol 58

tion to think about the unthinkable."[1] Crisis management is effective if it sustains, or quickly restores, core operations with minimal or no losses.[6] In the literature, causes of crises are generally couched in systems theory. Highly interactive, tightly coupled systems are more prone to crises.[3] Again, from the systems perspective, Pearson and Mitroff[1] noted that crises tend not to happen in isolation. In every crisis they examined there were elements compounding the crisis event. When it rains, it pours! Of course, management also faces the ever-present possibility of making a bad situation even worse.[7]

What can we do? Fortunately, we can learn a lot from the experiences of businesses and from scholars who have analyzed crises. Perhaps most important, we find that organizations can prepare for crises and that there are guidelines for successful responses. Many frameworks have been proposed for effective crisis management. The crisis management model highlights proactive as opposed to reactive responses to a crisis.[2] Pearson and Mitroff[1] provided a checklist of key actions in crisis management programs and grouped these activities into five categories: strategic actions, technical and structural actions, evaluative and diagnostic **actions**, communication actions, and psychological and cultural actions. Although the checklist reflects corporate efforts, pharmacy managers developing their own crisis management programs would find many features helpful. A six-stage approach was described by Augustine[7]: avoiding the crisis, preparing to manage the crisis, recognizing the crisis, containing the crisis, resolving the crisis, and profiting from the crisis.[7] Finally, Pearson and colleagues[4] listed five phases of crisis management: signal detection, preparation, damage containment, recovery, and learning and provided a self-assessment guide to preparedness. Drawing primarily on these sources, we have created a condensed set of pharmacy-applicable guide-

lines for crisis management. These guidelines fall into three categories, or stages: planning, acting, and learning (Figure 1).

Planning. Is it really possible, or practical, to plan for crises, given their nature (e.g., unpredictability and high ambiguity)? In view of the multitude of potential crises, how can management prepare for every possibility? The Mitroff et al.[2] model of crisis management reveals that detection of precrisis indicators is fundamental to proactive prevention. The lack of formal prevention places an unprepared management in the disadvantageous position of reacting to crises after they occur. Mitroff et al. make two other valuable points in this regard. First, even though management cannot expect to prevent all crises through planning, formal planning enables better responses to the crises that do occur. Second, organizations that believe that they are not at risk for a crisis tend to be very susceptible to crises. Planning, therefore, is the essence of proactive crisis management.

In our simplified scheme, planning includes both prevention of and preparation for crises. Crisis management can be brought into the pharmacy management routine through incorporation into the department's

formal strategic planning. Strategic management should include prioritizing possible crises according to their likelihood and potential impact. This screening should result in annual implementation plans addressing preparedness for targeted crises. As screening is repeated over time, the department can develop formal plans for a variety of potential crises. Attempting to prepare concrete plans for every possible crisis at one time should be avoided.

The creation and ongoing support of a crisis management team demonstrates management's commitment to preventing and preparing for crises. It also identifies an individual or individuals responsible for crisis planning and, if necessary, for the acting and learning phases of crisis management. The crisis management team should be formed before any crisis occurs. This will allow the team to evaluate current risk, identify likely or particularly damaging threats, develop selected crisis plans, and train managers and staff to respond to targeted situations. Recommended techniques for crisis team development and planning include the use of scenarios[4] and the inclusion of outsiders on the team.[1] Outsiders should include representatives from the other disciplines or departments with

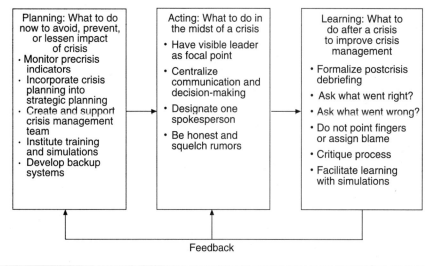

Figure 1. Crisis management process. Planning, acting, and learning form a cycle, with feedback completing the loop.

Planning: What to do now to avoid, prevent, or lessen impact of crisis
- Monitor precrisis indicators
- Incorporate crisis planning into strategic planning
- Create and support crisis management team
- Institute training and simulations
- Develop backup systems

Acting: What to do in the midst of a crisis
- Have visible leader as focal point
- Centralize communication and decision-making
- Designate one spokesperson
- Be honest and squelch rumors

Learning: What to do after a crisis to improve crisis management
- Formalize postcrisis debriefing
- Ask what went right?
- Ask what went wrong?
- Do not point fingers or assign blame
- Critique process
- Facilitate learning with simulations

Feedback

which the pharmacy would have significant interactions during a crisis.[3] With the inclusion of appropriate outsiders, even small pharmacy operations should be able to create crisis management teams with relevant expertise. Teams will also benefit from including newer members of the organization, as well as from improved managerial education.[3]

Maintaining a tightly knit crisis management team is essential. According to Weick,[8] pooled interdependent teams (often called crews) that come together to do their jobs but do not work together continuously over a period of time do not perform well in a crisis. Crews that assemble only infrequently to address pharmacy problems may lack the coordination skills necessary to perform effectively. In addition to this danger, much decision-making, even in normal circumstances, is emotion based; this is exacerbated in crises.[9] The training and planning that comes out of the crisis management team's activities are essential for overcoming the irrational and potentially dangerous decisions that sometimes occur in a crisis.

The preparation of backup systems (and even backups for the backups) is necessary for technology-driven operations. This applies not only to major technological equipment, such as robots and computer systems, but also to more basic devices, such as telephones and pagers. Measures are needed to communicate within and outside the institution if telephones and pagers are not functioning.

An important role of the crisis team (and of management) is the continual survey of the internal and external environments to detect early warning signs of potential crises and to recognize actual crises.[1,4,7] If the public or the hospital staff perceives a major flaw in the drug-use system (e.g., in availability, cost, preparation, distribution, or administration), that perception, accurate or not, can cause great harm. Gathering

data, observing the experiences of other health care providers, and playing devil's advocate are part of the team's function.

Despite an active program of monitoring, targeting, and training, crises will still occur. Planning should enhance the ability to respond effectively.

Acting. Top management must be highly visible during a crisis. Even if the director has little expertise in the problem at hand (e.g., a software failure), he or she can provide support and a sense of order and direction. Most of all, the director (or the director's designee) can become the focal point for decisions and communication. Consider the example of a crisis arising in the pharmacy service of a large institution. It is late in the day shift, and several managers rush to the main pharmacy. As the crisis begins to unfold, no one really has a complete picture of the problem or its cause yet. As nursing units telephone, pharmacists, technicians, and various managers are simultaneously presenting their own perceptions of events to different units. Unverified information, speculation, and rumors are flying. Moreover, the situation continues to change by the minute. Multiple individuals seek to take charge of some aspect of the situation, offering hypotheses and solutions (possibly conflicting) of their own to whomever is listening.

This situation, if not one of outright chaos, is certainly fraught with opportunities to make a bad situation worse. There are two primary points to make here. First, regardless of what shift is involved, one individual must be clearly in charge. On any shift, someone must be empowered to make decisions until top management or the crisis team arrives. In some cases, it may be over an hour until management support arrives. The time to designate persons for the decision-making role is during the planning stage, well before a crisis occurs. Training in crisis management, and in specific crisis scenarios,

should then become an integral part of their training.[9] In the event of a crisis, this leader can expect to be hit with a "tidal wave of information"[5] and must sort through it all to identify accurate information on which to base decisions. The crisis management team can be of great assistance in this process. Relying on training, crisis plans, and established information networks, the charge pharmacist or manager on duty will have important resources on hand to aid in decision-making. Even if rehearsed scenarios turn out not to be completely accurate, the decision-maker will have the advantage in addressing new situations.

The second point is the critical role of communication. As in decision-making, there must be one spokesperson for the pharmacy service. The planning phase should include developing channels of communication with nurse managers, institutional administrators, security personnel, computer support personnel, and others. These parties, in turn, should know who is authorized to speak for the pharmacy. It is the job of the pharmacy spokesperson to sift through all the rumors and misinformation and to fill in gaps to provide an accurate account of the situation as it is known at that moment. This includes keeping the pharmacy staff informed.

Learning. Pearson and colleagues[4] pointed to the learning stage as an opportunity to identify and evaluate what can be gained from the crisis. What went right? How can it be reinforced in future planning? What went wrong? How can this be remedied? What planning assumptions held, and which ones did not? Augustine[7] referred to the learning stage as "profiting from the crisis."

The assessment should be formal, with management and the crisis management team charged with documenting the findings and improving the crisis management process. It is tempting, after having survived a crisis, to let out one's breath and pro-

Reprinted with permission from ASHP: *Am J Health-Syst Pharm*; July 1, 2001, Vol 58

ceed with business as usual. In fact, participants in the crisis will tend to distance themselves from it.[4] There is also a tendency to make the learning stage an exercise in finger pointing.[1] Rather, assigning blame should be avoided and the focus placed on the systemic aspects. The formal structure of the debriefing is needed to resist these temptations.

Learning need not be limited to actual crises. Simulations are often effective alternatives to real-world learning. In the real world, the time lag between decision and outcome may preclude effective learning. Some decisions are too risky to try in the real world but can be explored in a simulation.[10] Computer simulations have been used to train radiologists and anesthesiologists in crisis management.[11,12] Similarly, system dynamics modeling can be used to create "flight simulators" to train pharmacy managers in crisis management.

Conclusion. The business literature provides a workable definition of a crisis, makes a strong case for advance preparation for crises, and suggests guidelines for dealing with the "wickedness" of crisis situations. How might Janice Parker's experience have been different had the pharmacy had strong, crisis-sensitive leadership and a seasoned crisis management team? Most of her questions would have been answered, and her energies would have been redirected to finding effective solutions. More important, she would then begin to address the systemic factors surrounding the crisis to reduce the likelihood of its recurrence.

References

1. Pearson CM, Mitroff II. From crisis prone to crisis prepared: a framework for crisis management. *Acad Manage Exec.* 1993; 7(1):48-59.
2. Mitroff II, Shrivastava P, Udwadia FE. Effective crisis management. *Acad Manage Exec.* 1987; 1(3):283-92.
3. Greening DW, Johnson RA. Do managers and strategies really matter? A study in crisis. *J Manage Studies.* 1996; 33(1):25-51.
4. Pearson CM, Clair JA, Misra SK et al. Managing the unthinkable. *Organ Dyn.* 1997; 26(2):51-64.
5. Stubbart CI. Improving the quality of crisis thinking. *Columbia J World Bus.* 1987; 22:89-99.
6. Pearson CM, Clair JA. Reframing crisis management. *Acad Manage Rev.* 1998; 23(1):59-76.
7. Augustine NR. Managing the crisis you tried to prevent. *Harv Bus Rev.* 1995; 73(6):147-58.
8. Weick KE. The collapse of sensemaking in organizations: the Mann Gulch disaster. *Admin Sci Q.* 1993; 38:628-52.
9. Duchon D, Ashmos D, Dunegan KJ. Avoid decision making disaster by considering psychological bias. *Rev Bus.* 1991; 13(1-2):13-8.
10. Sterman JD. Business dynamics: systems thinking and modeling for a complex world. Boston: McGraw-Hill; 2000.
11. Sica GT, Barron DM, Blum R et al. Computerized realistic simulation: a teaching module for crisis management in radiology. *Am J Radiol.* 1999; 172:301-4.
12. Gada DM. Improving anesthesiologist's performance by simulating reality. *Anesthesiology.* 1992; 76:491-4.

Pharmacy preparedness for incidents involving weapons of mass destruction

ANTHONY M. BURDA AND TODD SIGG

Introduction

Recent events, such as the Sarin gas attack in a Tokyo subway station in March 1995 and several anthrax hoaxes in the United States, have heightened concern among public health and law enforcement agencies that a real nuclear, biological, or chemical (NBC) attack may occur in this nation. The potential for a terrorist attack using a chemical or biological agent has many individuals involved with public health and safety, equipping themselves with information, contingency plans, and procedures to cope with such threats. Information from various governmental and other agencies is available concerning preparedness for a terrorist attack involving NBC weapons.[1-5] Instruction in this area is available via journal articles, Web sites, onsite and Internet training programs, seminars, and conferences.

Most references will provide practical discussion on issues such as local and statewide planning, onsite and hospital decontamination procedures, recognition and detection of NBC agents, diagnosis and pathophysiology of disease states, protocols for first responders, and a wide range of other public health issues.[6-10]

The objective of this article is to

Abstract: Recent worldwide terrorist acts and hoaxes have heightened awareness that incidents involving weapons of mass destruction (WMD) may occur in the United States. With federal funding assistance, local domestic preparedness programs have been initiated to train and equip emergency services and emergency department personnel in the management of large numbers of casualties exposed to nuclear, biological, or chemical (NBC) agents. Hospital pharmacies will be required to provide antidotes, antibiotics, antitoxins, and other pharmaceuticals in large amounts and have the capability for prompt procurement. Pharmacists should become knowledgeable in drug therapy of NBC threats with respect to nerve agents, cyanide, pulmonary irritants, radionucleotides, anthrax, botulism, and other possible WMD.

Index terms: Antidotes; Disaster planning; Biological warfare; Chemical warfare; Nuclear warfare
Am J Health-Syst Pharm. 2001; 58:2274-84

provide the pharmacy practitioner a concise summary and description of the types of pharmaceutical products that a health care facility pharmacy may be asked to provide as part of an overall response to an incident involving a weapon of mass destruction (WMD). These products may include, but are not limited to, antidotes, antibiotics, antitoxins, and other agents used in the symptomatic and supportive care of the poisoned patient. This list has been derived from a number of sources that describe the most common potential chemicals or biologicals that may be encountered in such a situation. Pharmacy managers are urged to check inventory for these products

and know where the nearest supplier (e.g., wholesaler, pharmaceutical manufacturer, etc.) is for each agent. It is important to know how these supplies can be obtained quickly in emergencies. Pharmacy managers often look to official sources (e.g., Joint Commission on the Accreditation of Healthcare Organizations, Food and Drug Administration, state health departments, etc.) for mandatory or suggested guidelines for the adequate stocking of antidotes and other pharmaceutical products needed when responding to community needs involving the use of WMD. Unfortunately, no such official "checklist" exists. Several studies have been published demonstrating inadequate

ANTHONY M. BURDA, R.PH., DABAT, is Chief Specialist, and TODD SIGG, PHARM.D., is Certified Specialist, Poison Information, Illinois Poison Center, Chicago.

Address correspondence to Mr. Burda at the Illinois Poison Cen-

ter, 222 South Riverside Plaza, Suite 1900, Chicago, IL 60606.

Originally published in the *Journal of Pharmacy Practice, Vol. 13, No. 2/April 2000.* Reprinted with permission. Copyright © 2000, Technomic Publishing Co., Inc.

Reprinted with permission from ASHP: *Am J Health-Syst Pharm*; December 1, 2001, Vol 58

stocking of poison antidotes used for a variety of toxicologic emergencies. These would include: digoxin immune Fab (Digibind) for cardiac glycoside poisoning, ethanol for toxic alcohol poisoning, pyridoxine hydrochloride for isoniazid overdose, etc.[11-16] The conclusions of these studies is that many health care facilities are unprepared for poisoning emergencies, let alone those involving WMD. Furthermore, small nonurban hospitals are more likely to be unprepared than larger urban, tertiary care facilities. In addition to monitoring inventory, pharmacy managers and pharmacy and therapeutics (P&T) committee members should be aware of their local or state governmental agencies that may support a depot of some of these pharmaceuticals. Often this information is classified and not readily available to individuals not serving on WMD readiness task forces or committees.

Although the likelihood of a terrorist event involving an NBC agent is greater in a large urban environment (e.g., large airport, sports stadium, shopping mall, etc.), pharmacists should avoid any complacency and support of the notion that "it can't happen here." One lesson learned from the bombing of a federal building in Oklahoma City a few years ago was that a terrorist attack could occur anywhere and at any time. Like other members of the health care delivery team, pharmacists must be prepared to share their expertise and resources when called upon in the event of an NBC incident.

The Nunn-Lugar-Domenici Domestic Preparedness Act of 1996 established a $250,000,000 program to train 120 cities in the U.S. in the principles of emergency and medical response to chemical and biological agents.[17] Headed by the Department of Defense (DOD), federal agencies involved with domestic preparedness programs include the Department of Energy (DOE), Federal Bureau of Investigation (FBI), Federal Emergency Management Agency (FEMA), and Environmental Protection Agency (EPA). Local government bodies are creating metropolitan medical response teams (MMRT) whose mission is to create a multiple level, technically diverse, professional response to any deliberate or accidental act involving an NBC agent within their jurisdiction. Antidote caches funded by federal grants to MMRTs will be intended for use by Emergency Medical Services (EMS) first responders for self-administration and to treat a number of casualties at the site of an NBC incident. The first 12 to 24 hours of any NBC emergency response will need to be managed by local resources prior to the arrival of DOD and other federal agencies. Every hospital that may receive NBC casualties should have a WMD plan as part of their disaster readiness.

Chemical agents

As defined by the U.S. Army, a chemical warfare agent is "a chemical substance intended for use in military operations to kill or seriously injure, or incapacitate humans or animals through its toxicologic effects."[18] Terrorists would find chemical agents attractive to use for several reasons. First, these poisons are extremely toxic. Second, they are readily available or easily synthesized. And third, pertinent toxicological information is easily accessible.

In many respects, emergency response systems and health care facilities will need to respond to a WMD chemical attack in the same fashion as a hazardous materials incident. The same principles regarding triage, decontamination, and allocation of resources that shape disaster plans related to hazardous materials will go into action during a WMD chemical attack.

Chemical agents are generally classified into several groups: blood agents, nerve agents, choking agents, and blistering agents. Each agent has been designated its own North Atlantic Treaty Organization (NATO) designation symbol (a military symbol), which is not its chemical formula. For example, the NATO designation symbol for cyanide is "AC," while its chemical formula is CN, whereas the NATO designation symbol for Mace is "CN."

An important principle to recognize concerning chemical agents is that the onset of symptoms is very rapid, typically within minutes of initial exposure. Therefore, prompt initiation of rescue, decontamination, medical attention, and antidotal therapy is critical in minimizing casualties. The Chemical and Biological Hotline 800-424-8802, based in Aberdeen, Maryland, serves as an emergency resource to all health care providers for technical assistance. Much of the following information has been adapted from a seminar presented by Dr. Howard Levitin[19] and the U.S. Army handbook, *Medical Response to Chemical Warfare and Terrorism.*[18]

Cyanide. In the form of an NBC agent, cyanide would most likely be encountered as hydrogen cyanide (AC) or cyanogen chloride (CK) gases. Ingestion of sodium or potassium cyanide salts may also have lethal consequences. An explosion of an industrial storage tank containing acetonitrile or acrylonitrile would pose a high risk of delayed cyanide toxicity. Cyanide toxicity is characterized by a rapid onset of dizziness, confusion, dyspnea, tachycardia, and hypertension, followed by coma, convulsions, bradycardia, hypotension, arrhythmias, and metabolic acidosis. Death may occur within minutes following significant exposures. Cyanide is classified as a "blood agent" by some WMD references.[18-19]

Nitrites in the cyanide antidote kit convert red blood cell (RBC) hemoglobin to methemoglobin. Methemoglobin combines with cyanide to form cyanomet-hemoglobin. In synergism with 100% oxygen, thiosulfate combines with cyanide via the rhodenese enzyme to form less toxic thiocyanate, which is eliminated in the urine. Two other pharmaceuticals, which serve as adjunctive therapy for cyanide poisoning, are injectable sodium bicarbonate to correct metabolic acidosis and benzodiazepines (e.g., diazepam or lorazepam) as anticonvulsants. Their availability is discussed later in this article. All of the average wholesale prices (AWP) are as listed in the *1999 Drug Topics Red Book*.[20]

1. Eli Lilly & Co. no longer manufactures the cyanide antidote package. It is now available from Taylor Pharmaceuticals, a Division of Akorn, Inc. Each package contains twelve amylnitrite pearls, two 10-mL vials of 3% Sodium Nitrite for Injection USP, and two 50-mL vials of 25% Sodium Thiosulfate for Injection USP.

   Taylor Pharmaceuticals
   Division of Akorn, Inc.
   P.O. Box 5136
   San Clemente, CA 92674
   800-223-9851
   AWP = $274.56
   Shelf life: 18 months
   Note: Lower prices are available under federal purchasing programs.

2. 3% Sodium Nitrite for Injection USP—300 mg/10-mL vials of Sodium Nitrite for Injection USP is available from:
   Hope Pharmaceuticals
   7626 East Greenway Road, Suite 101
   Scottsdale, AZ 85260
   800-755-9595
   AWP = $84.95
   Shelf life: 24 months

3. Amylnitrite pearls—Packages of twelve amylnitrite pearls are available from the following manufacturers:
   James Alexander Corp.
   845 Route 94
   Blairstown, NJ 07825
   908-362-9266
   AWP = $2.90
   —*and*—

Pharma-Tek, Inc.
P.O. Box 1920
Huntington, NY 11743-0568
800-645-6655
AWP = $6.25
Shelf life: 36 months

4. Sodium Nitrite Powder USP—Sodium Nitrite Powder USP is available from these sources. It can be used to extemporaneously prepare 3% Sodium Nitrite for Injection USP, although no referenced source could be found for compounding instructions. Suppliers will add additional charges for special packaging and shipping.
   A-A Spectrum Healthcare Products
   14422 South San Pedro Street
   Gardena, CA 90248
   800-772-8786
   500 gram AWP = $14.60
   —*and*—
   Ruger Chemical Co., Inc.
   P.O. Box 806
   Hillside, NJ 07205
   800-274-7843
   1 pound AWP = $8.40
   —*and*—
   Integra Chemical Co.
   710 Thomas Avenue SW
   Renton, WA 98055
   800-474-8993
   500 gram price per manufacturer = $34.62
   2500 gram price per manufacturer = $102.57
   Shelf life: 3–5 years

5. 25% Sodium Thiosulfate for Injection USP—50-mL vials of 25% Sodium Thiosulfate for Injection USP are available from the following suppliers:
   Hope Pharmaceuticals
   7626 East Greenway Road, Suite 101
   Scottsdale, AZ 85260
   800-755-9595
   AWP = $22.49
   —*and*—
   Prometic Pharma USA, Inc.
   5436 West 78th Street
   Indianapolis, IN 46268
   888-313-2520 or 317-334-5600
   AWP = $24.32
   —*and*—

American Regent Laboratories, Inc.
Subsidiary of Luitpold Pharm., Inc.
One Luitpold Drive
Shirley, NY 11967
800-645-1706
AWP = $22.50
Shelf life: 36 months; shorter for 10% solutions

Nerve agents. Nerve agents are organophosphates, which are potent inhibitors of acetylcholinesterase enzymes. Some examples of this group are Sarin (GB), Soman (GD), Tabun (GA), and VX. Some of the symptoms noted after significant exposures include the SLUDGE syndrome (Salivation, Lacrimation, Urination, Defecation, and Emesis), flaccid paralysis, apnea, and seizures. Serious poisonings are managed with three antidotal agents, atropine sulfate, pralidoxime chloride, diazepam or lorazepam.[18,19] Atropine sulfate blocks muscarinic receptor sites reversing bradycardia, bronchospasm, broncorrhea, vomiting, cramping, diarrhea, and miosis. Pralidoxime chloride (2-PAM) regenerates cholinesterase activity and reverses nicotinic toxicity demonstrated by muscle weakness, fasciculations, and respiratory depression. Diazepam or lorazepam, as anticonvulsants, are adjunctive measures to treat nerve agent induced seizures. Topical ocular homatropine or atropine can relieve miosis, pain, dim vision, and nausea.

1. Pralidoxime chloride (2-PAM, Protopam)—Protopam is available in 1-g vials only. It is manufactured by:
   Wyeth-Ayerst Laboratories
   Division of American Home Products Corp.
   P.O. Box 8299
   Philadelphia, PA 19101-8299
   800-666-7248
   AWP/6 vials = $384.76
   Shelf life: 5 years

2. Atropine Sulfate for Injection USP is available as a generic product from a variety of manufacturers. Some common forms are:

a. 0.4 mg/mL, 20-mL multidose vials (8 mg/vial)
   AWP/vial: from 84¢ to $1.33
   Shelf life: 24–36 months

b. Syringe sizes (0.1 mg/mL, 5-mL or 10-mL syringes)
   AWP/vial: from $4.54 to $6.95

c. 1 mg/mL, 1-mL single-dose vials
   AWP/25 vials: from $9.23 to $22.50
   Readers are advised to refer to the *Drug Topics Red Book*[20] or nearest pharmacy wholesaler for a complete list of companies.

3. Atropine Sulfate Powder USP is also available from several suppliers. This pharmaceutical grade powder may be used to prepare Atropine Sulfate USP for Injection extemporaneously in large amounts, although no referenced source could be found for compounding instructions. The manufacturers of this pharmaceutical grade chemical have provided no shelf-life guidelines. Additional charges are added for special packaging and shipping; prices are for 5-g quantities (unless otherwise indicated), available from:

   Amend Drug & Chemical
   83 Cordier Street
   Irvington, NJ 07111
   800-274-2636
   AWP = $12.00
   —and—
   Integra Chemical Co.
   710 Thomas Avenue, S.W.
   Renton, WA 98055
   800-474-8993
   Price per manufacturer = $19.27
   25 gram price per manufacturer = $73.96

4. Diazepam for Injection USP is available as a generic product from a variety of manufacturers. Some common forms are:

   a. 5 mg/mL, 2-mL prefilled syringes (10 mg/syringe)
      AWP for 10 units: from $25.06 to $38.18
      Shelf life: 24 months

   b. 5 mg/mL, 2-mL ampuls (10 mg/amp)
      AWP for 10 units: from $19.12 to $25.88

   c. 5 mg/mL, 10-mL multidose vial (50 mg/vial)
      AWP/vial: from $5.95 to $18.15

5. Lorazepam for Injection USP is available as a generic product from a variety of manufacturers. Some common forms are:

   a. 2 mg/mL, 1-mL single-dose vial (2 mg/vial)
      AWP/vial: from $9.74 to $11.41
      Shelf life: 18–24 months

   b. 2 mg/mL, 10-mL multidose vial (20 mg/vial)
      AWP/vial: from $26.09 to $101.65

   c. 4 mg/mL, 1-mL single-dose vial (4 mg/vial)
      AWP/vial: from $10.18 to $13.96

   d. 4 mg/mL, 10-mL multidose vial (40 mg/vial)
      AWP/vial: from $89.87 to $127.05

6. Military style auto-injectors containing atropine sulfate, pralidoxime chloride, and diazepam are available from Meridian Medical Technology, formerly Survival Technology, Inc.[21] These auto-injectors are manufactured in large quantities (25,000 units and 40,000 units). Small orders may be filled if the product is in Meridian's inventory; however, the shelf life may be shorter.

   a. Mark I kit (nerve agent antidote kit)
      Each kit contains one atropen and one combopen
      i. Atropen (atropine sulfate) 2 mg/0.7 mL
      ii. Combopen (pralidoxime chloride) 600 mg/2 mL
          Price: $17.00/kit
          Shelf life: 5 years

   b. Diazepam auto-injector
      Contents: 10 mg diazepam in 2 mL
      Price: $13.35
      Shelf life: 2 years

Per Meridian Medical Technologies: Please note that MMT requires the following information to accompany a purchase order (excluding the training kits which do not contain drug):

   i. Physician's prescription for all items.
   ii. A copy of the DEA registration certificate is also required if the purchase order (P.O.) includes the diazepam and/or morphine auto-injector(s).
   iii. Purchase order must include the following wording:
        "We certify that the items purchased under P.O.# ____ will be used only by _____. The material will not be sold to a third party, distributed or used for any other purpose."

Meridian Medical Technology, Inc.
10240 Old Columbia Road
Columbia, MD 21046
410-309-6830
Fax: 410-309-1475

Pulmonary or choking agents. Chlorine (CI) and phosgene (CG) are poisonous gasses, which were responsible for a large number of casualties during World War I. Today, chlorine and phosgene are industrial chemicals stored in special [industrial] tanks, and they are transported around the country in railroad tanker cars. As toxins, they act primarily as pulmonary irritants causing cough, shortness of breath, and dyspnea; however, it may be several hours before serious complications become evident (e.g., pulmonary edema). No specific antidote is available for treatment of these exposures. Symptomatic and supportive care may include administration of oxygen, other ventilation support, and bronchodilators, such as albuterol sulfate. Nebulized 3.75% sodium bicarbonate has provided dramatic symptomatic improvement in chlorine exposures, as noted in several anecdotal case reports.[22-24] This may be prepared by mixing 2 mL of 7.5%

Reprinted with permission from ASHP: *Am J Health-Syst Pharm*; December 1, 2001, Vol 58

Sodium Bicarbonate for Injection USP with 2 mL of sterile 0.9% sodium chloride. Antibiotics should be reserved for those patients with an infectious process documented by sputum gram staining and culture. Intravenous steroids may be indicated in those patients demonstrating latent or overt reactive airway disease.

1. Albuterol sulfate is available as a generic product in a variety of forms:
   a. Solution for nebulization, 0.09 mg/inhalation (17 grams)
      AWP/vial: from $12.50 to $22.95
      Shelf life: 18–36 months
   b. Solution for inhalation, 0.083%, 3-mL vials
      AWP for 25 vials: from $22.40 to $35.47
   c. Solution for inhalation, 0.5%, 20 mL multi-dose vial
      AWP/vial: from $11.95 to $16.50
2. 7.5% Sodium Bicarbonate for Injection USP (50 mL) is available in pre-filled syringes:
   AWP/syringe: from $2.89 to $18.58
   Shelf life: 18 months
3. Methylprednisolone Acetate for Injection USP is available as a generic product in several concentrations. Contact a pharmaceutical wholesaler or the *Drug Topics Red Book*[20] for latest prices.
   a. 20 mg/mL, 10-mL vials (200 mg/vial)
      AWP/vial: from $7.50 to $7.95
      Shelf life: 24–36 months
   b. 40 mg/mL, 5-mL vials (200 mg/vial)
      AWP/vial: from $7.20 to $12.95
   c. 80 mg/mL, 5-mL vials (400 mg/vial)
      AWP/vial: from $11.90 to $21.82

Blister agents. A number of potent alkylating agents may be used as chemical warfare agents. Examples include nitrogen mustard (HS), distilled mustard (HD), phosgene oxime (CX), and Lewisite (L). Toxicity produced by these agents includes blisters, vesiculations, eye injury, air-way damage, and bone marrow stem cell suppression. Blisters may form several hours after contact with the skin. Erythema may be treated with calamine or other soothing lotion or cream. Denuded skin areas should be treated with topical antibiotics such as silver sulfadiazine or mafenide acetate.[18] Systemic analgesics should be used liberally. Lewisite is the only blistering agent for which an antidote may be useful since it is an arsenic derivative. The antidote Dimercaprol (British Anti-Lewisite; BAL) is a chelating agent for arsenicals and other heavy metals.[18,25] BAL administration may reduce systemic toxicity of Lewisite. Although not commercially available, BAL skin and eye ointments may reduce the severity of lesions when applied soon after decontamination.[18] Since BAL is formulated in peanut oil, it must be given intramuscularly. BAL is available as 300 mg/3-mL vials in quantities of 10 from:

Taylor Pharmaceuticals
942 Calle Negocio, Suite 150
San Clemente, CA 92673
800-223-9851
AWP = $747.60
Shelf life: 5 years

Dimercaptosuccinic acid (DMSA, succimer, Chemet) has been used experimentally in animals for the treatment of Lewisite exposures.[26-30] This may be preferred in the treatment of multiple exposures because it is administered orally. Chemet is supplied in 100-mg capsules and is available in quantities of 100 from:

Sanofi Pharmaceuticals, Inc.
90 Park Avenue
New York, NY 10016
800-223-1062
AWP = $417.49
Shelf life: 24 months

Incapacitating agents. BZ (3-quinuclidinyl benzilate) and Agent 15 (the Iraqi equivalent of BZ) are anticholinergic agents, which incapacitate victims by causing delirium. Patients also demonstrate anticholinergic signs and symptoms (e.g., mydriasis, tachycardia, flushed skin, urinary retention, etc.).[18] Serious symptoms may be reversed by i.v. physostigmine (Antilirium), a reversible carbamate cholinesterase inhibitor. Neostigmine (Prostigmin) and pyridostigmine (Mestinon) are quaternary amines that do not cross the blood brain barrier and therefore will not reverse CNS symptomatology caused by these agents. Antilirium is available in 2-mL vials (1 mg/mL) in quantities of 10 vials from:

Taylor Pharmaceuticals
942 Calle Negocio, Suite 150
San Clemente, CA 92673
800-223-9851
AWP = $31.90
—*and*—
Faulding Pharmaceutical Co.
11 Commerce Drive, 3rd Floor
Cranford, NJ 07016
877-328-5346
AWP = $111.16
Shelf life: 24 months

Riot control agents. These agents are commonly known as CN (alpha-chloroacetophenone, Mace) or CS (ortho-chlorobenzylidene malononitrile) tear gas. Usually, the exposure effects of these agents are self-limiting. They include burning, itching, and watering of the eyes, burning and tingling of the skin, and respiratory discomfort. In most cases, no specific therapy is indicated other than basic measures such as movement of patient to fresh air, eye irrigation with water, and skin washing.

Nuclear agents

Although the detonation of a nuclear weapon is a concern with respect to global and international conflicts, it would be unlikely for a terrorist group to obtain, build, con-

Reprinted with permission from ASHP: *Am J Health-Syst Pharm*; December 1, 2001, Vol 58

ceal, or deliver such a weapon. Stealing and deploying radioactive material by a terrorist would most likely be designed to frighten people and create a major hazardous material clean-up crisis rather than cause many injuries.

Radiation emitted by radioactive materials can be characterized into three types: alpha particles, beta particles, and gamma rays. The health hazards of radiation are divided into acute or chronic exposure risks. Chronic exposures (i.e., a low dose over a long period of time) increase the risk of cancers and cataracts, while acute exposures produce nausea, vomiting, blood dyscrasias, and death. Since alpha and beta particles do not travel great distances, materials such as protective clothing easily block them. However, exposures due to inhalation or ingestion of alpha and beta particles pose the greatest potential for harm. Gamma rays are the most harmful because they travel great distances and require dense materials such as lead to block penetration of tissues.[19]

After exposure to a radiologic agent, patients may require treatment with either a chelator or a radionuclide blocker.[31] The following chelating agents for radionuclides are available through Radiation Emergency Assistance Center/Training Site (REAC/TS):

1. Insoluble Prussian Blue (ferric hexacyanoferrate) for cesium and thallium chelation therapy.[32]
2. Zinc-diethylenetriamine pentaacetic acid (Zn-DTPA) and calcium-DTPA (Ca-DTPA) for radioactive transuranic elements, including neptunium, plutonium, americium, curium, berkelium, and californium.[31,33-34]

REAC/TS trains, consults, and assists in the response to all types of radiation accidents or incidents. The center utilizes physicians, nurses, health physicists, radiologists, and emergency coordinators to provide 24-hour assistance at the local, national, or international level.

Other pharmaceutical chelators may be used for a variety of radionucleotide exposures and would be found in any well-stocked hospital pharmacy. These include d-penicillamine (Cuprimine), calcium disodium EDTA (Versenate), dimercaprol (BAL), succimer (Chemet), and deferoxamine (Desferal).[35] Colony stimulating factors may be considered in patients experiencing significant bone marrow suppression.

Radionuclide blocking agents saturate tissues with a nonradioactive element, which reduces the uptake of radioactive iodine. The most commonly used agents are potassium iodide tablets and Lugol's solution, both of which reduce uptake of ^{131}I into the thyroid tissue.[36] Most states with departments of nuclear safety will stock enough quantity of potassium iodide tablets to protect workers and emergency personnel involved in a nuclear reactor incident.

Lugol's solution is available from several suppliers:

AWP/480 mL: from $7.81 to $21.69
Shelf life: 2–5 years

Potassium iodide (Iosat), 130-mg tablets, are available in cases of 100 bottles (14 tablets/bottle) from:

Carter-Wallace, Inc.
P.O. Box 1001
Cranbury, NJ 08512
609-655-6147
AWP = $275.63
—and—
Anbex, Inc.
15 West 75th Street
New York, NY 10023
212-580-2810
AWP = $910.00
Shelf life: 60 months

For immediate assistance regarding a nuclear or radiological agent incident, contact the following:

1. Radiation Emergency Assistance Center/Training Site (REAC/TS) P.O. Box 117, MS-39 Oak Ridge, TN 37831-0117 Business hours: 865-576-3131 24-hour emergency line: 865-576-1005
2. The department of nuclear safety, for the state in which the incident occurred.
3. Health physicists affiliated with hospital nuclear medicine departments can serve as expert consultants for radiation incidents.

Biological agents

As NBC terrorist weapons, biological agents may be encountered as bacteria (e.g., anthrax), viruses (e.g., smallpox), or toxins (e.g., botulinum or ricin). This fact will explain the striking difference in the manner which victims will present to health care facilities. A catastrophe caused by a chemical weapon (e.g., nerve agent or cyanide) would be characterized by immediate death, or severe disablement of individuals at the site of the attack. First responders to such an incident would be paramedics, police, and other emergency personnel.

In contrast, with respect to biologicals, there is a delayed onset of signs and symptoms since incubation may take days. Emergency department clinicians and primary care practitioners would be the first to recognize and manage exposed patients. It is beneficial to health care facility professionals, including pharmacists, to be knowledgeable of these agents and their clinical effects. Knowledge of what medical and pharmaceutical interventions may be requested in a mass casualty event is crucial. It is beyond the scope of this article to delineate all the diagnostic clues, pathophysiology, laboratory monitoring, infectious disease control, guidelines for patient isolation, epidemiologic procedures, and public health ramifications of a bioterrorism event. Pharmacists, however, would wish to take note of this extensive list of pharmaceuticals (both oral and parenteral) that may be required in extraordinarily large amounts during an outbreak involving a biological weapon. Additionally, the duration of illness may be weeks to months thus creating an additional stress on the health care infrastructure. Once the cause of illness in a large number of patients has been identified as a biological agent, prompt availability and distribution of appropriate medication can greatly mitigate the destructive impact of the act of terrorism. It should be noted that special products, uncommonly used vaccines and antitoxins, would be provided via federal government storage and distribution programs. New therapies are also under development. Detailed information on diagnosis, patient management, vaccines, etc. may be obtained through COMMANDER US Army Medical Research Institute of Infectious Diseases[37] (USAMRIID) at 301-619-2833 during business hours, or at 888-USA-RIID, 24 hours/day. In the event of an emergency, contact the U.S. Army Response Center at 800-424-8802. Also, contact the Centers for Disease Control and Prevention (CDC) Bioterrorism Response Unit at 770-488-7100.

The following information is a very brief synopsis of 13 possible threats as biological agents. Much of this information has been adapted from an article in *JAMA*[1] entitled "Clinical Recognition and Management of Patients Exposed to Biological Warfare Agents," and teleconference materials provided by the CDC and Food and Drug Administration (FDA) entitled *Biological Warfare and Terrorism*.[37]

Bacteria. *Anthrax.* The etiologic agent causing anthrax is *Bacillus anthracis*, a gram-positive spore-forming bacillus. As a biological weapon, the spores of these bacteria would be aerosolized, with inhalation being the primary route of exposure. The clinical course is characterized by a necrotiz-

ing hemorrhagic mediastinitis. Initially symptoms may resemble a flu-like illness with fever, fatigue, and malaise, also vague chest pain and non-productive cough. Initial symptoms are followed by abrupt progression to dyspnea, stridor, diaphoresis, and cyanosis. Systemic complications of sepsis, shock, and meningitis may occur in up to half of the cases. Unfortunately, once symptoms occur, treatment is usually ineffective. Intravenous ciprofloxacin should be initiated at the earliest sign of anthrax. Other fluoroquinolones may be substituted; however, no animal studies exist for quinolones other than ciprofloxacin.[38] All natural strains of anthrax have been found to be sensitive to erythromycin, chloramphenicol, and gentamicin. Historically, penicillin G has been the drug of choice for anthrax. Chemoprophylaxis with oral ciprofloxacin or doxycycline in exposed individuals should be initiated and continued for four weeks or until three doses of anthrax vaccine are administered.[38] A licensed attenuated vaccine is available for prophylaxis. This vaccine stock is owned by the Department of Defense; in order to obtain it, contact USAMRIID at 301-619-2833. It is manufactured by:

Bioport Manufacturing
3500 North Dr. Martin Luther King Jr. Blvd.
Lansing, MI 48906
517-327-1500

Brucellosis. Human infection may be caused by four species of Brucella, which is a nonspore-forming gram-negative aerobic cocco-bacillus. Clinical manifestations include fever, chills, and malaise which may lead to cough and pleuritic chest pain. Other complications may include osteomyelitis, genitourinary infection, hepatitis, endocarditis, and central nervous system (CNS) infections. Drug therapy consists of antibiotic combinations. The treatment of choice is doxycycline and

rifampin; sulfamethoxazole/trimethoprim (SMZ/TMP) can be used as a substitute for rifampin. Severe systemic infectious complications may require the addition of streptomycin or other aminoglycoside agents. There are no approved vaccines or chemoprophylaxis treatments.

Cholera. This infection is caused by *Vibrio cholerae*, a gram-negative, nonspore-forming bacillus. Clinical manifestations include vomiting, abdominal distension, and pain, with little or no fever, followed rapidly by diarrhea. Fluid losses may be excessive with death caused by dehydration and shock. Antibiotic treatment may include tetracycline, ampicillin, and SMZ/TMP. Intravenous fluid/electrolyte solutions are necessary to treat dehydration. An FDA approved killed vaccine is available for prophylaxis. However, it provides only about 50% protection and lasts only six months.

Pneumonic plague. The gram-negative, nonspore-forming bacillus, *Yersinia pestis*, is responsible for both pneumonic and bubonic plague. Patients exposed to plague will have high fever, chills, malaise, cough with bloody sputum, headache, myalgia, and sepsis. Late in the course of illness, dyspnea, cyanosis, and respiratory failure may be noted. Effective antibiotic therapy includes streptomycin or gentamicin, chloramphenicol, and doxycycline. An FDA-approved vaccine is available for bubonic plague; however, its efficacy against aerosolized pneumonic plague is believed to be poor. Exposed individuals may be treated with doxycycline for chemoprophylaxis.

Q-Fever. Q-Fever is a rickettsial disease caused by *Coxiella burnetii*. The most common symptoms of Q-Fever are fever, chills, headache, fatigue, diaphoresis, malaise, anorexia, and myalgias. In some cases, cough with chest pain may be noted. Rare complications include hepatomegaly, splenomegaly, and jaundice. Effective therapies for Q-Fever include tetracycline, doxycycline, erythromycin, and azithromycin. Inactivated whole cell vaccine for Q-Fever prophylaxis is available, under investigational new drug (IND) status, in the U.S. Tetracycline or doxycycline may be given as chemoprophylaxis to exposed patients.

Tularemia. Tularemia is caused by *Francisella tularensis*, a gram-negative aerobic cocco-bacillus. It is also known as "rabbit fever" or "deer fly fever." Inhalation of tularemia organisms produces a typhoidal tularemia. Patients present with fever, weight loss, substernal discomfort, and nonproductive cough. The drug of choice is streptomycin. Other treatment options include gentamicin, tetracycline, and chloramphenicol; however, high relapse rates are associated with these other treatment options. A live attenuated vaccine is available under IND status for prophylaxis. Doxycycline or tetracycline may be used for chemoprophylaxis.

Viruses. *Smallpox.* The etiologic agent that causes smallpox is the *variola* major virus. Smallpox was declared eradicated by the World Health Organization in 1980. Much concern exists regarding the stockpiling of this infectious agent as a weapon of bioterrorism due to its high morbidity and mortality. Patients infected with *variola* present with fever, malaise, rigors, vomiting, headache, and backache. Dermal manifestations include appearance of a rash followed by lesions, which appear as macules, then papules, then eventually form pustular vesicles. By the second week, scabs are formed that leave depigmented scars upon healing. Patients are contagious until all the scabs are healed. All patients exposed to *variola* virus must be immediately vaccinated. Those U.S. citizens who were vaccinated against smallpox in the 1950s and 1960s are no longer protected against this virus.[39] The only smallpox vaccine in the United States is Wyeth-Ayerst's Dryvax, available by calling 800-666-7248. There is currently no chemotherapeutic agent

proven effective against smallpox. The U.S. Army and CDC maintain a supply of vaccinia immune globulin (VIG) which is used for post exposure prophylaxis. Contact the CDC at 404-639-3356 or USAMRIID at 301-619-2833 to obtain VIG.

Venezuelan equine encephalitis (VEE). Members of the Alpha virus genus of the Togaviridae family produce this encephalopathic syndrome. The usual mode of transmission is mosquitoes; however, aerosolization makes those pathogens a very effective WMD. Alpha virus will produce neurologic syndromes noted by fever, headaches, confusion, drowsiness, seizures, dysphasia, ataxia, myoclonus, cranial nerve palsies, photophobia, myalgia, and vomiting. No specific chemotherapeutic agents are indicated. Treatment is symptomatic and supportive care. Antipyretics and anticonvulsants may be used in severe cases. A live attenuated vaccine for VEE TC-83 is available for prophylaxis, while inactivated vaccines are under IND status.

Viral hemorrhagic fevers (VHF). The most widely known examples of this group are the Ebola and Marburg viruses. Common features of the VHF are myalgias, fever, and prostration. Mild symptoms include conjunctival injection, mild hypotension, flushing, and petechial hemorrhaging that may progress to shock. More severe symptoms include mucous membrane hemorrhage with maculopapule rashes and disseminated intravascular coagulation (DIC). No specific antiviral agents are effective against Ebola or Marburg viruses. Other related strains may respond to ribavirin. Many different pharmaceutical agents may need to be employed in the supportive management of hypotension, shock, and DIC. No vaccines or medicinals currently exist to protect against these viral illnesses.

Toxins. *Botulinum.* Botulinum toxin is a protein exotoxin produced

by *Clostridium botulinum*, an anaerobic gram-positive bacillus. There are seven types of botulism neurotoxins known as types A–G. Botulism poisonings are more commonly associated with improperly processed or canned foods. As a WMD, botulinum toxin may be inhaled from an aerosol or ingested in the form of sabotaged food. These toxins are the most toxic of all the NBC weapons. Clinical manifestations include blurred vision, mydriasis, diplopia, ptosis, photophobia, dysarthria, dysphonia, and dysphagia. Skeletal muscle paralysis follows, which presents as a symmetrical and descending progressive weakness resulting in respiratory failure. Patients are typically awake, alert, and afebrile. A trivalent equine antitoxin (types A, B, and E) for food-borne botulism is available from the CDC at eight urban quarantine sites: Atlanta, Chicago, Honolulu, Los Angeles, Miami, New York City, San Francisco, and Seattle. To obtain these antitoxins contact the CDC, 24 hours a day, at 404-639-2888 or during business hours at 404-639-2206. Connaught Laboratories, Ltd. manufactures this antitoxin for the CDC, one of only three suppliers in the world. A despeciated equine heptavalent antitoxin against all seven types was prepared and is under IND status. It should be noted that all horse serum based antitoxins pose the risk of anaphylaxis and serum sickness; therefore, skin testing is advised. A pentavalent (types A–E) toxoid is also available under IND status.

Ricin. This biological toxin is derived from the plant *Ricinus communis*, commonly known as the castor bean. After inhalation exposure, victims may experience fever, weakness, and cough, followed by hypotension and cardiovascular collapse. There is no available antitoxin. Treatment is supportive care only. Also, there is no available vaccine or other chemoprophylactic agent.

Staphylococcus enterotoxin B

Reprinted with permission from ASHP: *Am J Health-Syst Pharm*; December 1, 2001, Vol 58

(SEB). SEB is an exotoxin produced by *Staphylococcus aureus*, a gram-positive cocci. SEB is most commonly recognized as a cause of food poisoning as it is produced by bacterial growth in improperly handled foods. Inhalation of SEB in a biological warfare scenario may rapidly incapacitate its victims. Signs of exposure may include fever, chills, headache, myalgias, and non-productive cough, with severe problems including dyspnea, retrosternal chest pain, vomiting, and diarrhea. No specific antitoxin is available. Supportive therapies are directed towards adequate oxygenation and hydration. No vaccines for SEB are currently available.

Trichothecene (T-2) mycotoxins. Fungi of the genera *Fusarium, Myrotecium, Trichoderma,* and *Stachybotrys* produce these compounds. Clinical manifestations of exposure include skin irritation, pruritis, redness, vesicles, necrosis, sloughing of the epidermis, nose and throat pain, nasal discharge, fever, cough, dyspnea, chest pain, and hemoptusis. Serious cases are associated with prostration, weakness, shock, and death. There is no antidote or antitoxin. Treatment is supportive care. No vaccine or chemoprophylactic agent exists for T-2 mycotoxins.

The following are some of the aforementioned pharmaceutical products available for the treatment of patients exposed to biological warfare agents. If a variety of sizes and formulations are available for a particular pharmaceutical product, only the largest dose forms are listed. Readers are advised to refer to the *Drug Topics Red Book*[20] or nearest pharmaceutical wholesaler for a complete list of companies for the following products.

1. Ciprofloxacin is available in several different oral and parenteral dosage forms. These are available from:

Bayer Corporation
Pharmaceutical Division
400 Morgan Lane
West Haven, CT 06516-4175
800-288-8370
500-mg tablets (100 tabs) AWP = $399.47
750-mg tablets (100 tabs) AWP = $412.78
10 mg/mL, 120-mL bulk vial (1200 mg/vial) AWP/6 vials = $466.38
400 mg/200-mL premixed i.v. AWP/24 i.v.s = $720.29

2. Doxycycline hyclate is available from a number of generic suppliers in 100 mg tablets or capsules.
100-mg tablets or capsules AWP/100 tabs: from $8.76 to $45.90

3. Erythromycin is available in a large variety of salt forms and strengths.
500-mg tablets AWP/100 tabs: from $22.50 to $121.96

4. Penicillin V and G are available in a variety of formulations, both oral and intravenous.
500-mg tablets
10-million-unit vials
AWP/100 tabs: from $9.05 to $23.01
AWP/vial: from $6.40 to $40.55

5. Gentamicin sulfate is a powerful aminoglycoside antibiotic that is only used for systemic infections. It is available in a variety of formulations.
a. 40 mg/mL, 20-mL multidose vials (800 mg/vial) AWP/vial: from $7.10 to $12.64
b. 40 mg/mL, 2-mL single-use vials (80 mg/vial) AWP/25 vials: from $26.04 to $57.50

6. Streptomycin is a rarely used antibiotic; however, it has efficacy against several of the biological warfare agents. It is supplied in 1-g vials for injection. Streptomycin is available from:

Pharma-Tek, Inc.
P.O. Box 1920
Huntington, NY 11743-0568

800-645-6655
AWP/vial = $5.95

7. Chloramphenicol is another rarely used antibiotic. It can be obtained in vials or large quantities may be obtained in powdered form. This may be required to treat a large number of casualties.
a. 1000-mg vial, AWP/vial: from $6.51 to $6.65
b. 25-g USP powder, AWP: from $29.85 to $59.04

8. SMZ/TMP is another antibiotic that has efficacy against several of the biological warfare agents. The most commonly used formulation contains 800 mg of sulfamethoxazole and 160 mg of trimethoprim (Bactrim DS).
SMZ/TMP (800/160) tablets AWP/ 100 tabs: from $10.86 to $114.89

9. Rifampin is available in 300-mg capsules or in large quantities in powdered form.
a. 300-mg capsules, AWP/100 caps: from $162.93 to $197.46
b. 500-g USP powder, AWP: from $273.91 to $792.00

10. Tetracycline is available in 500-mg capsules or also in powdered form.
a. 500-mg capsules, AWP/100 caps: from $5.78 to $12.78
b. 100-g USP powder, AWP: from $56.70 to $59.40

Conclusion

With the increasing probability of an incident involving a WMD agent, many local, state, and federal agencies have initiated plans for appropriate and effective emergency medical response. Experts in the area of EMS, emergency medicine, infectious disease, and public health are becoming trained in the medical management of exposure to NBC agents.

Any large mass casualty scenario will demand the expertise and professional services of a hospital pharmacy. Therefore, pharmacists should equip themselves with knowledge of antidotes, antibiotics, antitoxins, and other supportive agents used to treat

Reprinted with permission from ASHP: *Am J Health-Syst Pharm*; December 1, 2001, Vol 58

casualties and how they may be obtained quickly in the event of an act of terrorism. Currently, there are no guidelines mandating minimum hospital inventory of the pharmaceutical products that may be needed. Pharmacy managers and P&T committee members are urged to participate in, or at least be familiar with, plans coordinated through local domestic preparedness programs.

---

[a] Drugs, dosages, and AWPs were current at the time of original publication. The AWPs quoted are from the year 2000.

References

1. Franz DR, Jahrling PB, Friedlander AM et al. Clinical recognition and management of patients exposed to biological warfare agents. *JAMA*. 1997; 278:399-411.
2. Danzig R, Berkowsky PB. Why should we be concerned about biological warfare? *JAMA*. 1997; 278:431-2.
3. Sharp TW, Brennan RJ, Keim M et al. Medical preparedness for a terrorist incident involving chemical or biological agents during the 1996 Atlanta Olympic games. *Ann Emerg Med*. 1998; 32:214-23.
4. Tucker JB. National health and medical services response to incidents of chemical and biological terrorism. *JAMA*. 1997; 278:362-8.
5. Anteau CM, Williams LA. The Oklahoma bombing: lessons learned. *Crit Care Nurs Clin North Am*. 1997; 9:231-6.
6. Richards CF, Burstein JL, Waeckerle JF et al. Emergency physicians and biological terrorism. *Ann Emerg Med*. 1999; 34:183-90.
7. Pesik N, Keim M, Sampson TR. Do U.S. emergency medicine residency programs provide adequate training for bioterrorism? *Ann Emerg Med*. 1999; 34:173-6.
8. Forrow L, Sidel VW. Medicine and nuclear war: from Hiroshima to mutual assured destruction to abolition 2000. *JAMA*. 1998; 280:456-61.
9. Zilinskas RA. Iraq's biological weapons: the past as future? *JAMA*. 1997; 278:418-24.
10. Lebeda FJ. Deterrence of biological and chemical warfare: a review of policy options. *Mil Med*. 1997; 162:156-61.
11. Dart RC, Stark Y, Fulton B et al. Insuffi-

cient stocking of poisoning antidotes in hospital pharmacies. *JAMA*. 1996; 276:1508-10.
12. Woolf AD, Chrisanthus K. On-site availability of selected antidotes: results of a survey of Massachusetts's hospitals. *Am J Emerg Med*. 1997; 15:62-6.
13. Chyka PA, Conner HG. Availability of antidotes in rural and urban hospitals in Tennessee. *Am J Hosp Pharm*. 1994; 51:1346-8.
14. Santucci KA, Shah BR, Linakis JG. Acute isoniazid exposures and antidote availability. *Pediatr Emerg Care*. 1999; 15:99-101.
15. Antidotes dangerously understocked in Colorado, Montana, and Nevada. *Am J Health Syst Pharm*. 1997; 54:16, 19. News.
16. Webster KS, Burda AM, Sigg T et al. Antidote preparedness of Illinois hospitals. *Pharmacotherapy*. 1999; 19:1229-30.
17. Preparedness and Response for Terrorist Incidents Amendment (Nunn-Lugar-Domenici Act) of 1996. Pub. L. No. 6250-12.
18. U.S. Army. Medical response to chemical warfare and terrorism. 3rd ed. Aberdeen Proving Ground, MD: Chemical Casualty Care Division, USAMRIID; 1998.
19. Levitin H. Hospital provider course—weapons of mass destruction: improving hospital-provider response to chemical, biological, and nuclear terrorism. Paper presented at the Metropolitan Chicago Healthcare Council. Chicago, IL; 1998 May 11-12.
20. Red Book. 103rd ed. Montvale, NJ: Medical Economics; 1999.
21. Departments of the Army, the Navy, and the Air Force, and Commandant, Marine Corps. Field Manual. Treatment of Chemical Agent Casualties and Conventional Military Chemical Injuries. www.nbc-med.org/SiteContent/MedRef/OnlineRef/FieldManuals/fm8_285/toc.htm.
22. Douidar SM. Nebulized sodium bicarbonate in acute chlorine inhalation. *Pediatr Emerg Care*. 1997; 13:406-7.
23. Bosse GM. Nebulized sodium bicarbonate in the treatment of chlorine gas inhalation. *J Toxicol Clin Toxicol*. 1994; 32:233-41.
24. Vinsel PJ. Treatment of acute chlorine gas inhalation with nebulized sodium bicarbonate. *J Emerg Med*. 1990; 8:327-9.
25. Arsenic. Vol 102. In: Peterson RG, Reigart JR, Kurt TL et al eds. Poisondex Health-Information System [CD-ROM]. Englewood, CO: Micromedex; 1999.
26. Aposhian HV, Carter DE, Hoover TD et

al. DMSA, DMPS, and DMPA—as arsenic antidotes. *Fundam Appl Toxicol*. 1984; 2(2 Pt 2):S58-70.
27. Aposhian HV, Mershon MM, Brinkley FB et al. Anti-lewisite activity and stability of meso-dimercaptosuccinic acid and 2,3-dimercapto-l-propanesulfonic acid. *Life Sci*. 1982; 31:2149-56.
28. Aposhian HV. Biological chelation: 2,3-dimercapto-propanesulfonic acid and meso-dimercaptosuccinic acid. *Adv Enzyme Regul*. 1982; 20:301-19.
29. Inns RH, Rice P. Efficacy of dimercapto chelating agents for the treatment of poisoning by percutaneously applied dichloro(2-chlorovinyl) arsine in rabbits. *Hum Exp Toxicol*. 1993; 12:241-6.
30. Inns RH, Rice P, Bright JE et al. Evaluation of the efficacy of dimercapto-chelating agents for the treatment of systemic organic arsenic poisoning in rabbits. *Hum Exp Toxicol*. 1990; 9:215-20.
31. Lincoln TA. Importance of initial management of persons internally contaminated with radionuclides. *J Am Ind Hyg Assoc*. 1976; 37:16-21.
32. Goans RE, Ricks RC, Townsend RD. *Radiogardase-Cs insoluble prussian blue (ferric hexacyanoferrate, $Fe_4[Fe(CN)_6]_3$).* Oak Ridge, TN: Radiation Emergency Assistance Center/Training Site; 1999 Nov.
33. Goans RE, Ricks RC, Townsend RD. *Ca-DTPA (trisodium calcium diethylenetriaminepentaacetate).* Oak Ridge, TN: Radiation Emergency Assistance Center/Training Site, 1999 Jul.
34. Goans RE, Ricks RC, Townsend RD. *Zn-DTPA (trisodium zinc diethylenetriaminepentaacetate).* Oak Ridge, TN: Radiation Emergency Assistance Center/Training Site, 1999 Jul.
35. Radiation. Vol 102. In: Hall AH, Dabney BJ, Markovchick V et al eds. Poisondex Health-Information System [CD-ROM]. Englewood, CO: Micromedex;; 1999.
36. Physicians' desk reference, 53rd ed. Montvale, NJ: Medical Economics, 1999:3185.
37. Biological warfare and terrorism: the military and public health response. Compiled by the US Army Medical Research Institute of Infectious Diseases for the CDC and the FDA. 1999 Sept 21-23. Satellite broadcast.
38. Inglesby TV, Henderson DA, Bartlett JG et al. Anthrax as a biological weapon: medical and public health management. *JAMA*. 1999; 281:1735-45.
39. Henderson DA, Inglesby TV, Bartlett JG et al. Smallpox as a biological weapon: medical and public health management. *JAMA*. 1999; 281:2127-37.

Reprinted with permission from ASHP: *Am J Health-Syst Pharm*; December 1, 2001, Vol 58

Addendum

Web sites with information on weapons of mass destruction

CDC Bioterrorism Preparedness and Response
    www.bt.cbc.gov

Chemical and Biological Defense Information Analysis Center (CBIAC)
    www.cbiac.apgea.army.mil

EmergencyNET
    www.emergency.com

FEMA Rapid Response Information System (RRIS)
    www.rris.fema.gov

Medical NBC Online Information Server
    www.nbc-med.org

National Disaster Medical System (NDMS)
    www.oep-ndms.dhhs.gov

Nuclear, Biological, and Chemical Weapons
    www.biochemweapons.com

The Terrorism Research Center
    www.terrorism.com/chembio/chembio.html

US Army Medical Research Institute of Infectious Diseases (USAMRIID)
    www.usamriid.army.mil

Editors' note: *At the time of publication, these Web site URLS were accurate.*

Reprinted with permission from ASHP: *Am J Health-Syst Pharm*; December 1, 2001, Vol 58

Citywide pharmaceutical preparation for bioterrorism

COLLEEN M. TERRIFF AND AMY M. TEE

Acts of bioterrorism can range from hoaxes to the release of agents that could cause mass casualties, and the threat is a concern both globally and locally.[1] For example, the Japanese religious cult Aum Shinrikyo, which released the chemical warfare agent sarin in a crowded Tokyo subway, is also believed to have an arsenal of biological weapons, including anthrax and botulinum toxin. Reportedly, members of Aum Shinrikyo traveled to Zaire in an effort to obtain the Ebola virus.[2] The cult may have spray tanks and aircraft available for disseminating their biological agents.

At Russia's State Research Center of Virology and Biotechnology, also known as VECTOR, laboratories have held quantities of smallpox, Ebola, and Marburg viruses and other viruses associated with hemorrhagic fever. Security at VECTOR has lapsed, key research scientists have left, those who remain are poorly paid, and viral materials may have been distributed to other parts of the world.[2,3]

In The Dalles, Oregon, *Salmonella*

Abstract: One community's efforts to become pharmaceutically prepared for an attack with biological agents is described.

In response to recent bioterrorist activities, including a local scare in 1999 involving anthrax, the pharmacy department at Deaconess Medical Center in Spokane, Washington, was asked to develop a plan for bioterrorism preparedness. A literature search was conducted, and resources, such as the Centers for Disease Control and Prevention, were contacted. For each biological agent, information was compiled about symptom onset, treatment, postexposure prophylaxis, patient isolation precautions, and the availability of antidotes at local hospitals. A procedure was developed for obtaining antidotes that might not be available or stocked in sufficient quantities. After being reviewed by appropriate authorities, the information was presented to area hospitals and trauma centers, drug wholesalers, hospital risk-management personnel, and emergency management personnel. In May 2000 dozens of emergency and medical personnel attended a day-long program on domestic preparedness. Citywide cooperation was obtained on how to respond to a mass exposure to a bioterrorism agent. The job of a pharmacist during a bioterrorism strike is to rapidly disseminate antidotes and information, provide dosage and vaccination schedules for both treatment and prophylaxis, and counsel patients.

Medical facilities in Spokane have cooperated to make the community more prepared for a bioterrorist attack.

Index terms: Antidotes; Anti-infective agents; Biological warfare; Disaster planning; Dosage; Dosage schedules; Drug distribution; Patient information; Pharmacists, hospital; Pharmacy, institutional, hospital; Public health; Vaccines

Am J Health-Syst Pharm. 2001; 58:233-7

typhimurium was used by the Rajneeshee religious cult to contaminate restaurant salad bars and a city water-supply tank.[4] About 751 people contracted salmonellal gastroenteritis during a one-month period.

Dissident nations, groups, and individuals have been turning to biological agents as a means of conducting warfare or terrorism. Many microorganisms and toxins are relatively easily acquired, and some can be mass-produced as aerosolized biological weapons. Inhalation of and other contact

COLLEEN M. TERRIFF, PHARM.D., is Assistant Professor, College of Pharmacy, Washington State University (WSU), and Clinical Pharmacist, Department of Pharmacy, Deaconess Medical Center (DMC), Spokane, WA. AMY M. TEE, PHARM.D., is Clinical Pharmacist, DMC.

Address reprint requests to Dr. Terriff at the Pharmacy Department, Deaconess Medical Center, 800 West 5th Avenue, Spokane, WA 99210, or to terriff@mail.wsu.edu.

The contributions of Julia Y. Pai, Pharm.D. (for compiling the information in the appendixes and table), Julie McCoy, Pharm.D. (for sharing information and knowledge), and James Nania, M.D. (for his direction and encouragement) are acknowledged.

Copyright © 2001, American Society of Health-System Pharmacists, Inc. All rights reserved. 1079-2082/01/0201-0233$06.00.

Reprinted with permission from ASHP: *Am J Health-Syst Pharm*; February 1, 2001, Vol 58

with these agents by large numbers of people could lead to mass casualties.[5-9] To date, except for the Rajneeshee attack with salmonella, major acts of bioterrorism have not occurred in the United States. Yet many experts say that the probability of a large-scale attack is greater today than ever before. It is probably not a case of if, but when. Public health and emergency officials believe it is increasingly important for our health care system to be prepared for a bioterrorist strike. Likewise, it is paramount that hospital emergency departments recognize the signs and symptoms of exposure to biological agents and initiate immediate and appropriate treatment.

Although many antidotes and vaccines can be obtained only from the Centers for Disease Control and Prevention (CDC), treatment for exposure to some infectious agents, such as anthrax, can be accomplished with antimicrobials that most hospital pharmacies currently have on their shelves.[5,6,8,10-12] The challenge is to ensure that there are sufficient quantities of these crucial drugs. In the event of bioterrorism, hospitals in the affected locale will need information on the following: the identified or presumed organism or toxin, the symptoms of exposure and time of onset, how to treat confirmed cases, what postexposure prophylaxis is needed, patient isolation precautions, and the local availability of necessary drugs, antidotes, and vaccines.

This report describes one community's efforts to become pharmaceutically prepared for an attack with biological agents. Differential diagnosis and signs and symptoms of exposure to various infectious agents will not be discussed; health care personnel can refer to their regional poison control center, their state health department, the CDC Office of Bioterrorism, or the Domestic Preparedness Chemical/Biological HelpLine (800-368-6498) for more information and assistance with triage.

Background

The health care system in Spokane, Washington, serves a regional population of approximately 410,000. A citywide network at four acute care hospitals (Sacred Heart Medical Center, Deaconess Medical Center, Holy Family Hospital, and Valley Hospital and Medical Center) and one rehabilitation center (St. Luke's Rehabilitation Institute) collaborates on such issues as formulary management, purchasing, information systems, adverse-drug-reaction reporting, and drug-utilization reviews.

In late 1998 CDC received numerous reports of alleged attacks involving the mailing of anthrax-contaminated letters to U.S. health clinics.[12] In February 1999 a letter, intended for Planned Parenthood of Spokane, was delivered to a dentist's office next door. Although the envelope was initially thought to contain anthrax, the threat was later found to be a hoax.

Initial program development

In response to Spokane's 1999 anthrax scare, the pharmacy department at Deaconess Medical Center developed an anthrax postexposure prophylaxis policy that incorporated CDC's recommendations for administration of vaccines and oral antimicrobials. In March 1999 a pharmacist presented this policy at a meeting of the hospital's emergency department interdisciplinary team, which included the department's director, nurse manager, physicians, nurses, charge secretaries, social worker, and pharmacist. After reviewing the recommendations, the interdisciplinary team requested that the pharmacy department develop a plan for bioterrorism preparedness. The initial focus was on biological warfare agents possibly associated with Y2K threats; the goal was to compile the information before December 31, 1999. This plan later evolved to include preparedness beyond Y2K.

A MEDLINE search was performed with the search term "bioterrorism" for the period from 1966 to April 1999 and then May 2000. Pertinent Web sites, such as CDC's home page, which includes the online versions of *MMWR Morbidity and Mortality Weekly Report* and *Emerging Infectious Diseases,* were searched for information, recommendations, and guidelines. For each biological agent, information was compiled about symptom onset, the treatment of symptomatic patients, postexposure prophylaxis, isolation precautions, the availability of antidotes at local hospitals and trauma centers, and references. Biological agents were ranked according to their likelihood of use, with anthrax, smallpox, and plague listed as the three most probable threats. In addition, information on drugs for prophylaxis and treatment was compiled in a table and preferred drugs were indicated. Inquiries regarding the availability of medications for treatment, prophylaxis, and vaccination were sent to CDC and local hospital pharmacy purchasing agents via fax or telephone. Finally, a procedure was developed for obtaining pharmacologic antidotes that might not be available or stocked in sufficient quantities.

In summary, during a mass exposure to a bioterrorism agent, the hospital emergency department would immediately contact the pharmacy department, which would contact other hospitals in the region and the drug wholesaler. Outside agencies, such as the regional poison control center, the health department, the U.S. Public Health Service, and CDC, would also be contacted.

Citywide cooperation

The information on bioterrorism was presented to the citywide pharmacy and therapeutics committee, the quality improvement and clinical outcomes subcommittee, the central infection-control committee, and one hospital's emergency department interdisciplinary team for feedback.

Reprinted with permission from ASHP: *Am J Health-Syst Pharm*; February 1, 2001, Vol 58

A completed three-page document, which included policies, procedures, and antidote information, was then distributed to area hospitals and trauma centers, drug wholesalers, hospital risk-management personnel, the city fire department's hazardous materials team, county emergency management personnel, and the local ambulance service.

In May 2000 dozens of emergency and medical personnel attended a day-long program on domestic preparedness, which provided assistance in planning for and responding to terrorist incidents involving nuclear, biological, and chemical weapons. Both this class and a tabletop exercise, in which a scenario involving sarin was discussed, were coordinated by the Spokane County Office of Emergency Management and by the U.S. Army Soldier and Biological Chemical Command. Attendees included hazardous materials personnel, law enforcement officers, medical and emergency management personnel (including physicians, nurses, ambulance workers, and a poison control center representative), state and federal officers (agents from the Federal Bureau of Investigation, the Washington State Department of Health, the U.S. Public Health Service, and the Federal Emergency Management Agency), and public information officers. The program was

invaluable for learning about our community's response potential and how to improve it.

Recommendations for the medical management of each specific biological organism or toxin were adopted by the citywide network (Appendix A), and a citywide policy for obtaining pharmacologic antidotes was established (Appendix B). The hospital and rehabilitation center pharmacy departments have pledged to work together and to contact each other for additional medications if necessary. Before January 1, 2000, the hospitals' drug wholesaler agreed to increase our local stock of available medications (Table 1) from a four-week to a seven-week supply. CDC, the Washington State Department of Health, and the U.S. Public Health Service have agreed to be available as critical resources during a bioterrorism incident by providing antidotes and expert advice.

During the tabletop exercise, it was learned that communities like Spokane may need to be self-sufficient for at least 24 hours after an incident, since it may take that long to obtain outside assistance. If financially feasible, some local stockpiling of certain antidotes, like antimicrobials, may be necessary. If the CDC Office of Bioterrorism is notified during a bioterrorism event, the director of CDC can activate the National Phar-

maceutical Stockpile Program. Within approximately 12 hours, antidotes, vaccines, and ventilators and other supportive medical supplies can be flown to the area. Also, immediate access can be provided to various vendors' inventories. Accurate and quickly accessible lists detailing local inventories of both medications and supplies are key to coordinating efforts with the outside and saving lives.

Future plans

The Spokane Citywide Disaster Committee, comprising representatives from local emergency departments and emergency medical services, recently decided to more aggressively address the issue of overall domestic preparedness, including readiness for nuclear and chemical attacks. Subcommittees were formed and charged with developing plans for five critical areas: education, medications, personal protective equipment, agency interfaces, and fiscal policy and procedures. The pharmacy work group, consisting of personnel from hospital pharmacy departments and Spokane's health department, fire department, and hazardous materials team, has the goal of providing current, simplified, and readily available information (for example, a list of bioterrorism resources [Appendix C]), educating

Table 1.
Medications Stocked for Treatment and Prophylaxis of Infection by Bioterrorism Agents

Medication	Preferred or Alternative	Infectious Illness[a]
Amoxicillin p.o.	Alternative	A (PEP)
Chloramphenicol i.v.	Alternative	A, P (treat)
Ciprofloxacin i.v.	Preferred	A (treat)
Ciprofloxacin p.o.	Preferred	A (PEP)
Doxycycline i.v.	Alternative	A, P, T (treat)
Doxycycline p.o.	Preferred	A, P, T (PEP); B (treat)
Erythromycin i.v.	Alternative	A (treat)
Erythromycin p.o.	Alternative	A (PEP)
Gentamicin i.m.	Alternative	A, P, T (treat)
Levofloxacin i.v.	Alternative	A (treat)
Levofloxacin p.o.	Preferred	A (PEP)
Penicillin i.v.	Alternative	A (treat)
Rifampin p.o.	Preferred	B (treat)
Streptomycin i.m.	Preferred	P, T (treat)
Tetracycline p.o.	Preferred	P, T (PEP); Q (treat)

[a]A = anthrax, PEP = postexposure prophylaxis, P = plague, treat = treatment, T = tularemia, B = brucellosis, Q = Q fever.

Reprinted with permission from ASHP: *Am J Health-Syst Pharm*; February 1, 2001, Vol 58

and training health care providers about domestic terrorism, and developing counseling pamphlets for victims who have been treated and released.

We plan to survey actual antidote quantities and select appropriate antidotes that have activity against multiple agents. The available quantities of supportive supplies, such as i.v. fluids, will also be assessed. Details about product expiration dates and storage requirements will be compiled. Required antidote quantities will be estimated on the basis of attendance figures for major local public events (sports events, concerts, parades, etc.). Finally, a budget will be drafted and presented to citywide health-system committees for discussion and may be sent to the Spokane County Office of Emergency Management so that federal assistance can be sought.

Discussion

Various recent acts of bioterrorism have made our community realize that we are unprepared for a bioterrorist strike of any scale. We have tried to address this by compiling facts concerning the infectious agents that might be used and the corresponding antidotes, drafting a policy for obtaining medications and supplies, and distributing this information to area hospitals and county officials.

Pharmacists play a vital role in planning for bioterrorism. They can provide up-to-date information on antimicrobial agents and vaccines, including availability, location, storage requirements, dosages, adverse effects, and administration routes. Calculating exactly what quantities of supplies will be needed for a bioterrorism disaster is challenging. Health systems' budgets are limited, and purchasing mass quantities of antidotes is usually prohibitively expensive. Pharmacists can help coordinate efforts to pool resources and share critical information.[14]

The job of a pharmacist during an actual bioterrorism strike is to rapidly disseminate antidotes and information, provide dosage and vaccination schedules for both treatment and prophylaxis, and counsel patients on the proper course of therapy, adverse effects, and follow-up care. Part of a hospital's disaster plan should include sending an extra pharmacist to the emergency department.

Experts are convinced that bioterrorism is a looming public health threat. It is imperative that communities nationwide implement preparedness plans.

Conclusion

Medical facilities in Spokane, Washington, have cooperated to make the community more prepared for a bioterrorist attack.

References

1. McDade JE, Franz D. Bioterrorism as a public health threat. *Emerg Infect Dis.* 1998; 4:493-4.
2. Henderson DA. Bioterrorism as a public health threat. *Emerg Infect Dis.* 1998; 4:488-92.
3. Fox JL. IOM report cites research needs for retaining smallpox virus. *Am Soc Microbiol News.* 1999; 65:392.
4. Torok TJ, Tauxe RV, Wise RP et al. A large community outbreak of salmonellosis caused by intentional contamination of restaurant salad bars. *JAMA.* 1997; 278:389-95.
5. Inglesby TV, Henderson DA, Bartlett JG et al. Anthrax as a biological weapon: medical and public health management. *JAMA.* 1999; 281:1735-45.
6. Inglesby TV, Dennis DT, Henderson DA et al. Plague as a biological weapon: medical and public health management. *JAMA.* 2000; 283:2281-90.
7. Henderson DA, Inglesby TV, Bartlett JG et al. Smallpox as a biological weapon: medical and public health management. *JAMA.* 1999; 281:2127-37.
8. Franz DR, Jahrling PB, Friedlander AM et al. Clinical recognition and management of patients exposed to biological warfare agents. *JAMA.* 1997; 278:399-411.
9. Henderson DA. The looming threat of bioterrorism. *Science.* 1999; 283:1279-82.
10. Drugs and vaccines against biological weapons. *Med Lett Drugs Ther.* 1999; 41:15-6.
11. Dixon TC, Meselson M, Guillemin J et al. Anthrax. *N Engl J Med.* 1999; 341:815-26.
12. Centers for Disease Control and Prevention. Bioterrorism alleging use of anthrax

and interim guidelines for management—United States, 1998. *MMWR.* 1999; 281:787-9.
13. Anthrax vaccine. *Med Lett Drugs Ther.* 1998; 40:52-3.
14. Macintyre AG, Christopher GW, Eitzen E Jr et al. Weapons of mass destruction events with contaminated casualties: effective planning for health care facilities. *JAMA.* 2000; 283:242-9.
15. Breman J, Henderson D. Poxvirus dilemmas—monkeypox, smallpox, and biologic terrorism. *N Engl J Med.* 1998; 339:556-9.

Appendix A—Recommended antidotes for bioterrorism agents

Anthrax

Onset of symptoms[8]: 1–5 days.

Treatment (symptomatic): For first-line treatment, ciprofloxacin 400 mg i.v. q 12 hr.[5,8,11-13] For second-line treatment, doxycycline 200 mg i.v. followed by 100 mg i.v. q 12 hr[5,8,11,12] OR penicillin 2 million units i.v. q 4 hr[11] plus streptomycin 30 mg/kg i.m. or i.v. daily (or gentamicin[11]). Supportive therapy for shock, fluid volume deficit, and airway adequacy may be indicated.[8]

Postexposure prophylaxis: In adults (including pregnant women), provide for 4 wk until 3 doses of vaccine are given or for 8 wk if vaccine is unavailable. For first-line prophylaxis, ciprofloxacin 500 mg p.o. b.i.d.[5,8,11,12] OR levofloxacin 500 mg p.o. daily.[12] For second-line prophylaxis in adults, doxycycline 100 mg p.o. b.i.d.[5,8,11,12] OR amoxicillin 500 mg p.o. q 8 hr (if susceptibility is confirmed).[5,12] In children, for first-line prophylaxis, ciprofloxacin 20–30 mg/kg/day p.o. in divided doses q 12 hr (maximum dosage, 1 g/day).[5,12] For second-line prophylaxis in children, doxycycline 2.5 mg/kg p.o. q 12 hr[12] OR amoxicillin adult dosage in children ³20 kg and 40 mg/kg/day in divided doses q 8 hr in children <20 kg.[5,12]

Isolation precautions: Standard precautions.

Comments: Vaccinate when antidote is given if the vaccine (obtainable from CDC) is available (for Bioport Corporation vaccine, give 0.5 mL s.c. as soon as possible after exposure, then at 2 and 4 wk[12,14]). Once symptoms appear, treatment is almost always ineffective.[8] Other therapeutic alternatives include erythromycin and chloramphenicol.[8]

Botulinum toxins

Onset of symptoms[8]: 1–5 days.

Treatment (symptomatic): Trivalent equine antitoxin for serotypes A, B, and E (available from CDC).[8]

Postexposure prophylaxis: None.

Isolation precautions: Standard precautions.

Comments: Risk of anaphylaxis; perform skin test for horse serum sensitivity before administering equine antitoxin. May also cause serum sickness.[8]

Brucellosis

Onset of symptoms[8]: 5–60 days (occasionally, months).

Treatment (symptomatic): Doxycycline 200 mg/day p.o. plus rifampin 600–900 mg/day p.o. ×

6 wk[8] OR doxycycline 200 mg/day p.o. × 6 wk plus streptomycin 15 mg/kg b.i.d. OR gentamicin 1.5 mg/kg q 8 hr i.m. for first 10 days.[10]

Postexposure prophylaxis: Doxycycline and rifampin × 3 wk.[8]

Isolation precautions: Standard; contact isolation if draining lesions present.

Plague

Onset of symptoms[8]: 2–3 days.

Treatment (symptomatic): For pneumonic plague, streptomycin 15 mg/kg i.m. b.i.d. × 10 days[1,3] OR gentamicin 1.5 mg/kg q 8 hr i.m. × 10 days[8,10] OR doxycycline 200 mg i.v. once, then 100 mg i.v. q 12 hr × 10–14 days.[8] For plague meningitis, chloramphenicol 25 mg/kg i.v., then 60 mg/kg/day in 4 divided doses.[10]

Postexposure prophylaxis: For first-line prophylaxis in adults (including pregnant women) and children, ciprofloxacin 500 mg p.o. b.i.d. OR doxycycline 100 mg p.o. q 12 hr × 7 days[6,8] OR (except in children and pregnant women) tetracycline 500 mg p.o. q.i.d. × 7 days.[8] Alternative: Chloramphenicol 25 mg/kg p.o. q.i.d.[6]

Isolation precautions: For pneumonic plague, droplet precautions until patient has been treated for 3 days.

Comments: Greer inactivated vaccine: 1 mL, then 0.2 mL at 1–3 and 3–6 mo (not protective against pneumonic plague).[6] Currently no vaccines are commercially available to the general public.

Q fever

Onset of symptoms[8]: 10–40 days.

Treatment (symptomatic): Doxycycline 100 mg p.o. q 12 hr × 5–7 days OR tetracycline 500 mg p.o. q 6 hr × 5–7 days.[8]

Postexposure prophylaxis: Start doxycycline 8–12 days after exposure × 5 days; start tetracycline 8–12 days after exposure × 5 days.[8]

Isolation precautions: Standard precautions.

Smallpox

Onset of symptoms[8]: 7–17 days.

Treatment (symptomatic): Cidofovir i.v. effective in vitro; dosage not known.[8,10,15] Also ribavirin i.v. (however, only p.o. and aerosolized formulations are available).[10,15]

Postexposure prophylaxis: Vaccinia immune globulin 0.6 mL/kg i.m. (give within 3 days of exposure; best if given within 24 hr).[8]

Isolation precautions: Airborne precautions.

Comments: If >3 yr since last vaccination, preexposure and postexposure vaccinations are recommended. Currently there are no vaccines commercially available to the general public.

Staphylococcal enterotoxin B

Onset of symptoms[8]: 1–6 hr.

Treatment (symptomatic): Ventilatory support and other supportive care.

Postexposure prophylaxis: None.

Isolation precautions: Standard precautions.

Comments: Vomiting and diarrhea may occur if toxin is ingested.

Tularemia

Onset of symptoms[8]: 2–10 days.

Treatment (symptomatic): Streptomycin 15 mg/kg b.i.d. i.m. × 10–14 days OR gentamicin 3–5 mg/kg/day i.m. × 10–14 days.[8]

Postexposure prophylaxis: Doxycycline 100 mg p.o. q 12 hr × 14 days OR tetracycline 2 g/day p.o. × 14 days.[8]

Isolation precautions: Standard precautions.

Comments: There is a live attenuated vaccine, but currently no vaccines are commercially available to the general public.

Viral encephalitides

Onset of symptoms[8]: Venezuelan equine encephalitis (VEE), 2–6 days; Eastern equine encephalitis (EEE) and Western equine encephalitis (WEE), 7–14 days.

Treatment (symptomatic): Supportive therapy (analgesics and anticonvulsants p.r.n.).

Postexposure prophylaxis: None.

Isolation precautions: Standard precautions.

Comments: There are vaccines for VEE, EEE, and WEE, but currently no vaccines are commercially available to the general public.

Viral hemorrhagic fevers (Congo–Crimean hemorrhagic fever, fevers caused by arenaviruses)

Onset of symptoms[8]: 4–21 days.

Treatment (symptomatic): Ribavirin 30 mg/kg i.v. initially, then 15 mg/kg i.v. q 6 hr × 4 days, then 7.5 mg/kg i.v. q 8 hr × 6 days (however, i.v. ribavirin not commercially available).[8]

Postexposure prophylaxis: None.

Isolation precautions: Contact precautions; additional precautions in cases of massive bleeding.

Comments: Aggressively manage secondary infections and hypotension.[8]

Appendix B—Spokane citywide policy on obtaining pharmacologic antidotes for bioterrorism exposures

Background

The threat of bioterrorism and biological warfare is increasing. Many microorganisms and toxins are easily acquired and mass-produced as aerosolized biological weapons. Contact of populations with these microorganisms has the potential to produce mass casualties that may overwhelm the public health system. It is critical that Spokane increase its preparedness for such attacks. Pharmacologic antidotes are available to treat many biological warfare agents (see attached chart [Appendix A]). However, hospital pharmacies may have an insufficient supply of necessary medications if many people are exposed. The attached chart includes information about treatment of confirmed cases, postexposure prophylaxis, isolation precautions, and local availability of agents.

The protocol below outlines the procedures for obtaining medications that may not be available or that may be stocked in insufficient quantities in the pharmacy.

Implementation

1. The pharmacy will be notified as soon as an exposure is known and will be given an estimate of how many patients may have been exposed.
2. The pharmacy will refer to the attached chart to determine which hospitals stock the necessary medications.
3. The pharmacy will call nearby hospitals and try to obtain the items. [Hospital names and telephone numbers listed]
4. The pharmacy will attempt to obtain the items from the wholesaler. [Wholesaler telephone number and after-hours pager number listed]
5. The pharmacy will obtain assistance from resources outside the local area:

Risk and Emergency Manager
Department of Health
[regional telephone number listed]

Emergency Coordinator
U.S. Public Health Service
206-615-2469

Centers for Disease Control and Prevention
    Emergency Response
770-488-7100

Poison Control Center
[regional telephone number listed]

Domestic Preparedness (partnership of
    federal agencies)
800-424-8802 (emergency)
800-368-6498 (nonemergency/information/
    planning)

Centers for Disease Control and Prevention
    Office of Bioterrorism, Preparedness,
    and Response
404-639-0385

Appendix C—Sources of information on bioterrorism preparedness

1. National Domestic Preparedness Office (partnership of federal agencies)
   Telephone: 800-368-6498
   Fax: 410-612-0715
   E-mail: cbhelp@sbccom.apgea.army.mil
   Web: http://dp.sbccom.army.mil
2. United States Army Medical Department, Medical NBC Information Server (www.nbc-med.org)
3. Johns Hopkins University Center for Civilian Biodefense Studies (www.hopkins-biodefense.org)
4. Centers for Disease Control and Prevention (publisher of *MMWR Morbidity and Mortality Weekly Reports* and *Emerging/Infectious Diseases*) (www.cdc.gov)
5. Centers for Disease Control and Prevention (Bioterrorism Preparedness and Response) (www.bt.cdc.gov)
6. American Society of Health-System Pharmacists Emergency Preparedness–Counterterrorism Resource Center (www.ashp.org/public/proad/emergency/em_prep.html)

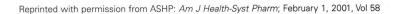

Reprinted with permission from ASHP: *Am J Health-Syst Pharm*; February 1, 2001, Vol 58

Bioterrorism preparedness: Answers for the health-system pharmacist

DAVID S. TEETER

Am J Health-Syst Pharm. 2002; 59:928-30

This presentation describes preparedness for bioterrorism in health care facilities, the findings of some applicable disaster research, and the role of and resources available to pharmacists and other health care professionals.

Preparedness in health care facilities. We who work in health care facilities often take them for granted; we forget about their vulnerabilities and limitations. Hospitals have a high density of people, many of whom are physically or mentally compromised. It is difficult for patients to tolerate the rapid moves and other changes that might be needed in an emergency. Hospitals are complex structures. They have miles of pipes and ducts, which are tempting targets for bioterrorists. Similarly vulnerable are the water and power supplies on which these facilities depend. Hospitals are important to the community, so if one shuts down, there could be a major problem.

Health care facilities and their staffs, patients, and visitors must be protected against the many threats they face. In planning such protection, the first step is to examine what is already in place. Hospitals have an employee health system, which would certainly be involved in immunization and chemoprophylaxis

for the staff. Hospitals have infection control policies, which could be used to monitor antimicrobial resistance in the event of an attack.

Implications of research findings. Social scientists have examined public perceptions about the threat of a disaster. Many Americans think, for example, that a crime such as someone putting anthrax spores into a heating and ventilation system is quite unlikely. If it does occur, they think, it will happen elsewhere, and if it happens here, it will not be that bad, and if it really is bad, there is nothing that can be done about it anyway. Over half the people living in California stated that they believed that an earthquake would never affect their lives—this despite the fact that much of California lies within a major earthquake zone. Disasters are low-probability events—they are not likely to happen to any one person or facility. So pharmacists may have a hard time convincing health care executives of the need for disaster preparedness.

Biological agents are relatively unlikely weapons of terrorism, but they can cause a great number of casualties. Experience shows that a bioterrorism attack is likely to be the work of a loner, cult, or militia group. The worst-case scenario is state-sponsored bioterrorism.

If a biological incident occurs, we will not have to advise people to come to the hospital—they will show up on their own in large numbers. In most mass-casualty incidents in the United States, over half the patients arrive without assistance from the emergency medical service (EMS). People do not wait to be picked up. They hurry to the nearest facility, even if a more appropriate one is not much farther. Volunteers will come, too. People might arrive and claim to be experts on infectious diseases or terrorism. The person on the hospital's doorstep could truly be an expert on infectious diseases—or an overzealous reporter who wants access to the facility.

The news media, in covering the story, is likely to provide some flawed information. During an anthrax hoax in Indianapolis, the first thing I heard out of a television reporter's mouth was misinformation about the supposed attack and the suspected biological agent.

In the event of bioterrorism, some people may break into pharmacies to obtain antimicrobials, but the type of chaos and mass antisocial behavior portrayed by Hollywood is unlikely.

Will health care providers fail to assume their professional roles in case of biological attack? This is

DAVID S. TEETER, PHARM.D., M.S., is Clinical Training Manager, Emergency Management, Strategic Healthcare Group, Veterans Affairs Medical Center, 1481 West Tenth Street, Indianapolis, IN 46202 (david.teeter@med.va.gov).

Presented at the ASHP Annual Meeting, Philadelphia, PA, June 5, 2000.

Reprinted with permission from ASHP: *Am J Health-Syst Pharm*; May 15, 2002, Vol 59

probably not a concern for pharmacists, who tend to show up for work unless they are on their deathbed, and is similarly unlikely to be a problem with other health care providers. But eventually practitioners are going to "burn out" and need replacement, and it will be important for the state and federal government to help bring in additional health care workers.

Health care professionals' role in preparedness. Effective disaster preparedness starts at the local level, because lives are saved by the actions and planning of local people. Practitioners must link up and get organized to deal with the unthinkable. No state or federal agency is going to be able to meet all the challenges of a large biological incident.

How do we manage an incident? There are two major phases, which overlap. The first one is to catch and stop the perpetrators. The Federal Bureau of Investigation (FBI) and the police are in charge of that. Before that phase is over, we are already dealing with the consequences of the event. The Federal Emergency Management Agency (FEMA) is in charge of managing those consequences. FEMA assigns the Public Health Service (PHS) responsibility for health and medical aspects, while the Red Cross has responsibility for sheltering and mass care. Many other federal partners (e.g., Department of Veterans Affairs, Department of Defense) support these agencies with people, equipment, and supplies.

Announced versus unannounced attack. Suppose someone announces that he or she has released anthrax spores into the ventilation system of a large public building. The FBI will first consider the possibility that the announcement is a hoax. However, even a hoax can disrupt the services of a community, including patient care.

In an unannounced attack, a terrorist releases a biological agent, say anthrax, and remains silent. Symptoms would not show up for days.

The lag in diagnosis has important clinical implications. If treatment for some forms of anthrax is started immediately after exposure, the chances of clinical success are quite good, but if treatment for inhalation anthrax is delayed until symptoms appear, then survival may be unlikely. With an unannounced attack, individual health care facilities are the first responders. The immediate challenge is to make an accurate diagnosis, which can be very hard. Then, once a biological weapon is suspected, the facility has to recognize that its patients may represent only part of a larger pool of victims and must alert local, state, and federal authorities.

Decontamination. When dealing with a biological attack that occurred a couple of days earlier, decontamination is generally not an issue. The approach seems to be shifting from hosing patients down to not decontaminating at all. If the patient is decontaminated, removing the clothing is going to take care of most of the problem. At one time, a dilute bleach (sodium hypochlorite) solution was thought to be the ultimate decontaminant. However, U.S. Army chemical warfare experts have good data indicating that soap and water may be best. A health care facility should decide whether to maintain fixed or portable sites for decontamination.

Planning. Comprehensive emergency management (CEM) represents the state of the art in planning for and managing emergencies in the United States. The four phases of CEM are preparing for emergencies, treating patients, facilitating a return to normalcy, and preventing or mitigating future emergencies. CEM improves how we do business and focuses on the big picture by including all hazards. It eliminates the need for separate plans for separate crises (e.g., bioterrorism, tornadoes, and lengthy utility outages). CEM is based on research, because it is best not to base actions on unsupported opinions when lives are at risk. CEM

includes dealing with the news media, mass fatalities, and the psychological impact of the event on the public and the staff. It discusses who is going to pay for everything, and it covers the roles and responsibilities of both the administrative and clinical staffs of the health care facility.

We need to take a realistic inventory of our capabilities. Pharmacists should meet with their wholesaler, review scenarios, and see what supplies can be obtained within 12, 24, and 36 hours. There may be resistance from some staff members, because they may think they are too busy, and from some managers, because preparedness costs time and money. Experts within the facility and the community should be identified.

We are all on too many committees, but I urge pharmacists to get involved with their facility's disaster-planning committee and with emergency-preparedness initiatives in the community. That does not mean that pharmacists have to be members and attend every meeting, but they should talk to the appropriate people and make themselves available. Preparedness must be made a priority. Pharmacists can offer their expertise to universities. I lecture on bioterrorism at both colleges of pharmacy in Indiana. The students say they have never thought about the topic but are glad to hear about it, and they start their careers knowing something about how to get help during a crisis.

Resources. Who are pharmacists going to call on if a bioterrorist act occurs? First are the local network, the EMS, pharmacist colleagues in other facilities, and the buying group. The regional poison control center can also help. Beyond local resources, pharmacists can look to their state agencies and local and state professional associations. The state health department will take the lead on recognizing that an event has occurred. There are also state emergency management groups and Na-

Reprinted with permission from ASHP: *Am J Health-Syst Pharm*; May 15, 2002, Vol 59

tional Guard civil-support teams that can rapidly determine if a biological incident has occurred. That determination will help the governor decide whether to call for federal help or to handle the situation with state resources only.

At the national level, the laboratory facilities of the Centers for Disease Control and Prevention (CDC) are invaluable in identifying biological agents. CDC recently signed a memorandum of understanding with the Department of Veterans Affairs to establish a national stockpile of vaccines and antimicrobials. This will help—but cannot replace—local planning. Supplies from the stockpile will not arrive immediately. The Occupational Safety and Health Administration will have something to say to a facility after a disaster if not enough personnel protective equipment (e.g., N95 respirators) was available. The U.S. Army Medical Research Institute for Infectious Diseases, in Fort Detrick, Maryland, has world experts on bioterrorism. FEMA is in charge of the federal response plan, which determines how the federal government directs resources to the affected state or states.

National pharmacy professional associations, such as the American Society of Health-System Pharmacists, are key resources.[a] Some 120 cities have received initial funding from the Domestic Preparedness Program, but it focuses on the "first-response community" (i.e., fire and rescue personnel and the police) and still falls short in meeting the needs of health care facilities. The Metropolitan Medical Response System (MMRS), managed by PHS, links public health services with health care facilities. The MMRS provides a framework that lets health systems prepare for biological or chemical terrorism. The Joint Commission on Accreditation of Healthcare Organizations will probably incorporate disaster preparedness into how it evaluates health care facilities.

Whenever there is a large or politically important public event, such as the Olympics, the federal government prepares disaster resources for release. If a disaster happens, these resources will be available. However, federal assets cannot be everywhere all the time. One of the world's largest sporting events, the Indianapolis 500, occurs in my hometown. The medical planning for the race is complex and extensive, but it is handled locally.

What pharmacists can do. Where we work determines what our role is in disaster preparedness. It does not matter if a pharmacist is employed by a health care facility, the pharmaceutical industry, or academia—there will be some type of role for that pharmacist to fill. For patients, our roles in a disaster will be pretty much what we do every day—counseling about compliance and adverse effects and providing general drug information. Pharmacists must ensure that they meet patients' needs and will have to be creative to meet these needs. A pharmacy director faced with hundreds of people coming in for medication after a bioterrorist act may want to use the hospital auditorium and have a physician, a public health official, and a pharmacist address the group. The pharmacist could emphasize the importance of taking the medicine as directed or the need to return in a week because a full month's supply cannot be dispensed immediately. Pharmacists will need to find ways to meet the tremendous demand for various medications and to advise prescribers about treatment options; they will get many telephone calls all at once asking what can be done and what the alternatives are.

Pharmacists, as health care professionals and as citizens, should become involved in planning a community's response to bioterrorism. They should also make advance provisions for their own families. Pharmacists on the frontline will be better able to focus on the task at hand knowing that the family is prepared, and family members will feel better knowing that Mom or Dad is also as safe as possible.

Conclusion. Having to cope with a biological attack is a small but definite possibility for any health care facility. Thorough planning takes a big effort but is a necessity of our time.

---

[a]See, for example, the extensive information available through ASHP's Emergency Preparedness–Counterterrorism Resource Center (www.ashp.org/public/proad/emergency/em_prep.html).

Expanding disaster preparedness to include bioterrorism

BARBARA M. POE

Am J Health-Syst Pharm. 2002; 59:926-7

This presentation discusses how bioterrorism differs from traditional disasters and how disaster planning must be expanded to include this newer class of threats.

"Traditional" disasters. I will first describe two events that belong within the traditional disaster-preparedness model: the Murrah Federal Building bombing in Oklahoma City in 1995 and the central Oklahoma tornado outbreak in 1999. We at Norman Regional Hospital were directly involved in the response to both disasters.

A few minutes after 9 a.m. on April 19, 1995, the Alfred P. Murrah Federal Building was destroyed by a bomb blast in what was to that date the largest terrorist attack in U.S. history. One hundred sixty-eight people were killed, and several hundred more were injured. The attack was a seminal event in prompting the federal government to rethink the nation's preparedness for terrorism.

The outbreak of tornadoes occurred on May 3, 1999, when multiple "super-cell" thunderstorms moved across Oklahoma. There were two F4 tornadoes and one F5 tornado. The highest wind speeds ever measured on the earth were recorded during the F5 event. Seventy-four of the 95 tornadoes that occurred in Oklahoma in 1999 took place on that one day. (By comparison, in 1997 and 1998 combined, there were a total of 90 tornadoes in Oklahoma.) The death toll in Oklahoma that day was 40—and we can thank an extremely talented group of meteorologists that the toll was not even higher. The injured numbered about 675, and the cost of the damage was estimated at $1.2 billion. Rescue workers said that the tornadoes' paths looked like bombed-out strips. Literally nothing was left standing in the wake of the F5 twister. Some 10,000 vehicles were destroyed that day in Oklahoma.

How bioterrorism and the response to it differ. I mention the Murrah Building bombing and the tornadoes because they are the types of events that traditional disaster planning addresses. For several reasons, a bioterrorist attack could necessitate a very different response.

Distinct versus indistinct characteristics. Traditional disasters have a distinct beginning and end, and there is immediately visible evidence of physical damage. These characteristics are important because they allow us to proceed from the event itself to its aftermath. We know that the event is over, and we can start putting our lives back together. This sense of closure would be far more elusive with a bioterrorist attack. We may not know when the attack begins and whether it is actually over, and it may be much harder to recognize and quantify the damage.

Intensity of the disaster response. The disaster response to the bombing and tornadoes was, from a health care perspective, intense while it lasted but relatively short-lived. By the morning after the day of tornadoes, things were pretty much back to normal in Oklahoma's health systems. The same can be said about the bombing: In just hours, relatively normal activity levels resumed. A bioterrorist attack may necessitate a more prolonged period of intense response.

Scope of the disaster. Traditional disasters in the United States often produce enormous physical damage and, at most, several hundred casualties. With a bioterrorist attack, there would probably be little or no physical damage, but there could be thousands of casualties. Local disaster plans could be implemented, but at some point a federal response would be necessary to begin moving resources to the area, because there is no way a community could fully handle most bioterrorist attacks on its own.

BARBARA M. POE, M.B.A., is Director, Pharmacy Services, Norman Regional Hospital, 901 North Porter, Norman, OK 73071.
Presented at the ASHP Annual Meeting, Philadelphia, PA, June 5, 2000.

Copyright © 2002, American Society of Health-System Pharmacists, Inc. All rights reserved. 1079-2082/02/0502-0926$06.00

Reprinted with permission from ASHP: *Am J Health-Syst Pharm*; May 15, 2002, Vol 59

Identity of the culprit. In a traditional disaster, the causative agent is immediately known. Because of the physical damage, disaster plan implementation is rapid at the local level. With a bioterrorist attack, we will have to rely on physicians, scientists, and law enforcement authorities to put the pieces of the puzzle together. This could be a slow process.

Inclusion of pharmacists in disaster preparedness. In December 1998, I participated in a tabletop exercise in Oklahoma City that involved emergency personnel from throughout the state. I had weaseled an invitation to the event and was the only pharmacist present. Most planners are not aware of how vital pharmacists can be in making disaster plans work and work well—especially in the case of bioterrorist attacks. Pharmacists who have not been included in such planning need to rattle some cages.

Psychological response of the populace. Should a bioterrorist attack occur, health care professionals will need to be prepared to deal with the public's fear and even panic. Properly trained health officials, including pharmacists, will be essential in allaying these reactions.

Public mobilization. After the Oklahoma City bombing and the state's tornado outbreak, officials were literally overwhelmed by the public's desire to help. It is unclear if that kind of a response would occur after a bioterrorist attack. Fear of placing one's own life in peril or spreading a contagion to loved ones could impede involvement by those who might otherwise readily volunteer.

Impact on civil liberties. The effect of a bioterrorist attack on civil liberties could range from the curtailment of travel to the imposition of martial law and would probably be much different from what we have been accustomed to with other disasters.

Concerns unique to pharmacy. We have become proficient at moving drug products along the supply chain from the manufacturer to the bedside. This strength could become a weakness during the pandemonium of a bioterrorist attack. Pharmacists should ask their wholesaler if it has a disaster or bioterrorism plan in place. My experience suggests that many wholesalers do not.

The golden 48 hours. In medicine we are accustomed to speaking of the "golden hour"—the time immediately after an event during which the most important treatment decisions and interventions must occur. Disaster preparedness requires capitalizing on a golden 48 hours. Between the event and the moment a state or federal official decides that full mobilization of disaster-response resources is needed, the pharmacist will be left to his or her own resources. That period could last anywhere from several hours up to 48 hours. Remember that we are talking about the potential for thousands of casualties. When I participated in the tabletop exercise in Oklahoma City, it became quite apparent that, within a very few hours, a lack of adequate pharmaceutical supplies would impede the ability to provide traditional care. Pharmacy has done such a good job of supplying drugs when needed that the effort it takes to move the product through the pipeline is not generally recognized outside pharmacy.

Security. During a bioterrorism disaster, it may be necessary to post armed guards at pharmacies. This is another detail that must not be overlooked in the preparedness plan.

Staffing. Pharmacy is struggling with a personnel shortage even during normal operations. Obviously, a large number of casualties will greatly exacerbate this problem. Creative solutions will be needed, such as shifting pharmacists and technicians to the locations in greatest need.

Conclusion. Terrorism has emerged as one of the most difficult problems of the post-Cold-War era. Because a terrorist attack can happen at any time, we must maintain a state of high readiness. Traditional disaster-preparedness models will need adjustment for bioterrorism scenarios, and pharmacists are key in making that adjustment. I close with these words from the Oklahoma City National Memorial: "We come here to remember those who were killed, those who survived, and those changed forever. May all who leave here know the impact of violence, and may this Memorial offer comfort, strength, peace, hope and serenity."

Reprinted with permission from ASHP: *Am J Health-Syst Pharm*; May 15, 2002, Vol 59

Therapeutic selection during an emergency response

MICHAEL J. MONTELLO AND TIMOTHY AMES

Abstract: Therapeutic selection in a postdisaster setting is described.

Therapeutic selection is the process of assessing a patient's pharmaceutical requirements and selecting the appropriate therapy. Although the primary criteria for drug selection during a disaster response are the same as in usual pharmacy practice, there is a shift in emphasis created by communication and transportation limitations and by changes in the patient's general living environment. The cost of agents is no longer viewed in terms of dollars but in the context of limited inventories. A disaster may exacerbate health problems or make adverse drug effects more common and problematic. Drug administration and patient compliance will be hampered. Pre-established guidelines for appropriate patient care should be reviewed and approved by a group of representative health care providers. General policies for pharmaceutical care should include guidelines for a formulary, prescription refills, dispensing limitations, and prescriber approval. Therapeutic selection should involve obtaining a medical history, selecting a drug regimen, educating and counseling the patient, and documenting the process. Pharmacists should use familiar procedures that they are comfortable with to minimize stress and optimize outcomes. Procedures should be flexible to adjust to circumstances and individual patient needs.

Therapeutic selection during a disaster response, although based on the same principles as traditional therapeutic selection, is more complex. Pharmacists will need to tailor their approach to the circumstances and to individual patient needs.

Index terms: Disasters; Dispensing; Documentation; Drugs; Formularies; Patients; Pharmaceutical care; Pharmacists; Prescribing; Prescriptions; Rational therapy
Am J Health-Syst Pharm.
1999; 56:236-40

CDR MICHAEL J. MONTELLO, M.S., is Deputy-Chief Pharmacy Officer, Disaster Medical Assistance Team-1, U.S. Public Health Service, Bethesda, MD. CPT TIMOTHY AMES, M.P.H., is Chief Pharmacy Officer, Disaster Medical Assistance Team-1, U.S. Public Health Service, Rockville, MD.

Address reprint requests to CDR Montello at the Cancer Therapy Evaluation Program, Division of Cancer Treatment and Diagnosis, National Cancer Institute, Executive Plaza North, Room 707, Bethesda, MD 20892, or to montellom@ctep.nci.nih.gov.

Reprinted with permission from ASHP: *Am J Health-Syst Pharm*; February 1, 1999, Vol 56

T he U.S. federal disaster response plan for health and medical services includes provisions for the overall public health response, preventive medicine, and the triage, treatment, transportation, and evacuation of patients.[1,2] Pharmacists in the Public Health Service (PHS) have participated in a number of emergency responses. Pharmacists have a variety of important administrative and clinical skills that are vital in these situations.[3] One of the most important clinical functions a pharmacist can perform during a disaster response is therapeutic selection.

Definition of therapeutic selection

Therapeutic selection is the process of assessing a patient's medication requirements and selecting the appropriate therapy to address the patient's needs. One must consider the therapeutic intent, patient characteristics, and the health care environment when selecting an agent. Simplified, the criteria for selecting a therapeutic regimen can be summarized by the following equation[4]:

Benefit of regimen + Danger of not treating the condition − Adverse events = Value of regimen

No matter the setting, a considerable amount of detail is required to adequately assess the value of a treatment regimen. The patient's comorbidities, concomitant medications, living environment, and finances must be considered. What is the cost of the agent? Does the patient have insurance? Questions about the health care environment should be addressed. Does the institution have a formulary?

Therapeutic selection during a disaster response

Although the primary criteria for selecting an agent in the traditional practice setting and during a disaster response are the same, there is typically a shift in emphasis during a disaster response. This shift is created by communication and transportation limitations and by alterations in the patient's general living environment. Road closures, power outages, and downed telephone lines can make consultation with other health care providers and replenishment of pharmaceutical supplies impractical or impossible. Inventory limitations create a restrictive environment. Given that patients are not charged for agents dispensed by federal response teams during a disaster, the cost of an agent is no longer measured in dollars but in terms of the current inventory. All things being equal, selection will likely be based on the quantity of an agent on hand rather than on the dollar value of the agent.

The patient's access to food, clean water, and shelter also affects therapeutic selection. Consider the following scenario: A pediatric patient has an earache. Augmentin (amoxicillin–clavulanic acid, SmithKline Beecham) and Bactrim (trimethoprim–sulfamethoxazole, Roche) are currently on formulary. The patient has limited access to food, potable water, and refrigeration, and no shelter. Both formulary options are problematic. The pharmacist must weigh the potential risks and benefits of both agents when selecting which product to dispense.

The altered living environment can also exacerbate health problems or make potential adverse effects more common and burdensome during a disaster. Consider the patient with well-controlled diabetes. Significant variations in blood glucose levels may result from dietary changes, dehydration, stress, exposure, and increased physical activity. Health care workers must consider the patient within both the predisaster and the postdisaster environment when making a therapeutic selection.

Ease of administration and compliance should be considered. Many patients will be too busy to remember to take a medication four times daily. Therefore, medications that have long half-lives or require less frequent administration are preferable. For example, for the treatment of sexually transmitted diseases or other infections, a single i.m. injection of an appropriate antimicrobial would be preferable to long-term oral antimicrobials. On the other hand, agents with a prolonged duration of action could be associated with adverse effects that persist for an extended period.

Pre-established policies for therapeutic selection

To ensure effective patient care and adequate control of the pharmaceutical inventory, pre-established guidelines for appropriate patient care during a disaster response should be reviewed and approved by a group of representative health care providers. Providers should review all policies before deployment of the response and periodically during deployment. The health care team should assess whether any of the policies should be modified. In general, policies should be flexible and should allow for adaptation to the unique circumstances of each disaster. General policies for pharmaceutical care should include guidelines for a pharmacy formulary, prescription refills, dispensing limitations, and prescriber approval.

Formulary. Identification of a standard pharmacy formulary is essential to ensuring quality patient care. The formulary should include representative agents for treating the major chronic diseases found in the United States (e.g., hypertension, diabetes mellitus, asthma). Appropriate acute care medications (e.g., analgesics, antimicrobials, cough and cold remedies) should also be included. Because of logistic concerns, the formulary should be limited. The inclusion of "me too" drugs should be minimized. Agents with multiple indications (e.g., ibuprofen, diphenhydramine) are ideal. The standard formulary may be supplemented according to the nature of the disaster or the demographics of the expected patient population.

Reprinted with permission from ASHP: *Am J Health-Syst Pharm*; February 1, 1999, Vol 56

Based on prior experience, it can be expected that, once deployed, the formulary will be in constant transition. Pharmaceutical companies, hospitals, government agencies, and charities often donate medications to disaster victims. There is frequently little control over the acquisition of medical supplies. Boxes of drugs, often short dated, will appear mysteriously. On the other hand, the pharmacist will often be unable to procure a specific antiepileptic or antiarrhythmic agent. Continuous monitoring of the formulary is of vital importance to therapeutic selection. Other prescribers should be notified as often as possible about any changes to the formulary.

Refills. Prescription refills are often the number one reason for patient visits to field clinics during a disaster and account for a substantial portion of a pharmacist's workload. Guidelines on the type of evaluation required for each refill should be established. For example, must all patients receive a complete physical evaluation (e.g., vital signs, laboratory work) before receiving a prescription refill, or can the pharmacist simply take a patient history before dispensing a refill? It should be clear who is responsible for performing any required physical evaluations.

Dispensing limitations. The quantity of medications dispensed will depend on the circumstances. Pharmacists should consider the agent's indication, the current inventory, and the anticipated re-establishment of the local health care system.

Prescriber approval. Authorized substitution of a therapeutically equivalent agent for the drug prescribed is considered to be therapeutic interchange. Given inventory limitations, the prescribed agent will often not be available. Must a pharmacist consult a physician before substituting a therapeutic alternative? If other prescribers are not available, often the only practical option is to make an unauthorized substitution of a therapeutically equivalent agent (i.e., therapeutic substitution).

Whether physician consultation is required may depend on the nature of the prescription and the agent prescribed. Most pharmacists would probably feel comfortable making a substitution with agents such as nonsteroidal anti-inflammatory drugs, cold preparations, and antilipemics but very uncomfortable making a substitution with drug classes such as antiarrhythmics and anticonvulsants. The pharmacist's comfort level will often depend on his or her prior experience. The health care team should establish general guidelines regarding which drug classes would require consultation and which classes would not.

A step-by-step approach to therapeutic selection

Therapeutic selection during a disaster response is not part of the average pharmacist's training, and literature on the subject is virtually nonexistent. A standard approach cannot be developed because of the volatile nature of disasters. During a disaster response it is important to remember that, although the surroundings may be unusual, pharmacists should use procedures they are comfortable with. Special "disaster procedures" should not be developed unless absolutely necessary. Performing familiar functions will minimize stress and optimize performance. The following practical step-by-step guidelines for therapeutic selection have been developed on the basis of prior experience.

Therapeutic selection in both the disaster setting and the traditional setting involves obtaining a patient history, making a therapeutic selection, providing patient education, and documenting the process. Depending on the circumstances, a physical assessment and prescriber consultation may also be obtained.

Patient history and assessment. The first step when making a therapeutic selection in a disaster setting is to obtain an in-depth and detailed patient history. In addition to the patient's medical history and information on drug allergies, a pharmacist should obtain information on the patient's current living conditions and determine the potential for patient education and compliance. The patient's medical chart or notes, if available, should be carefully reviewed for additional information.

During a disaster, patients' medications may be lost or destroyed. Often patients will approach the pharmacist with a handful of empty vials or a list of their current medications. The pharmacist should determine the indication, dosage, route, duration, efficacy, and toxicity for each medication. It is important to ask about other drugs (e.g., nonprescription drugs, illegal drugs) the patient may be taking. Most patients are somewhat reluctant to reveal any details about illegal drugs they are using, especially to a uniformed health care provider, but it does not hurt to ask.

Many drugs have multiple indications (e.g., propranolol, diazepam). The selection of a suitable alternative will depend on the indication of the agent in a particular setting. In most circumstances the alternative will be another agent in the same therapeutic class (e.g., atenolol instead of propranolol). Occasionally an agent in a different pharmacologic class might be an appropriate substitute. For example, diphenhydramine may be a suitable alternative to diazepam for sedation. Whenever possible, agents with similar mechanisms of action, toxicity profiles, and schedules should be selected.

The length of drug therapy should be considered. A patient who has been receiving a short course of prednisone after exposure to poison ivy would be treated differently from someone receiving long-term steroids for asthma. The prior effectiveness of a medication and any adverse effects should also be evaluated during therapeutic selection. The pharmacist should deter-

Reprinted with permission from ASHP: *Am J Health-Syst Pharm*; February 1, 1999, Vol 56

mine the patient's general medical condition before and after the disaster.

When assessing the patient's pharmaceutical needs, it is important to determine the patient's current living environment. A pharmacist must assess the patient's diet and access to shelter, clean water, refrigeration, and transport. Security of medications should also be considered. The loss of childproof locks on medicine cabinets could increase the risk of an accidental overdose and the propensity for vandalism. Unscrupulous individuals may seek prescription medications, especially narcotics, after a disaster. If possible, provisions should be made to minimize the risk of such events to patients and their families.

During the patient interview, the pharmacist should assess the potential for patient education. The pharmacist should consider any language barriers and the patient's mental capacity (e.g., age, whether mentally retarded). Substitution of a therapeutic alternative for a previously prescribed agent is dangerous if patients cannot be educated about potential changes in therapy. If family members are available, they should be involved in the conversation. Most patients will be under extreme stress, so it would not be unusual for someone to forget something important. The more individuals involved, the greater the likelihood that the proper information will be conveyed and retained.

Although there is no effective way to prospectively determine whether a patient will be compliant with therapy, the patient's chart or prescription vials will provide some clues. The date the last prescription was dispensed and the number of days' supply should be verified. It is important to keep in mind that some patients may have been noncompliant because of the disaster.

An appropriate physical assessment of the patient's condition should be made. If possible, laboratory data (e.g., blood glucose concentrations, electrolytes) should also be obtained. The level and complexity of the physical assessment and laboratory data will often depend on the workload, the size and composition of the health care team, and the patient's chief complaint.

Therapeutic selection. Whether the patient requires new pharmacologic therapy or continuation of therapy, the pharmacist must use whatever tools are available in making the appropriate selection. Medical charts or notes, if available, should be reviewed for potential contraindications. Pharmacists should also review available medical references, consult with other team members, and use their own clinical judgment. Of course, all decisions must be based on the current formulary.

A disaster does not lend itself to literature searches. It is not practical and is often quite difficult to maintain even a limited selection of medical references. Handbooks are very practical. Some personal recommendations include *Handbook of Clinical Drug Data* (Drug Intelligence Publications, Hamilton, IL), *Drug Information Handbook for the Allied Health Professional* (Lexi-Comp, Hudson, OH), *Harriet Lane Pediatric Handbook*, (Year Book Medical Publishers, Chicago, IL) and *Guide to Antimicrobial Therapy* (Antimicrobial Therapy, Dallas, TX). Photocopies of drug class reviews from *Drug Facts and Comparisons* (Facts and Comparisons, St. Louis, MO) are often very useful. *Martindale: The Extra Pharmacopoeia* (Pharmaceutical Press, London) may be a useful resource for foreign deployments. Consultation with other pharmacists or health care practitioners is advised whenever possible. However, there is no substitute for a pharmacist's practical experience in selecting an agent.

In most circumstances the choice of agent will be limited to what is currently available on formulary. If no suitable alternative is available, every attempt should be made to find a source of the item. Procurement of a nonformulary item will probably require considerable time and effort and in many circumstances may be impossible. If unable to obtain a specific agent, the pharmacist or health care team may have to decide whether to treat the patient with a less suitable alternative or provide no treatment. The decision will depend, among other things, on the severity of the illness. Pharmacists should remember the axiom "First do no harm."

Prescriber approval. How and when to seek prescriber approval for therapeutic selection will vary with the situation. The availability of prescribers, the state of communications, and the nature of the exchange should be considered. Workload and communication limitations may make consultation impractical in many circumstances. Ultimately the decision to solicit prescriber approval is going to be a judgment call.

Patient education and documentation. Substitution of an alternative therapeutic agent requires careful patient counseling. Failure to appropriately counsel a patient could have severe consequences. Patients have to be aware that an exchange has been made and have to know the reason. It should be made clear that this is only a temporary change and that only the minimum supply of medication is being dispensed to maintain the patient's care during the disaster. Patients should be instructed to return to their usual caregivers as soon as possible to resume their predisaster regimen. The pharmacist should outline what medications were originally prescribed, what medications are being used as alternatives, and why the new agent is a suitable alternative. All new instructions and warnings should be clarified. Any changes in schedule, frequency, or storage should be identified, and potential adverse effects should be clearly described.

Counseling skills are extremely important. The pharmacist should use open-ended questions and have patients repeat the directions to ensure that they fully understand all new instructions. It is important to provide as much documentation as possible and encourage patients to ask questions.

Reprinted with permission from ASHP: *Am J Health-Syst Pharm*; February 1, 1999, Vol 56

Pharmacists should be aware that patients may take the opportunity to obtain free medication even though they may have ample supplies at home. Unless supplies are especially tight, it is often simpler to dispense the medication without being concerned about what drugs the patient may or may not already have. It is virtually impossible to police this situation, and dispensing free medication to a patient is inconsequential compared with the losses many people may have experienced. However, it is important to explain in a nonaccusatory manner what patients should do if they happen to find a supply of their old medication. Patients must be instructed not to take their old and new drugs together. The pharmacist should explain in simple terms that this would result in therapeutic duplication and could potentially be harmful. Whenever possible, patients should be encouraged to continue with their predisaster regimens and to discard their new medications once they have located the old ones.

The process of therapeutic selection must be documented on the patient's chart or record, including what medications were originally prescribed, what medication is being used as an alternative, and both the old and new instructions. There should be a brief explanation of why the alternative was selected. References should be included if appropriate. There should be a record of whether prescriber approval was obtained. If a prescriber was not available for approval, a reason

should be stated briefly. The patient counseling session should also be documented.

The prescription label should include a brief statement clarifying that a therapeutic selection was made. The following wording is suggested: "As a result of the recent emergency, a therapeutic selection has been made. When possible, please return to your local pharmacy to continue with your previously prescribed medication."

Conclusion

Therapeutic selection during a disaster, although based on the same principles as traditional therapeutic selection, is more complex. Pharmacists will frequently be relied on to select appropriate drug therapy for a patient on the basis of the person's unique characteristics. Selection may not include physician consultation, and pharmacists should be prepared to apply their unique skills and clinical experience after a disaster.

References

1. The Federal Response Plan for Public Law 93-288. 1992 Apr.
2. Montello M, Ames T. The federal disaster response plan: health and medical services. *Fed Pract.* In press.
3. Ames T. The pharmacist's role in a disaster response. *Am J Health-Syst Pharm.* In press.
4. Melmon KL, Gilman AG, Mayer SE. Principles of therapeutics. In: Goodman and Gilman's the pharmacological basis of therapeutics. 6th ed. Gilman AG, Goodman LS, Gilman A, eds. New York: Macmillan; 1980:40-55.

2001 anthrax crisis in Washington, D.C.: Clinic for persons exposed to contaminated mail

Andrew S. T. Haffer, James R. Rogers, Michael J. Montello, Ellen C. Frank, and Craig Ostroff

During October 19–21, 2001, four workers from the U.S. Postal Service's Brentwood Processing and Distribution Center, in Washington, D.C., were hospitalized with inhalational anthrax, the most lethal form of anthrax. Two of these postal workers later died of their infections.[1] Postal workers and those who visited the Brentwood facility were potentially exposed to aerosolized anthrax spores when a letter contaminated with the bacterium passed through automatic mail-sorting equipment.

On October 21, 2001, teams from the Disaster Medical Assistance Team (DMAT) and the Commissioned Corps Readiness Force (CCRF), units of the U.S. Public Health Service (USPHS), were deployed to Washington to establish a clinic that would provide education and medication to workers and visitors to the Brentwood facility who may have been exposed. USPHS pharmacists performed critical roles in establishing and staffing this clinic.

Disaster plans are currently being developed or revised as a result of the

Abstract: An anthrax prophylaxis clinic is described.

In October 2001, four workers from the U.S. Postal Service's Brentwood facility in Washington, D.C., were hospitalized with inhalational anthrax; many others may have been exposed to anthrax spores. U.S. Public Health Service (USPHS) teams were deployed to establish an anthrax prophylaxis clinic that would provide education and medication to workers and people who visited the mail facility. The temporary clinic was set up at D.C. General Hospital and was staffed primarily by health care professionals from USPHS. The protocol at the clinic involved three major phases. Phase 1 consisted of gathering information from the patient and distributing educational materials. Phase 2 involved presentations by a physician and a pharmacist concerning anthrax, followed by a question-and-answer session. In phase 3, a pharmacist selected the most appropriate prophylactic agent, dispensed the medication, counseled the patient, and referred patients with flu-like symptoms or skin lesions to a physician. Two floor plans were used to maximize the number of patients seen per hour without jeopardizing patient care. The clinic operated 14 hours a day for 14 days. The 136-member health care team included 52 pharmacists, and medication was dispensed to more than 18,000 patients. The clinic may serve as a model for pharmacists and other professionals in designing and implementing disaster plans.

A multidisciplinary team established and operated a clinic to treat persons who may have been exposed to anthrax through contaminated mail.

Index terms: Ambulatory care; Anthrax; Biological warfare; Diagnosis; Disaster planning; Protocols; Team

Am J Health-Syst Pharm. 2002; 59:1189-92

anthrax crises that occurred in Washington, D.C.; Florida; New Jersey; and New York. We describe here a working protocol developed at the anthrax prophylaxis clinic in Washington. The concepts developed and used at the clinic may help pharmacists and other health care providers to design and implement their own treatment protocols in the event of future bioterrorism attacks.

Establishment and functioning of the clinic

A temporary anthrax prophylaxis clinic was initially established in a lo-

LCDR Andrew S. T. Haffer, Pharm.D., is Pharmacy Officer, PHS-1 Disaster Medical Assistance Team, U.S. Public Health Service (USPHS), and Regulatory Review Officer, Division of Drug Marketing, Advertising, and Communications, Food and Drug Administration (FDA), Rockville, MD. LCDR James R. Rogers, Pharm.D., is Deputy Chief Professional Officer—Pharmacy, PHS-1 Disaster Medical Assistance Team, USPHS, and Regulatory Review Officer, Division of Drug Marketing, Advertising, and Communications, FDA. CDR Michael J. Montello, Pharm.D., is Chief Professional Officer—Pharmacy, PHS-1 Disaster Medical Assistance Team, USPHS, and Head, Protocol and Information Office, Cancer Therapeutics Evaluation Program, National Cancer Institute, Rockville. LCDR Ellen C.

Frank, B.S.Pharm., is Pharmacist, Commissioned Corps Readiness Force, USPHS, and Chief, Project Management Staff, Division of Special Pathogen and Immunologic Drug Products, FDA. LT Craig Ostroff, Pharm.D., is Pharmacy Officer, PHS-1 Disaster Medical Assistance Team, USPHS, and Regulatory Management Officer, Division of Pulmonary and Allergy Drug Products, FDA.

Address correspondence to LCDR Haffer at the Division of Drug Marketing, Advertising, and Communications, HFD-042, Food and Drug Administration, 5600 Fishers Lane, Room 17B-17, Rockville, MD 20852 (haffera@cder.fda.gov).

This article represents the opinions of the authors and does not necessarily reflect the policy of the U.S. Public Health Service.

Reprinted with permission from ASHP: *Am J Health-Syst Pharm*; June 15, 2002, Vol 59

cal District of Columbia government building. On the second day of the mission, a more permanent location for the clinic was established at D.C. General Hospital. The clinic was staffed by officers from the DMAT and CCRF teams and by other USPHS officers. Health care professionals and support personnel from D.C. General Hospital, the District of Columbia Department of Health, the Centers for Disease Control and Prevention (CDC), and the Department of Health and Human Service's Office of Emergency Preparedness (OEP) also provided support. The team included pharmacists, physicians, nurses, mental health professionals, other health care workers, and management support personnel.

The health care professionals combined their expertise and resources to develop a working protocol for establishing, staffing, monitoring, and assessing the clinic. Pharmacists were involved in all aspects of the mission and performed many key functions within the clinic. In addition to dispensing medication and counseling patients, pharmacists participated in educational sessions, screened patients, selected appropriate therapeutic agents, and provided logistical support.

The protocol at the clinic involved three major phases: patient receiving and collection of patient information, education about anthrax and treatment options, and distribution of the most appropriate prophylactic medication for each individual (Figure 1).

Receiving. On arrival at the clinic, people were brought to a receiving area where general information was collected, such as their names and the locations of potential exposure. Individuals were quickly assessed to determine if they were at risk (i.e., whether they had entered the Brentwood facility or had come into contact with mail from it or any other affected location). Printed educational materials about anthrax, prophylactic therapy, and psychological

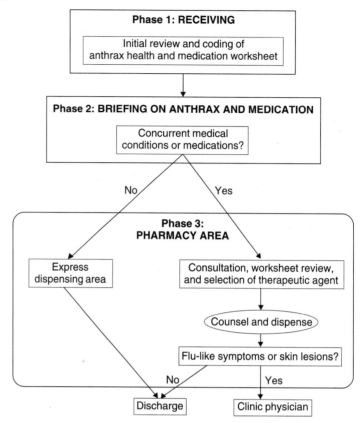

Figure 1. Flow chart for patient receiving, counseling, and treatment in the anthrax prophylaxis clinic.

issues were provided to each person. The printed materials gave a telephone number and Web-site address that patients could refer to for additional information about anthrax and their medication. An anthrax health and medication worksheet was distributed so that the medical history could be quickly assessed.[2] The medical support staff and postal authorities were also available to answer procedural questions and facilitate completion of the forms.

The worksheet was developed at the clinic as a tool for rapidly assessing each individual for appropriate therapeutic selection and education. Patients answered 16 yes-or-no questions about their current health status (including presence of flu-like symptoms or skin lesions), concurrent medical conditions, and drug–drug, drug–food, and drug–disease interactions that might affect treat-

ment selection. All worksheets were immediately reviewed by a nurse and assigned a 1 if all questions were answered no, indicating no concurrent medical conditions or medications, or a 2 if any questions were answered yes, indicating the presence of concurrent medical conditions or medications.

Briefing on anthrax and medication. After the patients completed the worksheets, groups of approximately 50 each were assembled in a briefing area. The briefing included a short presentation by a physician on anthrax and what to expect while visiting the clinic. After the physician's presentation, a pharmacist briefly discussed drug therapy, including dosage schedule, interactions, adverse effects, and other medication-related information. The physician and the pharmacist then answered questions, of which there were many. The most frequently reported con-

Reprinted with permission from ASHP: *Am J Health-Syst Pharm*; June 15, 2002, Vol 59

cerns included the risk of developing inhalational anthrax or of transferring anthrax to family members, what to do with potentially contaminated clothing, and interactions between alcohol and the anthrax-prophylaxis medication. The briefing helped alleviate some of the patients' stress and anxiety. (Mental health professionals were also available at the briefing to address psychological issues.)

Pharmacy area. Individuals with a code of 1 (i.e., those with all "no" answers on the worksheet) were triaged to an "express" dispensing area to receive prophylactic medication and were discharged. The express dispensing area was staffed by nurses who dispensed medication and provided general information. Patients in this area did not require in-depth consultation, because their worksheets did not signal a contraindication, potential interaction, or concurrent medical condition. The written information and the oral briefing were considered sufficient interventions.

Individuals with a code of 2 (i.e., those with at least one affirmative response) were triaged to the pharmacy area for consultation with a pharmacist. The pharmacist met with each patient, reviewed the worksheet, and prescribed and dispensed one of three antimicrobials (ciprofloxacin, doxycycline, or amoxicillin). The pharmacist concluded with a brief discussion of drug–drug, drug–food, and drug–disease interactions and other medication-related issues, depending on the individual's needs. Patients with flu-like symptoms or skin lesions were directed to a clinic physician. Those who preferred not to see a clinic physician were referred to their personal primary care provider.

Therapeutic interchange was left to the discretion of the pharmacist on the basis of predetermined criteria established in consultation with physicians and current CDC recommendations. CDC suggested either ciprofloxacin or doxycycline as the drug of choice for postexposure prophylaxis against inhalational anthrax when antimicrobial susceptibility was unknown.[3] Initially, ciprofloxacin was determined to be the drug of choice and was dispensed to all patients, unless the pharmacist determined that an alternative agent was necessary. After several days, testing by CDC demonstrated that the strain of the anthrax bacterium was susceptible to doxycycline. Doxycycline was made the prophylactic drug of choice because of its comparable effectiveness, more favorable safety profile, and availability from multiple sources.

All individuals were initially dispensed a 10-day supply of antimicrobials. CDC determined that 10 days was a reasonable time for prophylaxis to cover the normal incubation period after inhalational exposure to anthrax spores. This 10-day period also allowed CDC sufficient time to fully test each postal facility to determine who needed a prolonged (60-day) prophylactic regimen. Certain employees from the Brentwood facility were determined to be at a higher risk of exposure and were asked to return to the clinic for an additional 50-day supply of medication (to complete a full 60-day regimen).

Antimicrobials dispensed at the clinic were provided by CDC's National Pharmaceutical Stockpile Program (NPSP).[4] The medications were delivered in bulk from NPSP "push packages." Push packages consist of 50 tons of preassembled supplies, pharmaceuticals, and medical equipment ready for delivery to a mass-casualty area within 12 hours. The pharmacists who staffed the pharmacy area of the clinic repackaged and labeled the bulk antimicrobials for dispensing.

Design of the clinic

The design of a temporary clinic is largely determined by space limitations and the number of individuals to be treated. Two floor plans were utilized at the D.C. General Hospital clinic site to maximize the number of patients seen per hour without jeopardizing patient care. The first floor plan (Figure 2) was developed to process large numbers of patients (>100 per hour). Hospital corridors and rooms were used in such a way that many people could pass through the clinic in an orderly manner. The receiving area was a hallway lined with chairs. Patients then moved to a classroom or a larger hallway, where the briefing was conducted. Each briefing area contained approximately 50 chairs. With the briefing concluded, patients were directed to the pharmacy area. The pharmacy area had 20 desks that were used as individual counseling and dispensing stations and a long table designated as the express dispensing area. A secure room in the pharmacy area was used to store medications during normal clinic hours.

The second floor plan was developed to handle up to 100 patients per hour. This design had only two areas for all three phases of clinic operation. A hallway lined with chairs served as the receiving area. The briefing and dispensing functions both took place in a classroom.

CDC and OEP are reviewing the experience of the anthrax prophylaxis clinic at D.C. General to determine how its operations could be improved. They are particularly interested in determining if this type of operation can be scaled up to treat 100,000 to 1,000,000 patients. A consensus statement on this topic is expected later in 2002.

Discussion

The anthrax prophylaxis clinic was initially designed to treat several thousand potentially exposed postal workers from the Brentwood facility. However, the clinic was expanded as the number of potentially exposed people increased, and this necessitated adjustments in both resources and staffing. The clinic operated 14 hours a day, 7 days a week, for 14 days.

Reprinted with permission from ASHP: *Am J Health-Syst Pharm*; June 15, 2002, Vol 59

Figure 2. Designs of anthrax prophylaxis clinics capable of handling >100 patients per hour (A) and 100 patients per hour (B).

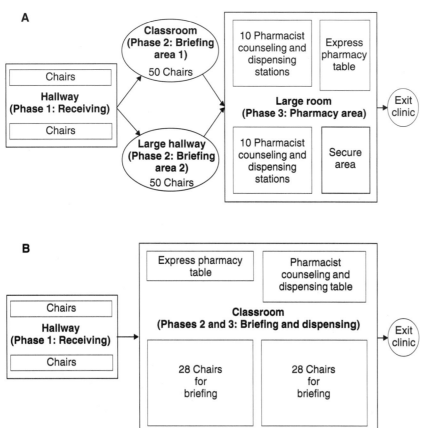

failures and improvements needed to prepare for possible future operations.

The experience at the anthrax prophylaxis clinic at D.C. General Hospital illustrates the vital role pharmacists can play in temporary clinics set up to educate, screen, treat, and counsel patients who may have been exposed to harmful microorganisms. A pharmacist at such a clinic may be required to assume responsibility for patient education, screening, protocol development, dispensing, counseling, and drug selection. Therapeutic selection is not performed by pharmacists as part of their routine professional activities; however, as demonstrated by our response to the bioterrorism attack in Washington, D.C., pharmacists can proficiently perform such a function during times of crisis.

Conclusion

A multidisciplinary team established and operated a clinic to treat persons who may have been exposed to anthrax through contaminated mail.

References

1. Centers for Disease Control and Prevention. Evaluation of *Bacillus anthracis* contamination inside the Brentwood Mail Processing and Distribution Center—District of Columbia, October 2001. *MMWR.* 2001; 50:1129-33.
2. Montello MJ, Ostroff C, Frank EC et al. 2001 anthrax crisis in Washington, D.C.: pharmacists' role in screening patients and selecting prophylaxis. *Am J Health-Syst Pharm.* 2002; 59:1193-9.
3. Centers for Disease Control and Prevention. Update: investigation of anthrax associated with intentional exposure and interim public health guidelines, October 2001. *MMWR.* 2001; 50:889-93.
4. Centers for Disease Control and Prevention. National pharmaceutical stockpile. www.bt.cdc.gov/documentsapp/nationalstockpile/nationalstockpile.asp (accessed 2001 Dec 14).

Over the two-week period, the clinic was staffed by 52 pharmacists—more than a third of the 136-member health care team. The clinic dispensed medication to 18,051 patients. During the busiest times, as many as 250 patients an hour received education and drugs. Processing time per patient ranged from 20 to 55 minutes, depending on patient volume, staffing, and patient medical issues.

The clinic can be used as a model for pharmacists and other health care professionals in designing and implementing disaster plans. When designing a bioterrorism response protocol, it is important to consider that

- Patient volume, available staff, and available space may vary greatly;
- The health care staff may consist primarily of volunteers;
- Resources will have to be closely monitored and reallocated as needed;
- Good records of daily activities must be maintained;
- Regular briefings will be needed to address changes in processes, new information, and problems; and
- A debriefing must be held at the end of the mission to discuss successes and

Reprinted with permission from ASHP: *Am J Health-Syst Pharm*; June 15, 2002, Vol 59

2001 anthrax crisis in Washington, D.C.: Pharmacists' role in screening patients and selecting prophylaxis

MICHAEL J. MONTELLO, CRAIG OSTROFF, ELLEN C. FRANK, ANDREW S. T. HAFFER, AND JAMES R. ROGERS

On October 15, 2001, a member of the staff of U.S. Senate Majority Leader Thomas Daschle opened an anthrax-contaminated letter in the Hart Senate Office Building.[1] In the weeks that followed, additional letters laced with anthrax spores were identified, and at least 22 people developed either cutaneous or inhalational anthrax.[2] Many of the afflicted were postal workers assigned to the U.S. capital region. Thousands of other federal and nonfederal personnel may have been exposed.

Agencies of the U.S. Public Health Service (USPHS), including the Centers for Disease Control and Prevention (CDC) and the Office of Emergency Preparedness, planned and implemented a rapid response to the crisis.[3] One of the primary missions of USPHS during this crisis was distributing prophylactic antimicrobials to individuals determined to be at risk for anthrax exposure. USPHS personnel stationed in a clinic

Abstract: Pharmacists' development and use of a worksheet facilitating their rapid selection of patient-appropriate prophylactic antimicrobials in an anthrax clinic is described.

A clinic housed at D.C. General Hospital, in Washington, D.C., treated most of the people—many of them postal workers—who may have been exposed to anthrax in that city during the 2001 anthrax crisis. A form was needed to assist pharmacists in the rapid selection of prophylactic antimicrobials and in patient education and counseling. A team of pharmacists collaborated on the development of a form tailored to the clinical and logistical needs of the operation. The questions on the form were based largely on the two antianthrax agents most likely to be used, ciprofloxacin and doxycycline, and were designed to identify the circumstances that would most frequently require a medication change or a modification of patient education. Yes-or-no check boxes allowed pertinent data to be captured most efficiently. A positive response to any question triggered a personal interview and assessment by a pharmacist. A treatment algorithm was also developed to ensure consistent pharmacist selection of agents in the face of potentially changing policies and staff. The worksheet questions sought to establish treatment objectives, document allergies and concomitant therapies, and identify patients who were pregnant or lactating.

Pharmacists developed a patient-screening worksheet that helped determine their choice of treatment for people who may have been exposed to anthrax in Washington, D.C., during the 2001 anthrax crisis.

Index terms: Ambulatory care; Anthrax; Biological warfare; Ciprofloxacin; Diagnosis; Disaster planning; Doxycycline; Pharmacists; Protocols; Quinolones; Tetracyclines
Am J Health-Syst Pharm. 2002; 59:1193-9

housed at D.C. General Hospital, in Washington, D.C., treated most of these people. A tool to assist pharmacists in the rapid selection of the appropriate prophylactic antimicrobials and in patient education and counseling regarding the selected therapy was needed. An anthrax

CDR MICHAEL J. MONTELLO, PHARM.D., is Chief Professional Officer—Pharmacy, PHS-1 Disaster Medical Assistance Team, U.S. Public Health Service (USPHS), and Head, Protocol and Information Office, Cancer Therapeutics Evaluation Program, National Cancer Institute, Rockville, MD. LT CRAIG OSTROFF, PHARM.D., is Pharmacy Officer, PHS-1 Disaster Medical Assistance Team, USPHS, and Regulatory Management Officer, Division of Pulmonary and Allergy Drug Products, Food and Drug Administration (FDA), Rockville. LCDR ELLEN C. FRANK, B.S. PHARM., is Pharmacist, Commissioned Corps Readiness Force, USPHS, and Chief, Project Management Staff, Division of Special Pathogen and Immunologic Drug Products, FDA. LCDR ANDREW S. T. HAFFER, PHARM.D., is Pharmacy Officer,

PHS-1 Disaster Medical Assistance Team, USPHS, and Regulatory Review Officer, Division of Drug Marketing, Advertising, and Communications, FDA. LCDR JAMES R. ROGERS, PHARM.D., is Deputy Chief Professional Officer—Pharmacy, PHS-1 Disaster Medical Assistance Team, USPHS, and Regulatory Review Officer, Division of Drug Marketing, Advertising, and Communications, FDA.

Address correspondence to CDR Montello at PHS-1 Disaster Medical Assistance Team, 6130 Executive Boulevard, Executive Plaza North, Room 6118, Rockville, MD 20852 (montellom@ctep.nci.nih.gov).

This article represents the opinions of the authors and does not necessarily reflect the policy of the U.S. Public Health Service.

Reprinted with permission from ASHP: *Am J Health-Syst Pharm*; June 15, 2002, Vol 59

health and medication worksheet was developed to meet this need. This article describes the development of the worksheet and how pharmacists used it to help screen patients and select prophylaxis.

General development of the worksheet

Early in the crisis, an existing CDC patient-screening form was tried but found to be too complex—and then, after a quick revision, too superficial. A team of pharmacists collaborated on another revision tailored to the clinical and logistical needs of the operation. The objectives were to

1. Capture patient data for assessment and therapeutic selection,
2. Maximize comprehensibility for the public (by writing the form at an eighth-grade reading level),
3. Promote swift identification of patients with complex medical problems and those requiring intensive education or especially careful therapeutic selection,
4. Facilitate rapid assessment of whether objectives for therapeutic selection and patient education were being met,
5. Reinforce oral education of patients,
6. Minimize delays in patient processing without compromising therapeutic selection and education,
7. Record patient history, agent selection, comments, and other ancillary information (e.g., quantity of medication dispensed).
8. Collect epidemiologic data,
9. Serve as a quality assurance and quality control tool, and
10. Support training of health care workers.

The result was the anthrax health and medication worksheet (Figure 1). Clinic pharmacists considered it superior to its predecessors, and patients found it much easier to use. Throughout the mission, revisions of the worksheet continued to be made when necessary.

While the worksheet served as a valuable screening tool, it was not the only method of presenting, discussing, or capturing data on the provision of anthrax prophylaxis and patient education. All people who came to the clinic were given a 15- to 30-minute lecture that covered most of the frequently asked questions about anthrax and preventive agents.[3] Time was set aside during each presentation for people to ask questions or express concerns. In addition, each individual had the opportunity to meet personally with a health care provider, typically a pharmacist, to discuss any personal or medical matters related to the event.

The policy on agent selection was somewhat fluid. A flexible treatment algorithm was needed in case the drug of choice was changed. At the time of the crisis, ciprofloxacin was the only drug approved by FDA for anthrax treatment and prophylaxis. CDC recommended either ciprofloxacin or doxycycline hyclate as first-line therapy.[4] Therefore, the treatment protocol used ciprofloxacin as the drug of choice and doxycycline as a secondary agent when necessary (Appendix A). Amoxicillin was used only if there was a contraindication to both ciprofloxacin and doxycycline. Once susceptibility test results were available, the agent of choice was modified as necessary. Doxycycline soon became the preferred agent because its spectrum of activity was similar to ciprofloxacin's, it was safer, and it was available from multiple sources.

The worksheet facilitated rapid identification of the most appropriate therapy for each patient and of the patient's educational needs. The questions were based largely on the two antianthrax agents most likely to be used, ciprofloxacin and doxycycline, and were designed to identify circumstances that would most frequently require a medication switch or a modification of patient education. Yes-or-no check boxes allowed

pertinent data to be captured most efficiently and served to identify individuals with more complex needs. A positive response to any question triggered a personal interview and assessment by a pharmacist, possibly leading to a change in therapy or a special emphasis on education.

Development of the treatment algorithm

During the mission, pharmacists discussed with one another their experiences and particularly complicated cases. A consensus on therapeutic selection began to form. A treatment algorithm was developed to ensure a consistent approach to agent selection in the face of possible changes in agent-selection policies and in the pharmacy staff. Similar questions were grouped to facilitate rapid completion of the document by patients and allow the provider to efficiently weigh all pertinent factors when deciding on a treatment. The algorithm was further refined as part of the postoperation debriefing. The final algorithm is shown in Appendix B.

Establishing treatment objectives. The first set of questions on the worksheet established whether the patient required definitive treatment, prophylaxis, or no therapy. Asymptomatic individuals who had completed the full anthrax vaccination series within the previous year did not require any therapy but were given the option of receiving prophylactic antimicrobials. In clinical studies designed to evaluate the efficacy of the anthrax vaccine, 83% of people had a vaccine-induced immune response (indirect hemagglutination) two weeks after the first dose, and 95% had an even stronger response (a fourfold increase in antibody titer) after three doses.[5] Since a direct correlation between antibody titer and protection from anthrax remains unproven, the authors believed that the more prudent approach was to provide antimicrobial prophylaxis to

Reprinted with permission from ASHP: *Am J Health-Syst Pharm*; June 15, 2002, Vol 59

Figure 1. Anthrax health and medication worksheet.

Name: _____		Today's Date: _____	
Date of Birth: _____		Social Security Number: ___ - ___ - ___	
Have you ever received the anthrax vaccine?		Yes ☐	No ☐
Do you have flu-like symptoms (fever, aches, chills, cough)?		Yes ☐	No ☐
Do you have a skin lesion or sore that appeared or got worse recently?		Yes ☐	No ☐

Medication Information

Are you allergic to any medications?	Yes ☐	No ☐
Name(s) of medications: _____		
Do you currently take any medications?	Yes ☐	No ☐
Name(s) of medications:		
_____		
Do you take vitamins or supplements (calcium, iron, zinc, magnesium, multivitamins)?	Yes ☐	No ☐
Do you use antacids (Tums, Maalox, Mylanta, Rolaids, Pepto-Bismol)?	Yes ☐	No ☐

Disease Information

Do you have or have you had epilepsy (seizures)?	Yes ☐	No ☐
Do you have or have you had liver disease or hepatitis?	Yes ☐	No ☐
Do you have or have you had kidney disease?	Yes ☐	No ☐

Dietary Information

Do you drink two or more drinks WITH CAFFEINE per day (coffee, tea, colas, etc.)?	Yes ☐	No ☐
Do you eat dairy products (milk, yogurt, cheese, ice cream)?	Yes ☐	No ☐
Do you drink orange juice WITH EXTRA CALCIUM?	Yes ☐	No ☐

Females Only

Are you breast-feeding?	Yes ☐	No ☐
Is it possible you are pregnant?	Yes ☐	No ☐
Do you take birth-control pills?	Yes ☐	No ☐

For Pharmacist Use Only

Agent/directions selected:
Ciprofloxacin 500 mg BID ☐   Doxycycline 100 mg BID ☐   Amoxicillin 500 mg TID ☐
Ciprofloxacin_____ ☐   Doxycycline _____ ☐   Amoxicillin _____ ☐
Qty Dispensed: 10 Day Supply ☐   50 Day Supply ☐   60 Day Supply ☐   R.Ph. Signature: _____
Notes:

anyone who did not complete the vaccination series.

A patient with signs and symptoms that were consistent with cutaneous or inhalational anthrax and were temporally related to the exposure event received prophylactic therapy and was routed to a primary care provider for further assessment. All symptomatic patients were instructed to see a primary care provider immediately. These patients were given the option of seeing a USPHS physician at the clinic for a brief screening or their personal physician for a more extensive evaluation. The provision of prophylactic therapy to these individuals represented a prac-

Reprinted with permission from ASHP: *Am J Health-Syst Pharm*; June 15, 2002, Vol 59

tical attempt to streamline clinic operations and minimize the reprocessing of previously screened patients. To minimize interference with antimicrobial susceptibility testing, these individuals were cautioned not to take any prophylactic medications until after they had consulted a physician.

Documenting allergies and concomitant therapies. The second set of questions allowed gathering of detailed information on drug allergies and concomitant treatments that could affect therapeutic selection. Because of the potential interactions of ciprofloxacin or doxycycline with cations like calcium, aluminum, and magnesium, specific questions regarding vitamin and mineral supplements and antacids were included in the questionnaire. In general, therapy was not changed if patients answered yes to either of the questions about minerals and antacids. However, patients were counseled to avoid taking minerals or antacids with ciprofloxacin or doxycycline.

A positive response on the worksheet regarding allergies or allergic reactions elicited further investigation. If a patient was suspected to have a true allergy to the drug of choice or other agents in the same class, a suitable alternative agent was prescribed. If the patient had not tolerated, but not been allergic to, the drug of choice or similar drugs, the pharmacist decided whether an alternative agent was warranted.

The drug interaction assessment was quite complex. The pharmacists familiarized themselves with the most common and most severe drug interactions involving ciprofloxacin, doxycycline, and amoxicillin.[6,7] The approach to agent selection and counseling for patients receiving concomitant drug therapy is summarized in Appendix C. None of the antianthrax agents were considered absolutely contraindicated for use in combination with other medications.[6,7] In practice, however, it was not uncommon for a pharmacist to

exercise caution and use an alternative agent. All patients were instructed to see a physician to discuss whether any further modifications to their drug therapy were necessary.

Patients already receiving antimicrobial therapy proved challenging in screening for drug interactions. Pharmacists had to determine the specific indication, the treatment start date, the duration of therapy, and the susceptibility (if any) of the anthrax strain to the currently used antimicrobial. If the agent was included in the CDC anthrax prophylaxis guidelines or if susceptibility test findings were available, the patient was instructed to complete the current course of therapy. If necessary, additional antimicrobials were dispensed to complete the prophylactic regimen.

Assessment of appropriate antimicrobial therapy for other indications (urinary-tract infections, upper-respiratory-tract infections, etc.) was beyond the scope of the operation. Therefore, for the patient currently receiving antimicrobial therapy that did not meet CDC anthrax prophylaxis guidelines or yield a positive result in susceptibility tests, pharmacists dispensed the appropriate preventive agent and instructed the patient to consult a physician before beginning treatment. The District of Columbia's health department was available to assist community health care providers in selecting appropriate therapy.

Several medical conditions contraindicated treatment with the drug of choice or at least created the need for extra caution. Ciprofloxacin is known to lower the seizure threshold.[6,7] Patients with epilepsy or who were taking antiepileptic drugs typically received doxycycline. Ciprofloxacin is excreted almost exclusively by the kidneys,[6,7] and recommendations are available for adjusting ciprofloxacin dosages on the basis of serum creatinine concentration. Since this laboratory value was unlikely to be

available during the crisis, patients who indicated they had renal disease were given doxycycline, which is metabolized primarily by the liver.

The worksheet included dietary questions to remind pharmacists to reinforce patient education. Every patient was informed of dietary restrictions; this occurred during group counseling and one-on-one sessions with a pharmacist. Most patients indicated that they consumed caffeine or dairy products. Therefore, the form was designed to promote patient education without detracting from rapid assessment and appropriate therapeutic selection. Check boxes for responses in the form's dietary section were offset so that they did not line up with the other check boxes. This formatting helped providers deemphasize this section during the initial assessment and focus on questions that could result in a switch to a secondary agent.

Pregnancy and lactation. CDC's anthrax prophylaxis guidelines allow for the use of either ciprofloxacin or doxycycline in pregnant or lactating women. Before the results of any susceptibility testing were known, both ciprofloxacin and doxycycline were dispensed to pregnant or lactating women, and they were instructed to consult their obstetrician before starting to take the drugs. Once susceptibility test findings were available, these patients were prescribed amoxicillin because of its demonstrated safety in pregnant women.[7] Most antimicrobials can decrease the effectiveness of oral contraceptives. Thus, all women of childbearing age receiving oral contraceptives were advised to use an alternative method of contraception during the course of therapy.

Additional information. Space was provided at the bottom of the worksheet for pharmacists to write notes about agent selection, directions given, quantity dispensed, unique patient issues, and justification for a decision to use an alternative drug.

Reprinted with permission from ASHP: *Am J Health-Syst Pharm*; June 15, 2002, Vol 59

Discussion

While the anthrax health and medication worksheet was designed to capture the key information that might guide agent selection or patient education, it was not intended to generate an exhaustive list. Other factors arose relatively frequently that affected agent selection; many of these related to patient preference for a particular dosage form. Also, the worksheet was not designed to address pediatric matters. The affected population consisted almost entirely of adults. CDC's anthrax prophylaxis guidelines do include recommendations for children. It is unclear what modifications to the worksheet, if any, would be required to meet the needs of children.

The screening form, developed and refined by pharmacists, was effective for assessing patients' medical history. This tool was used by pharmacists to quickly determine appropriate medical treatment with reasonable assurance that the most important medical concerns had been addressed. The details of the worksheet were based on pharmacists' knowledge of drug therapy and disease management. These skills were used effectively to provide medical care during a crisis.

Conclusion

Pharmacists developed a patient-screening worksheet that helped determine their choice of treatment for people who may have been exposed to anthrax in Washington, D.C., during the 2001 anthrax crisis.

References

1. Cable News Network. Daschle: 'They were trying to kill someone.' www.cnn.com/2002/us/03/26/anthrax.investigation/index.html (accessed 2002 Apr 26).
2. Centers for Disease Control and Prevention. Update: investigation of bioterrorism-related anthrax and adverse events from antimicrobial prophylaxis. *MMWR.* 2001; 50:973-6.
3. Haffer AST, Rogers JR, Montello MJ, et al. 2001 anthrax crisis in Washington, D.C.: clinic for persons exposed to contaminated mail. *Am J Health-Syst Pharm.* 2002; 59:1189-92.
4. Centers for Disease Control and Prevention. Update: investigation of anthrax associated with intentional exposure and interim public health guidelines, October 2001. *MMWR.* 2001; 50:889-93.
5. Centers for Disease Control and Prevention. Use of anthrax vaccine in the United States: recommendations of the Advisory Committee on Immunization Practices (ACIP). *MMWR.* 2000; 49 (RR-15):7.
6. McEvoy GK, ed. *AHFS drug information 2001.* Bethesda, MD: American Society of Health-System Pharmacists; 2001.
7. Drug interaction facts. St. Louis, MO: Facts & Comparisons; 2001.

Appendix A—Suggested antimicrobial prophylaxis after confirmed or suspected exposure to *Bacillus anthracis*[5]

Any one of the following agents may be used:

1. Ciprofloxacin 500 mg (as the hydrochloride) orally twice daily in adults or 10–15 mg/kg/day orally in divided doses every 12 hours in children;
2. Ofloxacin 400 mg orally twice daily in adults; not recommended in children;
3. Doxycycline 100 mg (as the hyclate) orally twice daily in adults; 5 mg/kg/day orally in divided doses every 12 hours in children;
4. Penicillin V: Not indicated in adults; 50 mg (as the potassium salt) per kilogram per day orally in divided doses four times daily in children;
5. Amoxicillin 500 mg (as the trihydrate) orally three times daily in adults; 80 mg/kg/day orally in divided doses two or three times daily in children.

Prophylaxis should continue until exposure to *B. anthracis* has been excluded. If exposure is confirmed and vaccine is available, prophylaxis should continue for four weeks and until three doses of vaccine have been administered; if vaccine is not available, prophylaxis should continue for 30–60 days. Use of tetracyclines and fluoroquinolones in children has potential adverse effects, including staining of teeth and cartilage damage, respectively. However, these risks must be weighed against the risk of developing anthrax. If potential exposure has occurred, treatment of children should begin as soon as susceptibility of the organism to penicillins has been confirmed. Data on the pediatric use of ofloxacin or other fluoroquinolones (except ciprofloxacin) are limited.

Reprinted with permission from ASHP: *Am J Health-Syst Pharm*; June 15, 2002, Vol 59

Appendix B—Algorithm for selection of prophylactic agent based on anthrax health and medical worksheet[a]

	Question	Agent if Response Is Yes	Comments
1.	Have you received the anthrax vaccine?	No agent if schedule is complete. If schedule is incomplete, dispense ciprofloxacin, doxycycline, or amoxicillin.	[a]Determine when anthrax vaccine was received and how much of the schedule was completed. Recommended vaccination schedule: s.c. injection at 0, 2, and 4 wk, then 6, 12, and 18 mo. An annual booster injection is necessary if immunity is to be maintained.[5]
2.	Do you have flu-like symptoms (fever, aches, chills, cough)?	Ciprofloxacin, doxycycline, or amoxicillin	Determine the nature of the complaint and its duration. Dispense antianthrax agent but recommend that the individual not take a first dose until he or she has seen a primary health care provider. If signs or symptoms and temporal relationship are consistent with anthrax, schedule immediate medical follow-up.
3.	Do you have a skin lesion or sore that appeared or got worse recently?	Ciprofloxacin, doxycycline, or amoxicillin	Determine the nature of the complaint and its duration. Dispense antianthrax agent but recommend that the individual not take a first dose until he or she has seen a primary health care provider. If signs or symptoms and temporal relationship are consistent with anthrax, schedule immediate medical follow-up.
4.	Are you allergic to any medications?	If the patient is allergic to (or intolerant of) the drug of choice, switch to secondary medication.	Validate that an allergic reaction has occurred. Discontinue the antianthrax agent and contact a primary health care provider if there are any signs or symptoms consistent with an allergic reaction.
5.	Do you currently take any medications?	Ciprofloxacin, doxycycline, or amoxicillin unless contraindication (Appendix C)	See Appendix C.
6.	Do you take vitamins or supplements (calcium, iron, zinc, magnesium, multivitamins)?	Ciprofloxacin, doxycycline, or amoxicillin	Give ciprofloxacin or doxycycline 2 hr before or 2 hr after vitamin or supplement.
7.	Do you use antacids (e.g., Tums, Maalox, Mylanta, Rolaids, Pepto-Bismol)?	Ciprofloxacin, doxycycline, or amoxicillin	Give ciprofloxacin or doxycycline 2 hr before or 2 hr after antacid.
8.	Do you have or have you had epilepsy (seizures)?	Doxycycline or amoxicillin	Ciprofloxacin is contraindicated (lowers seizure threshold and interacts with phenytoin). Doxycycline is indicated, but phenytoin, carbamazepine, and barbiturates decrease serum doxycycline concentrations (see Appendix C).
9.	Do you have or have you had liver disease or hepatitis?	Ciprofloxacin or amoxicillin	Determine the nature of any hepatic injury or dysfunction. Doxycycline's half-life is prolonged in liver disease (significance unknown).
10.	Do you have or have you had kidney disease?	Doxycycline or amoxicillin	Determine the nature of any renal injury or dysfunction. Doxycycline is unaffected by renal disease. Ciprofloxacin is excreted primarily by the kidneys. Ciprofloxacin dosage guidelines for renal impairment are available in the package insert.
11.	Do you drink two or more drinks with caffeine per day (coffee, tea, colas, etc.)?	Ciprofloxacin, doxycycline, or amoxicillin	Determine the amount of caffeine consumed per day. If the drug of choice is ciprofloxacin, recommend reducing the caffeine intake. Ciprofloxacin inhibits the metabolism of xanthines (e.g., caffeine). If the drug of choice is ciprofloxacin and caffeine consumption raises concern, give doxycycline.
12.	Do you eat dairy products (milk, yogurt, cheese, ice cream)?	Ciprofloxacin, doxycycline, or amoxicillin	Give ciprofloxacin 6 hr before or 2 hr after dairy products.
13.	Do you drink orange juice with extra calcium?	Ciprofloxacin, doxycycline, or amoxicillin	Give ciprofloxacin 6 hr before or 2 hr after calcium-fortified orange juice.
14.	Are you breast-feeding?	Ciprofloxacin, doxycycline, or amoxicillin	If possible, the drug should be taken immediately after breast-feeding to reduce risk to the newborn. Amoxicillin is the drug of choice once positive susceptibility test data become available. Until susceptibility test results are available, ciprofloxacin and doxycycline are the drugs of choice during breast-feeding.
15.	Is it possible you are pregnant?	Ciprofloxacin, doxycycline, or amoxicillin	Amoxicillin is the drug of choice once positive susceptibility test data become available. Until susceptibility test results are available, ciprofloxacin and doxycycline are the drugs of choice during pregnancy.
16.	Do you take birth-control pills?	Ciprofloxacin, doxycycline, or amoxicillin	Advise patient to use an alternative method of contraception. Ciprofloxacin, doxycycline, and amoxicillin can decrease the effectiveness of birth-control drugs.

[a]Ciprofloxacin and doxycycline are the drugs of choice until susceptibility test data become available. Amoxicillin may be used *only* if there are contraindications to ciprofloxacin or doxycycline.

Reprinted with permission from ASHP: *Am J Health-Syst Pharm*; June 15, 2002, Vol 59

Appendix C—Drug interactions involving antianthrax agents

Antianthrax Agent and Interacting Drug	Use Another Antianthrax Agent?	Comments
Ciprofloxacin		
Antacids	No	Antacids containing aluminum, magnesium, or calcium decrease oral absorption of ciprofloxacin, resulting in decreased bioavailability of ciprofloxacin. Give ciprofloxacin 2 hr before or 2 hr after antacids.
Probenecid	Yes	Probenecid interferes with renal tubular excretion of ciprofloxacin, resulting in a 50% increase in systemic ciprofloxacin concentrations and a prolonged serum half-life. Switch to an alternative antianthrax agent (e.g., doxycycline). If other antianthrax agents are contraindicated, dispense ciprofloxacin and adjust the dosage.
Warfarin	No	Prolongation of prothrombin time and hematemesis may occur. Use combination with caution. Monitor prothrombin time.
Iron, zinc, or calcium supplements	No	Mineral supplements or multivitamins containing iron, zinc, or calcium decrease oral absorption of ciprofloxacin, resulting in decreased bioavailability of ciprofloxacin. Administer ciprofloxacin 2 hr before or 2 hr after mineral supplements.
Other antiinfectives	Possibly	Assess for therapeutic duplication, synergism, or antagonism. Determine the intent and duration of use of the other antiinfective. Dispense ciprofloxacin and recommend that the patient discuss therapeutic options with a primary care provider.
Theophylline	Yes	Ciprofloxacin alters theophylline's pharmacokinetics, resulting in elevated theophylline concentrations and increased risk of theophylline toxicity. Switch to an alternative antianthrax agent (e.g., doxycycline). If there are contraindications to other antianthrax agents, dispense ciprofloxacin, adjust the theophylline dosage, and monitor serum drug levels.
Sucralfate	No	Sucralfate decreases oral absorption of ciprofloxacin, resulting in decreased bioavailability of ciprofloxacin. Administer ciprofloxacin 2 hr before or 2 hr after sucralfate.
Oral contraceptives	No	Decreased bioavailability and effectiveness of oral contraceptives. Advise the patient to use an alternative method of contraception.
Doxycycline		
Antacids	No	Antacids containing aluminum, magnesium, or calcium decrease oral absorption of doxycycline, resulting in decreased bioavailability of doxycycline. Administer doxycycline 2 hr before or 2 hr after antacids.
Iron, zinc, or calcium supplements	No	Mineral supplements or multivitamins containing iron, zinc, or calcium decrease oral absorption of doxycycline, resulting in decreased bioavailability of doxycycline. Administer doxycycline 2 hr before or 2 hr after mineral supplements.
Warfarin	No	Prolongation of prothrombin time and hematemesis may occur. Use combination with caution. Monitor prothrombin time.
Other antiinfectives	Possibly	Assess for therapeutic duplication, synergism, or antagonism. Determine the intent and duration of use of the other antiinfective. Dispense doxycycline and recommend that the patient discuss therapeutic options with a primary care provider.
Oral contraceptives	No	Bioavailability and effectiveness of oral contraceptives decrease. Advise the patient to use an alternative method of contraception.
Barbiturates, phenytoin, or carbamazepine	Possibly	Serum half-life and serum concentrations of doxycycline decrease. Switch the patient to an alternative antianthrax agent if there is no other contraindication. If other antianthrax agents are contraindicated, dispense doxycycline.
Amoxicillin		
Oral contraceptives	No	Bioavailability and effectiveness of oral contraceptives decrease. Advise the patient to use an alternative method of contraception.
Probenecid	No	Probenecid interferes with renal tubular excretion of penicillins, resulting in a 30–60% increase in systemic penicillin concentrations and a prolonged serum half-life. This interaction has been used to therapeutic advantage.
Allopurinol	No	Rash is more frequent when allopurinol and amoxicillin are administered together. It is unclear if the rash is associated with increased allergenicity. Inform the patient of the increased risk of rash. If a rash develops, the patient should discontinue amoxicillin immediately and inform a primary care provider.
Other antiinfectives	Possibly	Assess for therapeutic duplication, synergism, or antagonism. Determine the intent and duration of use of the other antiinfective. Dispense amoxicillin and recommend that the patient discuss therapeutic options with a primary care provider.

Reprinted with permission from ASHP: *Am J Health-Syst Pharm*; June 15, 2002, Vol 59

Pharmacist participation in the management of incidents involving hazardous materials

DAVID B. LEVY, JOSEPH A. BARONE, JOHN J. RAIA, JOHN M. YORK, AND DAVID P. VOGEL

Abstract: The role of the pharmacist as a hazardous materials consultant is described.

Pharmacists in a university-affiliated teaching hospital are contacted by either emergency medical services or the emergency department to assist in the management of incidents involving toxic hazardous materials. These incidents can range from major chemical spills or leaks to long-term exposures involving generalized, nonspecific symptoms. An advanced pharmacy resident in emergency medicine is the primary pharmacy contact for hazardous materials consults. The services provided by the clinical pharmacist include identification of the hazardous materials involved, initiation of special precautions for rescue-squad and hospital-based personnel, clinical assessment of the toxicologic problem, and formulation of therapeutic recommendations. Teaching programs have been developed for pharmacy, nursing, and medical students, hospital employees, and emergency-response agencies. Pharmacy participation in the management of hazardous materials incidents has been well received by emergency department physicians and nurses, as well as by rescue personnel. During the period between January 1 and July 1, 1986, the pharmacy was consulted on 66 hazardous materials incidents. Since pharmacists have traditionally been used as information resources for clinical toxicology questions, it follows that their participation can extend into the field of environmental toxicology, specifically involving hazardous materials.

The pharmacist's input as a hazardous materials consultant in our institution has been well received, and we believe that pharmacy departments can play an important role in the management of incidents involving hazardous materials.

Index terms: Chemicals; Education; Emergency services; Identification; Pharmacists, hospital; Pharmacy, institutional, hospital; Pharmaceutical services; Toxicity, environmental

Am J Hosp Pharm. 1987; 44:549–56

The pharmacist's role as a toxicology consultant has evolved over the years to encompass both public service and professional practice functions in poison centers, emergency departments, or other hospital areas.[1-13] Pharmacists are thought to be well suited for this role because of their extensive training in pharmacology, and in some cases, toxicology.[5,13-23] Considerable contributions have been made by clinical pharmacists in assisting physicians, other health professionals, or the lay public with the management and therapy of poisonings or drug overdoses.[7,13,24-32]

The discipline of clinical toxicology has expanded to also include the management of untoward effects resulting from exposure to hazardous materials and other chemical substances present in the environment. Public interest has also focused on the immediate and long-term consequences of internal or external exposure to toxic chemicals.[1]

The Department of Transportation defines hazardous materials as substances that pose an unreasonable risk to health, safety, and property when transported in commerce. A hazardous material (HAZMAT) incident is defined as any discharge involving bioconcentrative, highly flammable, extremely reactive, toxic, irritating, corrosive, or infectious materials that places human life in jeopardy, whether it be caused by a fire, a motor vehicle accident, or an industrial leak.[33]

Dealing with accidents involving hazardous materials requires specially trained individuals working in a "HAZMAT team." HAZMAT teams, in general, are of three basic types: industrial teams, commercial teams, and public safety agency teams. Almost every major chemical manufacturing and processing firm in this country (e.g., Du Pont, Union Carbide, Exxon) has personnel on call to respond to incidents involving the company's

DAVID B. LEVY, PHARM.D., is Clinical Specialist in Emergency Medicine, Detroit Receiving Hospital and University Health Center, Detroit, MI, and Adjunct Assistant Professor of Clinical Pharmacy, Wayne State University College of Pharmacy and Allied Health Professions, Detroit; at the time this report was written, he was Advanced Resident in Emergency Medicine, Robert Wood Johnson University Hospital, New Brunswick, NJ. JOSEPH A. BARONE, PHARM.D., is Assistant Professor and Director of Clinical Programs, Rutgers University College of Pharmacy, Piscataway, NJ, and Assistant Director for Academic Affairs, Robert Wood Johnson University Hospital. JOHN J. RAIA, PHARM.D., is Assistant Professor of Clinical Pharmacy, Rutgers University College of Pharmacy, and Pharmacy Clinician, Robert Wood Johnson University Hospital. JOHN M. YORK, PHARM.D., is Post-Doctoral Fellow in Industrial Clinical Pharmacy Practice, Rutgers University College of Pharmacy. DAVID P. VOGEL, M.S., is Director of Pharmacy Services, Robert Wood Johnson University Hospital, and Assistant Professor of Clinical Pharmacy, Rutgers University College of Pharmacy.

Address reprint requests to Dr. Levy at Detroit Receiving Hospital and University Health Center, Department of Pharmacy Services, 4201 St. Antoine, Detroit, MI 48201.

Copyright © 1987, American Society of Hospital Pharmacists, Inc. All rights reserved. 0002-9289/87/0301-0549$02.00.

Reprinted with permission from ASHP: *Am J Health-Syst Pharm*; March 1987, Vol 44

products. Commercial response teams are private, for-profit firms that respond to HAZMAT incidents or provide related services for any employer. In the public sector, control and containment of chemical accidents and management of victims has been left up to individual municipalities and hospitals. Public safety agency teams are most commonly composed of local fire or health department personnel and, being the first responding agency, may request assistance from one of the previously mentioned HAZMAT teams.[33]

The public-safety HAZMAT team in our area was the first of its type to be developed in the state. The team is funded by the county department of health and is staffed by environmental health specialists on 24-hour call for emergencies. The HAZMAT team responded to nearly 300 dangerous chemical spills or leaks during 1985 in our county alone. During the past year the HAZMAT team added a clinical pharmacist as a consultant. Pharmacy involvement in this area has grown out of the responsibilities associated with a pharmacy-based emergency medicine residency program and the interest of the emergency medicine resident and his faculty preceptors. The objective of this paper is to describe the function and discuss the impact of the pharmacist as a consultant and educator for the management of HAZMAT situations.

Description of Facility

The practice site, a 416-bed university-affiliated hospital, is the primary teaching site for the schools of medicine, nursing, and pharmacy. The emergency department is staffed by attending physicians and medical and surgical residents. Approximately 30,000 patients annually are treated in the emergency department, which serves as the primary base station for the county emergency medical services.

Description of Emergency Medical Services

Emergency medical services, which are provided by paramedics and emergency medical technicians, are the responsibility of a separate department within the hospital. The 911 phone system comes directly into the emergency department, and two mobile intensive-care units and one basic life-support unit are dispatched from the emergency department. These units respond to approximately 13,000 emergencies per year. County-wide telemetry (paramedic–physician base contact) communication is also established through the dispatch center at the hospital. The proximity of the department of emergency medical services, the emergency department, and the pharmacy department has been a major asset to the pharmacy consultant's participation in poisoning, drug overdose, and HAZMAT cases. The unique location of the dispatch center within the emergency department has led to the rapid notification of responsible personnel and has facilitated expedient transmission of information. All dispatchers are trained emergency medical technicians and have had extensive training in advanced medical dispatch.

Description of Clinical Pharmacy Services

The pharmacy department has provided clinical services to the emergency department since 1982, and in 1984 an advanced residency program in emergency medicine was established. The residency program was designed to expand the knowledge and experience of the clinical pharmacist in the emergency medicine environment. The resident's major responsibilities include research and clinical service duties in the emergency department.

Clinical service duties include participation in work rounds, response to cardiopulmonary resuscitation and trauma codes, initiation and evaluation of clinical pharmacy consults, and provision of clinical toxicology and general drug information to hospital staff. The resident's main responsibilities involve assisting the physician with the management of poisonings and drug overdoses (e.g., with salicylates, acetaminophen, antipsychotics, antidepressants, and drugs of abuse such as cocaine, heroin, and glutethimide). Patients are initially evaluated and managed in the emergency department, and then brought to the respective intensive-care units for further observation and follow-up care. Pharmacy resident consultation with the pediatric and medical residents and staff attending physicians is common and is initiated in the emergency department. Identifying the offending substance and providing current antidotal and therapeutic management information for the specific poisoning or overdose are the main purposes of the consult. The pharmacy department also provides staff pharmacist coverage for both of these intensive-care units. When a poisoned or overdosed patient is admitted to pediatric or medical intensive care, the pharmacy resident relays pertinent information to the pharmacist assigned to that unit. Daily morning rounds are made by the pharmacy resident and the clinical pharmacy preceptors on all patients admitted during the previous 24 hours that may require pharmacy intervention. Patient charts are reviewed and necessary follow-up is relayed to the appropriate satellite staff pharmacist.

Research training is also a component of the residency program. In addition to participating in ongoing research projects, the resident is expected to develop and complete an individual research proposal. The previous resident participated in various studies evaluating the effects of multiple-dose activated charcoal on toxic ingestions and developed his own protocol evaluating the use of sublingual nifedipine in the prehospital setting for hypertensive emergencies. The resident also partici-

Reprinted with permission from ASHP: *Am J Health-Syst Pharm*; March 1987, Vol 44

pates in monthly research meetings of the state-wide Emergency Medical Group. This corporation provides emergency medicine physicians to many of the emergency rooms across the state.

Pharmacy Participation in HAZMAT

In the past year, the institution has had increased involvement as a referral center for victims of HAZMAT incidents. As a result, the pharmacy resident and other pharmacy supportive personnel have developed an active role in the management of these patients. The pharmacy resident has been placed on a call list, along with the paramedic field and operations supervisors, for any suspected HAZMAT incident. The resident is the primary pharmacy contact for a HAZMAT consult. If the resident is unavailable, the faculty preceptor is contacted. Both can be contacted via long-distance pager. When the resident or faculty preceptor is not available, emergency drug information and consultation are available 24 hours per day from staff pharmacists in the pharmacy department.

In the event of a chemical spill or leak, the county HAZMAT team is notified in one of two ways: (1) by simultaneous dispatch to the scene with the fire and police agencies or (2) by request of a public service agency upon discovery of a HAZMAT substance. If information needs to be obtained or relayed about the HAZMAT incident, direct communication with the HAZMAT team is made through the emergency medical services dispatch center at our hospital. Once information about the type of incident is relayed to the dispatcher, the pharmacy resident is summoned by pager if any information on drugs or chemicals is needed. The type of information initially needed involves the health and safety of the rescuers, the local inhabitants, and surrounding property. The first priorities are positive identification of the materials involved and initiation of special precautions for onsite personnel. This entails knowing whether the chemical or chemicals involved require full or special protective clothing, evacuation (and if so, the distance necessary), or decontamination of personnel and equipment.

An example of a chemical needing such investigation is hydrogen peroxide. Many people think of this as an innocuous multipurpose medicinal product, which it is in a concentration of 3%. Yet the danger inherent in this chemical is based upon its concentration. HAZMAT reference books (Appendix A) classify hydrogen peroxide as a corrosive oxidizer, which means higher concentrations can dissolve common metals and can result in spontaneous ignition if allowed to contact combustible materials. An evacuation radius of 2500 feet is suggested if a concentration >52% is exposed directly to flame, because the container can rupture violently. An incident involving a high concentration

of hydrogen peroxide was one of the HAZMAT consults. The scenario was a dual tanker truck containing 55% hydrogen peroxide. The truck overturned on the turnpike and the fuel tank of the cab ruptured. The turnpike was closed for a mile in either direction until the spill could be contained. There were no injuries.

The county HAZMAT team has a number of text resources at their disposal. Yet because of the small size of their vehicle and the amount of space consumed by essential HAZMAT equipment (e.g., storage drums, breathing apparatus, absorbent rolls), many references are unavailable onsite. The pharmacy has access to many of the reference materials that aid in obtaining this information. Data gathering is done through various HAZMAT reference texts (Appendix A). If these sources are not sufficient, a phone list is reviewed for the appropriate agency or individual to contact (Appendix B). Ultimately, the manufacturer will be identified and a medical or scientific representative will assist in eliciting pertinent information.

A separate but equally important aspect of managing the HAZMAT incident involves the rapid transfer of information from the reference person to the rescuers. Once the chemical has been positively identified, the pertinent information must be given to the proper individuals to expedite control of the hazard and to minimize casualties. Information regarding the safety and decontamination of exposed individuals is first given to the emergency medical services dispatcher, who relays it directly to the officer in charge (OIC) at the scene of the incident. The OIC may be a member of the HAZMAT team, a fire captain or battalion chief, a police officer, or a paramedic. It is the OIC's responsibility to make sure the information is relayed to the proper individuals at the scene and that necessary measures are carried out. Once the OIC has been notified, the emergency department staff physician and charge nurse are informed, either by the pharmacy resident or the emergency medical services dispatcher, for adequate preparation before receiving any victim(s).

In addition to major chemical accidents, the pharmacy resident is asked to consult on individual patients admitted to the emergency department for generalized, chronic, or nonspecific complaints possibly related to chemical exposure. In most of these cases, background research is needed to assimilate information regarding the patient's reasons for seeking treatment. The resident gathers pertinent medical and epidemiological information in a busy and usually understaffed emergency department. Data collection includes a complete patient interview and review of current symptoms and complaints. A history of the chemical exposure is also obtained. When the patient cannot provide sufficient information, it is then necessary to contact the place where the exposure occurred and

Reprinted with permission from ASHP: *Am J Health-Syst Pharm;* March 1987, Vol 44

attempt to assess the potential toxicity. This is done by identification and confirmation of the offending agent(s) and the extent of the exposure. This contact is useful in discovering if other individuals have had similar complaints and ensuring that no other people are in potential danger. Once the history and type of exposure are confirmed, recommendations regarding proper treatment of the patient are then made to the emergency department physician. The resident is also involved with follow-up for these patients, both in the hospital and on an outpatient basis.

Teaching is also a major emphasis in our program. The pharmacy resident gives informal and formal lectures on HAZMAT and clinical toxicology topics to medical, pharmacy, nursing, dental, paramedic, and physician-assistant students on emergency medicine rotation. There are also regularly scheduled inservice-education sessions for emergency department staff nurses, physicians, inhouse emergency medical services personnel, and pharmacy personnel. The recent increase in chemical accidents prompted the pharmacy resident to participate with the emergency medical services education department in teaching emergency response personnel (police, firefighters, paramedics) the toxicological and pharmacological aspects of HAZMAT. Additional courses are being developed for special training of local emergency service personnel in the proper management of these situations. The pharmacy resident and faculty preceptor have attended these courses to gain a working knowledge of field operations and management techniques. The pharmacy resident is working with the emergency medical services education department in integrating hospital HAZMAT management and information-seeking techniques into these courses.

Recently, the "Worker and Community Right to Know Law" was passed in our state. This act is designed to provide a comprehensive program for ensuring the safety, health, and welfare of employees in work environments containing hazardous chemicals. Some of the pharmacy staff at our institution have become involved in teaching hospital employees about these hazardous chemicals and in compiling material safety data sheets from manufacturers and hazardous-substance fact sheets from the state department of health. These data sheets contain information necessary for recognizing the hazards of a particular material, the safe conditions for handling it, the emergency procedures for containing or neutralizing it, and the emergency first-aid measures needed for exposure. Pharmacists, because of their backgrounds in pharmacology, toxicology, chemistry, and pharmacotherapeutics, are ideal candidates for providing this service. The teaching activities have strengthened the working relationships with the emergency department staff and have helped other health professionals better understand the role of the clinical pharmacist in this setting.

Disaster Planning

In conjunction with teaching and consulting, the pharmacy resident has become involved in the development of a disaster plan for HAZMAT incidents and has been invited to serve on both the internal and external disaster committees. The internal committee functions to prepare for in-hospital disasters (e.g., radiation leaks, fires). This committee includes members from hospital security, administration, nursing, building maintenance, radiology, emergency medical services, the emergency department, pharmacy, and the laboratory. The external committee is primarily involved in planning for multiple-casualty incidents (e.g., plane crash, natural disasters, building collapse). It consists of many of the same individuals from the internal disaster committee, along with community representatives (e.g., fire department training officer, police department liaison, department of public health officer, and large corporation representatives).

Along with committee work, the pharmacy resident has participated in both community-sponsored and inhouse disaster drills and HAZMAT accident simulations. The resident takes part in the evaluation of emergency response agencies and hospital personnel regarding their performance in chemical identification, containment of the hazardous substance, and any decontamination procedures. Pharmacy involvement in disaster planning has been documented in the literature, and participation has been well received at our institution.[9,34-5]

Discussion

Between January 1 and July 1, 1986, the pharmacy department was consulted on 66 HAZMAT incidents. Table 1 lists HAZMAT cases that required pharmacy assistance. Formal policies and procedures are being written by emergency medical services and the emergency department to incorporate a clinical pharmacist as part of the emergency toxicology team.

The impact of pharmacy participation in HAZMAT cases has been positive, in that the information relayed to the HAZMAT team, emergency medical services, and emergency department personnel regarding patient management or decontamination has been received favorably. Formal introduction of the resident onto the on-call list is evidence of this. As the number of clinical referrals increases, more personnel may be needed to expand the service.[36] As the number of pharmacy HAZMAT consults increases, the number of staff formally trained will need to be expanded. Educa-

Reprinted with permission from ASHP: *Am J Health-Syst Pharm;* March 1987, Vol 44

tional programs on HAZMAT management will be developed for interested staff pharmacists.

The resident and preceptor have attended state,

Table 1.
Hazardous Materials Pharmacy Consults between January 1 and July 1, 1986

HAZMAT Incident	No. Incidents	No. Patients Treated
Chemical Fires		
Rocket fuel explosion (cyclotetramethylene–tetranitrosamine, ammonium perchlorate) on government testing site	1	4
Chemical refinery fire involving 41 toxic chemicals	1	52
Acetylene torch explosion in automobile repair shop	1	2
Photo factory fire involving 15 toxic chemicals	1	8
Numerous house fires involving stored flammable substances	6	34
Total	10	100
Industrial Spills and Leaks		
Lithium bromide leak in hospital air-conditioning system	1	3
Tetrahydrofuran spill in warehouse	1	2
Nitric acid spill in warehouse	1	5
Nitrogen oxide spill in warehouse	1	12
Pyridine liquid leak in university chemistry laboratory	1	5
Liquid nitrogen leak in chemical refinery	1	0
Hydrogen sulfide gas leak in oil refinery	1	60
Propargyl alcohol, methylethylketone, methylbutylketone tanker leak on major highway	1	4
Kerosene tanker spill on local road	2	1
Hydrogen peroxide spill on turnpike	1	0
Gasoline spill on local road	7	2
Total	18	94
Home- or Work-Related Exposures		
Asbestos inhalation exposure	8	8
Arsenic and chromium inhalation exposure	1	1
Tear gas, dermal and inhalation exposure	4	4
Carbon monoxide inhalation exposure	8	15
Battery fume inhalation resulting in lead exposure	1	1
Alkaline floor finish (potassium hydroxide, ammonium hydroxide, ethanolamine) inhalation exposure	1	2
Paint thinner-induced hepatitis resulting from inhalation exposure	1	1
De-icing chemical dermal exposure	4	4
Caustic soda dermal and oral exposure	4	4
Acrylic enamel ingestion and dermal exposure	2	2
Organophosphate ingestion and dermal exposure	2	5
Kerosene ingestion	2	2
Total	38	49

county, and local courses sponsored by various agencies on HAZMAT topics. The topics range from practical and tactical considerations for emergency response personnel to identification and recognition of individual hazardous materials. The resident has also had field experience and observed field operations with the local HAZMAT team and the New York City Fire Department's Hazardous Materials Response Unit ("HAZMAT 1").

The cost incurred in providing HAZMAT consultation has been difficult to estimate since much of this activity has been integrated into the clinical service component of the residency. Thus far, the only costs incurred have been related to the purchase of text and reference books and tuition for educational seminars. The major benefit of this program is that it provides a level of preparedness that helps to ensure the safety and well-being of staff and patients. The other benefit to the institution is that it provides a cadre of individuals who are in a position to evaluate potential health hazards associated with a hazardous materials incident and to provide information for effective management of such incidents to community agencies.

Efforts have also been made to keep the state poison control center apprised of the increasing involvement of the hospital in HAZMAT cases. In fact, the faculty preceptor for the emergency medicine pharmacy residency program is a member of the state poison center advisory committee. The preceptor has functioned as a liaison between our evolving HAZMAT consulting service and the state center in an attempt to formulate a consolidated HAZMAT information system.

It is our impression that pharmacists are in a unique position to assist the proper authorities with the necessary toxicologic information required in chemical spills and accidents. Because obtaining the information in a timely fashion is vital, an organized information retrieval system is the key to a successful consulting service. HAZMAT data can be obtained from many texts and references. In addition, on-call agencies are available to assist with cases.[37] In our contact with outside agencies such as CHEMTREC, the Chemical Referral Center, the Department of Environmental Protection, the National Response Center, and others, we have encountered a helpful support network. These various national information or response centers have shown a great deal of interest in working with pharmacists. It is our opinion that pharmacy involvement in the HAZMAT field will continue to be met favorably and will provide an opportunity for pharmacists to expand their current roles in toxicology. Since pharmacists have been used as information resources for clinical toxicology questions, it follows that their participation will extend into the area of environmental hazards.

Reprinted with permission from ASHP: *Am J Health-Syst Pharm;* March 1987, Vol 44

Conclusion

In our institution, the pharmacist has been used as a resource person for toxicology information related to HAZMAT incidents. The pharmacist's input as a HAZMAT consultant has been well received, and it is our impression that pharmacy departments can play an important role in the management of such situations.

References

1. Autian J. The hospital pharmacist and toxicology. *Am J Hosp Pharm.* 1970; 27:136-9.
2. Oderda GM, Litovitz T, Verhulst HL. The pharmacist's role in toxicology. *Am Pharm.* 1984; NS24(Feb): 40-4.
3. Winek CJ. A role for the hospital pharmacist in toxicology and drug blood level information. *Am J Hosp Pharm.* 1971; 28:351-6.
4. Roberts RW, Russell WL. A pharmacy-based toxicology service. *Drug Intell Clin Pharm.* 1978; 12:665-70.
5. Curtis EG, Patel JA. Pharmacy-based analytical toxicology service. *Am J Hosp Pharm.* 1977; 34:823-6.
6. Czajka PA, Skoutakis VA, Wood GC et al. Clinical toxicology consultation by pharmacists. *Am J Hosp Pharm.* 1979; 36:1087-9.
7. Inniss CN. A poison consultation system: University of Michigan Medical Center. *Clin Toxicol.* 1970; 3:205-9.
8. Elenbaas RM, Waeckerle JF, McNabney WK. The clinical pharmacist in emergency medicine. *Am J Hosp Pharm.* 1977; 34:843-6.
9. Troutman WG. Pharmacist in emergency medicine: poison information. *Can J Hosp Pharm.* 1981; 34(Jan-Feb):9-11.
10. Skoutakis VA, Wood GC. Pharmacy-based clinical toxicology services. *Clin Toxicol Consult.* 1979; 1:3-14.
11. Johnson P. Poison information specialist: new career opportunity. *Tomorrow's Pharm.* 1982; 4(Mar):7-8.
12. Powell MF, Solomon DK, McEachen RA. Twenty-four hour emergency pharmaceutical services. *Am J Hosp Pharm.* 1985; 42:831-5.
13. Manoguerra AS. The poison control center—its role. *Am J Pharm Educ.* 1976; 40:382-4.
14. Kinnard WJ. The role of the pharmacist in the control of acute poisoning. *Clin Toxicol.* 1971; 4:659-63.
15. Bagley JI. Poison prevention: the pharmacist in the spotlight. *Am Drug.* 1982; 185(Jan):56-8.
16. Troutman WG. The pharmacist and poisoning. *Am J Hosp Pharm.* 1978; 35:1351. Editorial.
17. Weaver LC. The importance of pharmacology and toxicology to the pharmacist in the delivery of improved patient care. *Am J Pharm. Educ.* 1971; 35:728-34.
18. Stewart RB, McKenzie M, Rutledge M. Acute drug intoxications: their value in the education of pharmacy students. *Am J Pharm Educ.* 1974; 38:75-80.
19. Veltri JC, Temple AR, Bradford DC. Terminal behavioral objectives for teaching clinical toxicology to clinical pharmacists. *Am J Pharm. Educ.* 1976; 40:385-95.
20. Autian J. Challenge of environmental problems to the pharmaceutical sciences: toxicology and environmental health. *Am J Pharm. Educ.* 1973; 37:262-6.
21. Coutts RT. Poisoning and its emergency treatment. *Can Pharm J.* 1978; 111(Nov): 383-4.
22. Autian J, Wood G. The role of toxicology in the pharmacy curriculum. *Am J Pharm. Educ.* 1976; 40:378-82.
23. Oderda GM. Current therapeutic concepts: clinical toxicology. *J Am Pharm Assoc.* 1974; NS14(Nov):626-40.
24. Groleau M. At your service without prescription: poisonings. *Can Pharm J.* 1985; 118(Aug):372-3.
25. Bijan A, Easom JM. Poison control: the pharmacist's role in handling and preventing poisonings. *NARD J.* 1984; 103(Mar):61-5.
26. Trudeau TW, Braden FM. A pharmacy-coordinated year-round poison control program. *J Am Pharm Assoc.* 1976; 16(Dec):664-5.
27. Sketris I, Gillis MC, MacNeil TJ et al. Effects of a poison education program in primary school. *Can Pharm. J.* 1984; 117(Aug):361-4.
28. Steiner GA, Swanson LN, Henderson HR et al. Evaluation of clinical pharmacy services on a polydrug detoxification unit. *Drug Intell Clin Pharm.* 1978; 12:80-7.
29. Comstock EG. Clinical toxicology 1971: where to now? *Hosp Pharm.* 1971; 9(Dec):4-5.
30. Shelly DW, Doering PL, McKenzie MW. Community pharmacist as poison expert: documenting the standards of practice. *Am Pharm.* 1985; NS25(Feb):30-4.
31. Kernaghan SG. Poison prevention: pharmacists wanted. *Hospitals.* 1973; 47(May 16):155-8.
32. Cramer R. Assistance from community pharmacists in identifying generic drug products. *Am J Hosp Pharm.* 1985; 42:1937-8.
33. Cashman JR. On site with a hazardous materials team. *Paramed Int.* 1979; 4(Aug):53-7.
34. Moore TC. Administrative approach to disaster preparedness in the pharmacy. *Am J Hosp Pharm.* 1979; 36:1337-41.
35. Bragdon RL, Gousse GC, Piwarzyk P et al. Regional disaster planning for hospital pharmacies. *Am J Hosp Pharm.* 1982; 39:913-5.
36. Anon. New industrial hygiene field offers pharmacists careers. *Am Drug.* 1981; 183(Feb):36.
37. Bresnitz EA, Rest KM, Miller N. Clinical industrial toxicology: an approach to information. *Ann Intern Med.* 1985; 103:967-72.
38. California Department of Health Services. Health effects of toxic substances: a directory of references and resources. Berkeley, CA: California Department of Health Services, Community Toxicology Unit; 1985.

Appendix A—Selected Hazardous Materials Reference Texts[a]

Chemical Hazards of the Workplace. Proctor NH, Hughes JP. Philadelphia, PA: J. B. Lippincott; 1978.

The Condensed Chemical Dictionary. 10th ed. Hewley GG. New York: Van Nostrand Reinhold Company, Inc.; 1981.

Dangerous Properties of Industrial Materials. Sax NI. New York: Van Nostrand Reinhold Company, Inc.; 1984.

Documentation of the Threshold Limit Values for Chemical Substances in the Workroom Environment. 4th ed. *Supplementation Documentation 1984,* American Conference of Governmental Industrial Hygienists. 6500 Glenway Avenue, Bldg D-5, Cincinnati, OH 45211.

Emergency Handling of Hazardous Materials in Surface Transportation. Bureau of Explosives, Association of American Railroads. 1920 "L" Street, N.W., Washington, DC 20036; 1981.

Emergency Response Guidebook. Research and Special Programs Administration, U.S. Department of Transportation. DOT P 5800. 2 Washington, DC: Superintendent of Documents, U.S. Government Printing Office; 1984.

Hamilton and Hardy's Industrial Toxicology. 4th ed. Finkel AJ. Boston: John Wright-PSG, Inc.; 1983.

Handbook of Toxic and Hazardous Chemicals. Marshall Sittig. Park Ridge, NJ: Noyes Data Corporation; 1981.

Hazardous and Toxic Effects of Industrial Chemicals. Marshall Sittig. Park Ridge, NJ: Noyes Data Corporation; 1979.

Hazardous Chemicals Data Book. Weiss G. Park Ridge, NJ: Noyes Data Corporation; 1980.

Material Safety Data Sheets from GE. General Electric Company, 120 Erie Blvd., Dept. 20, Schenectady, NY 12305.

Occupational Diseases: A Guide to Their Recognition. Key MM et al, eds. (NIOSH Publication No. 77-181.) Washington, DC: U.S. Government Printing Office; 1977.

Reprinted with permission from ASHP: *Am J Health-Syst Pharm;* March 1987, Vol 44

Occupational Health Guidelines for Chemical Hazards. Mackison FW, ed. U.S. Department of Health and Human Services, Public Health Service, Centers for Disease Control, National Institute for Occupational Safety and Health. Washington, DC: U.S. Government Printing Office; 1981.

Pesticides Studied in Man. Hayes W Jr. Baltimore: Williams and Wilkins; 1982. *Recognition and Management of Pesticide Poisonings,* 3rd ed. Morgan DP. U.S. Environmental Protection Agency. EPA-540/9-80-005. Washington, DC: Superintendent of Documents, U.S. Government Printing Office; 1982.

Pocket Guide to Chemical Hazards. NIOSH/OSHA. Washington, DC: DHEW (NIOSH) Publication No. 78-210. U.S. Government Printing Office; 1981.

Registry of Toxic Effects of Chemical Substances (RTECS). Lewis R, Tatken R, eds. U.S. Department of Health and Human Services, Public Health Service, Centers for Disease Control, National Institute for Occupational Safety and Health. (DHHS [NIOSH] Publication No. 83-107-3.) Washington, DC: U.S. Government Printing Office; 1981.

A System for Prevention, Assessment, and Control of Exposures and Health Effects from Hazardous Sites. U.S. Centers for Disease Control; 1984. (For copies, write the Chronic Diseases Division, Centers for Disease Control, 1600 Clifton Road, Atlanta, GA 30333.)

---

[a] Adapted from reference 38. Used with permission of California Department of Health Services, Community Toxicology Unit.

Appendix B—Selected Hazardous Materials Information Agencies[a]

American Cancer Society

Local chapter

ACS offers public and professional education on prevention, detection, diagnosis, and treatment of cancer. Educational materials include information on carcinogens in the workplace and on nutrition and cancer.

Center for Occupational Hazards

5 Beekman Street, New York, NY 10038
Phone: (212) 227-6220, 8:30 a.m.–7:00 p.m., Monday–Friday

This center is a national clearinghouse for research and education on hazards in the visual arts, performing arts, educational facilities, and museums. The center responds to questions on hazards of specific materials, ventilation, respirators, and other precautions; provides referrals to industrial health physicians; and distributes over 60 books, pamphlets, articles, and data sheets to disseminate information on art hazards.

Chemical Referral Center (CHEMINFO)

Chemical Manufacturer's Association
2501 "M" Street, N.W.
Washington, DC 20037
Phone: (800) 262-8200, 8:00 a.m.–9:00 p.m., Monday–Friday

CHEMINFO is a non-emergency information center open to the public for general chemical information. The center provides general health and safety data, e.g., identification or disposal information for household products. The center can access company consultants for specific individual product or material information.

Chemical Transportation Emergency Center (CHEMTREC)

2501 "M" Street, N.W.
Washington, DC 20037
Phone: (800) 424-9300, (202) 887-1100, 24 hours/day

CHEMTREC provides immediate emergency response information for controlling hazards created by hazardous materials spills, leaks, fires, accidents, and other emergencies when the identity of the material is known. The center is equipped to provide precautionary information, to assist in substance identification, and to notify manufacturers and shippers of an incident involving their product; manufacturers and shippers can then offer assistance and expertise. The center also activates other industrial and commercial response teams.

Consumer Product Safety Commission, United States

Local branch
Phone: (800) 638-2772, 8:00 a.m.–5:00 p.m., Monday–Friday

The Commission provides information on health and safety effects related to consumer products and has direct jurisdiction over long-term and chemical hazards in consumer products.

Environmental Protection Agency

Local branch, 8:00 a.m.–4:30 p.m., Monday–Friday

The EPA responds to information requests on acute and long-term health effects of industrial hazardous materials. Its basic function is to provide information on EPA regulations and programs. Archives are available for reference use on a wide range of issues, including air and water pollution and toxic substances such as polychlorinated biphenyls, asbestos, pesticides, and radiation.

Food and Drug Administration, United States

Local branch

The FDA inspects manufacturing plants and warehouses and collects samples of foods, drugs, cosmetics, and therapeutic devices to analyze these for adulteration and misbranding. Its responsibilities also extend to sanitary preparation and handling of foods, waste disposal on interstate carriers, and enforcement of the Radiation Control Act as related to consumer products. Epidemiological and other investigations are conducted by FDA to determine causative factors or possible health hazards involved in adverse reactions or hazardous materials accidents.

Health Agencies

Local branch

Health agencies frequently serve as good information or referral sources especially on hazards particular to their jurisdictions. They may also provide help to local citizens. *Local directors of environmental health* are frequently involved in emergency and regulatory actions relative to toxic substance control. These actions might include inspection programs for underground storage of hazardous materials, emergency response, and implementation of community right-to-know ordinances. *Local health officers* have broad authority and responsibility to protect the health and safety of the public within their jurisdictions. This authority includes power to take action in emergency and nonemergency situations involving toxic chemicals.

National Health Information Clearinghouse (NHIC)

U.S. Public Health Service
P.O. Box 1133, ODPHP
Washington, DC 20013-1133
Phone: (800) 336-4797, 9:00 a.m.–5:00 p.m., Monday–Friday

NHIC publishes a series of resource guides, one of which is a listing of selected federal health information clearinghouses and information centers. This agency helps the general public and health professionals locate health information through identification of health information resources and an inquiry and referral system. Health questions are referred to appropriate health resources that, in turn, respond directly to inquirers. NHIC does not provide medical advice, diagnosis, or physician referrals.

National Institute for Environmental Health Sciences (NIEHS)

Dr. Edward Gardner, Jr., Program Director
·Research Grants Programs

Reprinted with permission from ASHP: *Am J Health-Syst Pharm;* March 1987, Vol 44

Extramural Program
P.O. Box 12233
Research Triangle Park, NC 27709
Phone: (919) 541-7723, 8:00 a.m.–4:30 p.m., Monday–Friday

NIEHS is the principal federal agency for biomedical research on the effects of chemical, physical, and biological environmental agents on man's health and well-being. The institute supports efforts to identify potentially hazardous environmental agents through the development, testing, and validation of biological test systems that can be used to measure and predict human toxicity from exposure to environmental factors. NIEHS is interested in research applications concerned with the use of laboratory or clinical tests that will aid in the detection and measurement of toxicity to man from chemical exposure at levels that do not produce overt acute symptoms but that may produce detectable damage years later.

National Institute for Occupational Safety and Health (NIOSH)

Local branch

NIOSH investigates health and safety hazards upon request in all kinds of workplaces. After identifying and evaluating the hazards, NIOSH recommends procedures for prevention or control. NIOSH also does research on selected industries.

National Pesticide Telecommunication Network

Texas Technical University Health Science Center
School of Medicine
Department of Preventive Medicine
Lubbock, TX 79430
Phone: (800) 858-7378, 24 hours/day

This network provides information on such things as pesticide toxicity, health effects, residue data, and efficacy. Referral services are available. Specific information is available on herbicides, fungicides, insecticides, and rodenticides.

National Response Center (NRC)

United States Coast Guard Headquarters
2100 2nd Street, S.W., Rm 2611
Washington, DC 20590
Phone: (800) 424-8802 or (202) 426-2675, 24 hours/day

NRC functions in accordance with the National Contingency Plan to plan for coordinated pollution response by federal and state government agencies. NRC receives initial reports of oil and chemical spills and rapidly passes the information to the predesignated federal on-scene coordinator for action. Technical information such as hazard assessments and movement forecasting is available to federal on-scene coordinators. NRC also provides support to the National Response Team (representatives of 12 federal agencies that plan for and provide guidance during major oil and hazardous substance spills). These 12 agencies are the Environmental Protection Agency, U.S. Coast Guard (Department of Transportation), Department of Agriculture, Department of Commerce, Department of Defense, Department of Energy, Department of Health and Human Services, Department of the Interior, Department of Justice, Department of Labor, Department of State, and the Federal Emergency Management Agency.

Office of Emergency Services (may be the state police in some states)

This agency responds to inquiries from local government and emergency personnel and serves as the central notification point for hazardous materials accidents throughout the state. It notifies other state agencies that are qualified to give technical assistance and information regarding hazardous materials incidents.

Poison Control Center

Local center

Poison centers offer comprehensive drug, poison, and chemical information, referral, and treatment suggestions around the clock. These centers are staffed by specially trained nurses, pharmacists, and physicians.

Radiologic Assistance Program, U.S. Department of Energy

Upton, Long Island, NY 11973
Phone: Region I: Northeast U.S.: (516) 282-2200, 24 hours/day

The U.S. Department of Energy (DOE) Radiological Assistance Program (RAP) makes DOE resources available and provides emergency assistance to state and local agencies to control radiological hazards, protect the public health and safety, and minimize loss of property. A response to a request for federal radiological monitoring and assessment assistance may take many forms, ranging from advice given by telephone to a large federal operation at the site of a serious incident.

Toxic Substances Control Assistance Office

401 "M" Street, S.W.
Washington, DC 20037
Phone: (800) 424-9065, 8:30 a.m.–5 p.m., Monday–Friday

This office is primarily a regulatory agency for establishing guidelines for chemical manufacturers. Technical information is provided on polychlorinated biphenyls and asbestos. It also provides the necessary focus and leadership to ensure that adequate public health protection is being given.

Union Carbide Hazardous Emergency Leak Program (H.E.L.P.)

P.O. Box 4488
Charleston, WV 25304
Phone: (800) 822-4357, 24 hours/day

Union Carbide views its H.E.L.P. system as working in tandem with CHEMTREC. While CHEMTREC is essentially an informational resource, the H.E.L.P. team can provide trained experts at the scene of an emergency. The four phases in which the H.E.L.P. teams operate are analysis, containment, on-scene repairs, and cleanup. This service is offered across the country.

United States Agency for Toxic Substances and Disease Registry

Atlanta, GA.
Phone (emergency response): (404) 452-4100 or (404) 329-2888, 24 hours/day

This is the newest agency of the Public Health Service, U.S. Department of Health and Human Services. It coordinates those provisions of the Comprehensive Environmental Response, Compensation, and Liability Act (CERCLA) of 1980 that relate to public health and worker safety and health and that are carried out through appropriate components of the Public Health Service. Specifically, the agency is charged with protecting the public from exposure to hazardous substances. The agency arranges for program support to ensure adequate response to public health emergencies declared under the authority of CERCLA.

---

a Adapted from reference 38. Used with permission of California Department of Health Services, Community Toxicology Unit.

Weapons of Mass Destruction Events With Contaminated Casualties
Effective Planning for Health Care Facilities

Anthony G. Macintyre, MD

Lt Col George W. Christopher, USAF, MC

COL Edward Eitzen, Jr, MC, USA

LTC Robert Gum, MC, USA

Scott Weir, MD

Craig DeAtley, PA-C

CDR Kevin Tonat, DrPH, MPH, USPHS

Joseph A. Barbera, MD

Biological and chemical terrorism is a growing concern for the emergency preparedness community. While health care facilities (HCFs) are an essential component of the emergency response system, at present they are poorly prepared for such incidents. The greatest challenge for HCFs may be the sudden presentation of large numbers of contaminated individuals. Guidelines for managing contaminated patients have been based on traditional hazardous material response or military experience, neither of which is directly applicable to the civilian HCF. We discuss HCF planning for terrorist events that expose large numbers of people to contamination. Key elements of an effective HCF response plan include prompt recognition of the incident, staff and facility protection, patient decontamination and triage, medical therapy, and coordination with external emergency response and public health agencies. Controversial aspects include the optimal choice of personal protective equipment, establishment of patient decontamination procedures, the role of chemical and biological agent detectors, and potential environmental impacts on water treatment systems. These and other areas require further investigation to improve response strategies.

JAMA. 2000;283:242-249   www.jama.com

THE PERCEIVED THREAT OF chemical or biological weapons directed against the US civilian population has increased substantially.[1-3] The designation of these weapons, along with nuclear materials and high explosives, as "weapons of mass destruction" emphasizes their potential catastrophic effect on the health of a large population. Comprehensive communitywide management programs for civilians exposed to chemical or biological warfare agents are still under development and many response issues have not been fully addressed. Health care facilities (HCFs) are an integral yet often overlooked component of the overall community response.

Although response requirements differ for chemical and biological agent releases, in both cases there might be situations necessitating the removal of the agent from exposed individuals (decontamination). We discuss the planning of an effective HCF response to incidents that require decontamination of

For editorial comment see p 252.

exposed persons. Such a response must be coordinated within the entire community response framework, as in the incident command system, the most widely accepted command and control model for emergency response in the United States.[4] Events that are likely to challenge the decontamination capability of a HCF include 2 types of worst-case scenarios, chemical and biological.

With the release of a chemical weapon in a populated area, casualties may present en masse with little or no advance notification. The chemical agent deployed could be a traditional militarized agent (such as the vesicant mustard) or a more readily obtainable industrial hazardous material. As shown in the Tokyo sarin attack, a significant number of exposed individuals may find their own means of

transportation to the HCF unassisted by emergency medical services (EMS).[5] These patients will not have undergone triage or decontamination, and the least injured will often present first. The HCF must have the ability to immediately decontaminate and treat those who are ill from the agent.[6] Some persons may have

Author Affiliations: Institute for Crisis, Disaster and Risk Management (Dr Barbera) and Department of Emergency Medicine (Drs Macintyre and Weir and Mr DeAtley), George Washington University Medical Center, Washington, DC; US Army Medical Research Institute of Infectious Diseases, Fort Detrick, Md (Lt Col Christopher and COL Eitzen); US Army Center for Health Promotion and Preventive Medicine—Europe, Landstuhl Army Regional Medical Center, Landstuhl, Germany (LTC Gum); and the Office of Emergency Preparedness, US Public Health Service, Rockville, Md (CDR Tonat).
Corresponding Author and Reprints: Anthony G. Macintyre, MD, 2140 Pennsylvania Ave NW, Washington, DC 20037 (e-mail: emdagm@gwumc.edu).

©2000 American Medical Association. All rights reserved.

Reprinted with permission from: *JAMA*; January 12, 2000, Vol 283, No.2

experienced very little exposure to the agent, or none at all. They may still require decontamination because exposure cannot be ruled out. Symptoms may be accompanied by anxiety and may be diverse and confusing.[5,7] Residual chemical agents on those exposed may pose a risk of secondary spread to the HCF and its workers by contact or vaporization.[8,9]

In a biological attack, an infectious agent may be released surreptitiously and discovered after the incubation period, when patients present with illness. However, if a biological attack is announced or discovered publicly as it is occurring, it could result in large numbers of patients suddenly presenting for services. In contrast with chemical agents, most biological agents (except mycotoxins) are not dermally active or volatile. Reaerosolization of infectious particles is theorized to be a low but possible risk.[10] Therefore, decontamination to lessen the effects of primary exposure and to prevent secondary exposure is less important than with chemical agents, but may be necessary.[11,12] The procedure could be as simple as taking a shower and changing clothes (exposure to mycotoxins would call for procedures similar to those used for chemical agents, including extensive patient decontamination).[13] A sudden biological event may require administration of prophylactic medications and vaccines and could place extraordinary demands on medical and public health staff and facilities.[14-16] We do not address the epidemiological investigation and large-scale measures needed to control infection in the event a mass exposure to infectious agents is recognized in a delayed fashion. Plans for HCF response to these types of events are under development.[11,17]

BACKGROUND

Until recently, any threat to civilians from hazardous materials (HAZMATs) primarily has come from industrial events.[18] While unintentional releases are relatively common, they generally cause few serious toxic exposures per event.[19] HAZMAT response guidelines have been developed and implemented for managing these incidents.[20]

The unintentional release of militarized chemical agents from US military depots has been another civilian concern. In response, a major preparedness initiative, the Chemical Stockpile Emergency Preparedness Program, has been implemented in communities surrounding the depots.[21] The response system has never been activated.[22] No similar community preparedness program for biological release has been developed, since the US military ceased maintaining biological weapons in 1972.[23,24]

The newly perceived threat entails the deliberate use of chemical and biological weapons against civilians. In many instances, these weapons are relatively easy to produce, inexpensive, and can be deployed covertly. Most significantly, the widespread terror caused by the use of these weapons could complicate response needs.[25,26]

The toxic and psychological threats posed by chemical terrorism were demonstrated by the 1995 sarin attack in the Tokyo subway system.[5,27] The assault resulted in 11 deaths and more than 5000 emergency medical evaluations, of which 73.9% had no identifiable clinical injury.[28] The majority of those exposed apparently had either a subclinical exposure or psychogenic symptoms. No chemical attacks of this nature have been reported in the United States.

No successful biological attack has occurred in the United States with an aerosolized agent, but other crimes and hoaxes involving biological agents have occurred.[29-31] The potential psychological effects of bioterrorism were demonstrated by the 1997 B'nai B'rith incident in Washington, DC.[32] A Petri dish found in the mail room of the B'nai B'rith headquarters was labeled to indicate the presence of *Bacillus anthracis* and *Yersinia pestis*. Responders and incident managers were unaware that nonaerosolized, agar-based organisms pose no inhalation or cutaneous exposure hazard (it was later proven that neither organism was present). As a result, an expensive scene-control operation took place, causing fear and inconvenience among those potentially exposed. Other recent biological hoaxes

have also disrupted communities across the country.[33]

CURRENT CAPABILITY

As the potential threat of civilian exposure increases, the new challenge for the medical emergency response community will be managing contaminated mass casualties, some of whom may be ill. Many HCFs are poorly prepared for the decontamination requirements of even small-scale HAZMAT incidents,[34,35] as demonstrated by the temporary closures of well-run, full-service emergency departments after presentation of only 1 or 2 contaminated patients in 1997.[36] The most comprehensive HCF response plans to date were designed to cope with specific individual chemical or biological agents and radioactive nucleotides.[37]

Development of HCF response plans has been hampered by many factors. Foremost is the lack of civilian experience with mass casualty events of a chemical or biological nature. Many civilian plans are derived from the experiences of prehospital HAZMAT response teams or military defense procedures that may not be appropriate.

The HAZMAT approach assumes that responders will enter a highly toxic environment near the source of release (away from an HCF). Maximum protection is provided for a few workers rescuing a small number of patients, usually without time pressure for decontamination. The primary objectives are scene containment and environmental protection. In line with these assumptions, the Occupational Health and Safety Administration (OSHA) has mandated the use of a "Personal Protection Level based upon site hazards."[38] However, site hazards are more easily defined at the point of release than at the HCF, where patient care is conducted. Thus, current OSHA guidelines may be inappropriate for HCFs. Traditional HAZMAT products, such as decontamination tents, trailers, and isolation rooms, are expensive, require prolonged setup time, or are inadequate for large numbers of patients.[39]

Military countermeasures for chemical and biological weapons are also inappropriate for civilian use without modi-

©2000 American Medical Association. All rights reserved.

Reprinted with permission from: *JAMA*; January 12, 2000, Vol 283, No.2

fication. Military personnel are a more homogenous population, generally physically fit, mentally disciplined, and equipped for chemical warfare. Because they are designed for operations in very toxic environments, military contingency plans can be complex.[40] Incorrect civilian use of military protective equipment and decontamination procedures may be hazardous, as with the use of military-style gas masks by Israeli civilians during Gulf War missile attacks. Fatalities resulted from improper mask use.[41,42]

The US government has recently begun addressing civilian preparedness deficits. A 1995 presidential initiative funded the prototype for Metropolitan Medical Strike Teams,[43] which were composed of specially trained local personnel were organized to help communities respond to events. This effort has been revised to include a systems approach and has been renamed Metropolitan Medical Response Systems (MMRS). The overall goal of the MMRS program is to link first-response, public health, and health care systems. As a component of the MMRS, HCFs will remain responsible for initial management of contaminated patients. To date, 47 urban areas have received funding for development of an MMRS and more communities are expected to receive similar support.

The Nunn-Lugar-Domenici congressional legislation allocated federal funds to the Department of Defense to upgrade the capabilities of civilian first responders, including HCF personnel.[44] This Domestic Preparedness Program is being conducted serially in 120 metropolitan areas by the US Army Soldier and Biological Chemical Command.[45] This program is intended to provide operational-level preparedness, with educational tracts for community response entities, including emergency management, law enforcement, fire, and medical personnel. The current program for hospital personnel has lacked detailed operational methods.[46,47] A large-scale chemical agent exercise in New York City, conducted after hospital personnel had participated in the Domestic Preparedness Program, demonstrated that hospitals would still have difficulty managing patient decontamination.[48]

The federal government has established a National Domestic Preparedness Office (NDPO) under the auspices of the Department of Justice to act as a clearing house during responses to domestic chemical and biological terrorist incidents. The NDPO will handle information pertinent to law enforcement, emergency medical response, medical, and public health sectors.

Federal preparedness initiatives have been paralleled by private industry's development of chemical and biological agent response products and training programs. Self-described expert consultant groups offer risk analysis and training for various components of local emergency response, including HCFs. Some programs market equipment packages supplied by vendors working in conjunction with the consultants.[49] Most offer operational guidelines based on traditional HAZMAT procedures. As yet, no published large-scale exercise or response experience has validated these programs.

PROPOSED HCF CONCEPT OF OPERATIONS

Owing to the complexity of a civilian event involving chemical or biological weapons, HCFs should begin by delineating priorities that guide their preparedness process. These objectives should be established in coordination with the other members of the community involved in emergency response. The priorities of the HCF could be ranked in this order: (1) protection of the current patients, staff, and facility; (2) provision of the best possible medical care for contaminated patients presenting to the institution for care; and (3) environmental protection external to the HCF. In a large-scale event, containment of wastewater will probably be impossible, though no consensus has yet been reached on this controversial point. This issue should be addressed through comprehensive planning that includes local environmental and water authorities.

Certain assumptions can be made to simplify planning. One is that the exposure site is remote from the HCF (ie,

the HCF is receiving patients but is not within the primary release area). Otherwise, facility evacuation or "sheltering in place" may be indicated. Key components of the model preparedness plan are illustrated in the FIGURE.

Event Recognition

In an unannounced event, it is essential to recognize contaminated patients before their entrance into the facility. Security personnel must be trained in early recognition and should be stationed at the hospital entrances. Security personnel should immediately notify management personnel when they suspect a problem, and they should be prepared to protect themselves by donning personnel protective equipment (PPE). Even so, it is reasonable to expect some contaminated individuals may gain entrance into the facility. These situations should be handled on a case-by-case basis with a rational approach. It will not be necessary to completely seal off the facility or a department in most circumstances.[50]

Activation of Plan

The alert mechanism should be expeditious: PPE must be immediately accessible to decontamination and patient care personnel, and the decontamination facility should be operational within 2 to 3 minutes.

Management

The principles of the incident command system should be incorporated into the HCF's emergency preparedness plan.[51] The use of this system will enable HCF staff to fully integrate their activities with community emergency response assets, since it is widely used by fire, EMS, and police personnel as well as many state and federal agencies. Although initial response efforts will be centered in the decontamination and treatment areas, other HCF departments will play vital roles. For instance, security officers must direct the flow of casualties and vehicles to prevent facility compromise and must prevent unauthorized access to the decontamination and treatment areas.

©2000 American Medical Association. All rights reserved.

Reprinted with permission from: *JAMA*; January 12, 2000, Vol 283, No. 2

Personnel from departments including emergency, critical care services, plant operations, pharmacy, supply services, infectious disease, respiratory therapy, laboratory, and toxicology must be targeted for education and training in the response plan.

A widespread chemical or biological incident will result in extended operational periods. Staff should be coordinated to provide relief from physically taxing activities such as patient decontamination. Providing food and hydration in a hygienic manner will enhance staff performance. Psychological support for staff should be available.

Personnel caring for contaminated patients should be properly outfitted in PPE. Specific data to determine the appropriate level of hospital worker protection remains limited, and a recent extensive review on chemical and biological terrorism published by the Institute of Medicine is inconclusive on this issue.[52] Level C PPE consists of a nonencapsulated, chemical-resistant suit, gloves, and boots, with a full-face air purifier cartridge mask (powered or nonpowered). This gear should afford adequate respiratory protection for outdoor exposure to contaminated chemical casualties who have survived transport to the HCF.[21,53] For HCF workers conducting decontamination of patients acutely contaminated with infectious biological agents, level D protection (standard work clothes) plus latex gloves, eye splash protection, and N-95 respiratory masks (used in many hospitals for protection against tuberculosis) should be adequate.[54,55] If responders are concerned about reaerosolizing an agent during clothing removal, a high-efficiency particulate air (HEPA) filter mask could be added. If the agent class for a sudden release cannot be identified, level C PPE with an organic vapor/HEPA filter cartridge mask is recommended.

Training is essential for the correct use of PPE. Work times and conditions must be monitored while personnel are using PPE to prevent fatigue or heat stress. Personnel should be rotated if decontamination operations are prolonged. Once patients have been decontami-

nated, they may be handled by staff using universal precaution guidelines.

Crowd control will require firm, authoritative direction from hospital security and, if available, police or the National Guard. Since PPE face masks muffle the voice, loudspeakers should be provided to personnel directing contaminated patients. Signs designating functional areas and providing patient instructions should be in place.

Primary Triage

All exposed and potentially exposed individuals should receive an initial brief triage, performed by medical personnel in PPE, before decontamination. They should then be directed to 1 of 2 areas, nonmedical decontamination or medical decontamination. The uninjured, those with minor injuries requiring no medical intervention during decontamination, and the majority of ambulatory patients will be assigned to nonmedical decontamination. These individuals may require nonmedical assistance with washing themselves (eg, unaccompanied children, persons in wheelchairs, and those with other special needs). Those with injuries or illness poten-

tially requiring medical intervention will be assigned to medical decontamination by staff.

Throughout the decontamination process, attention must be given to symptoms of exposure to chemical or biological agents that may indicate early life-threatening deterioration (eg, a sore throat or mild shortness of breath after exposure to pulmonary or laryngeal irritants).

Patient Sign-in/Identification and Securing Property

A brief sign-in process should capture name and date of birth (full registration can occur after decontamination and should be consistent with the community patient tracking system). A number on a log can be assigned to each patient, who would receive 2 identically numbered plastic bags and a nonpermeable wristband. Clothing would be placed into the larger clear, impervious bag. Separation of valuables into the second, smaller bag would enhance the security of these items. A meticulous, practical method of cataloging belongings will ensure their return and possibly assist in forensic investigations.

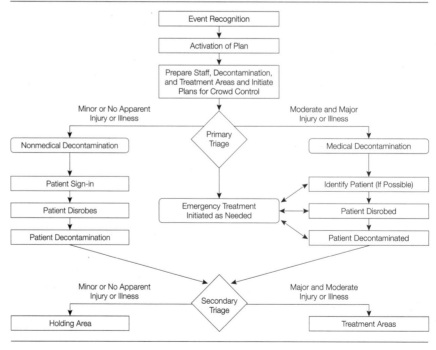

Figure. Health Care Facility Response Plan for Chemical or Biological Weapons Release

©2000 American Medical Association. All rights reserved.

Reprinted with permission from: *JAMA*; January 12, 2000, Vol 283, No.2

Patient Decontamination

The HCF should possess partially fixed or preconstructed decontamination facilities that can be activated immediately. This facility should be designed to occupy little storage space and not disrupt routine operations while in use. The Israeli model, developed during the Gulf War, consists of showers permanently fixed to the ceiling structure of an open-air parking garage or the side of a building.[56] The George Washington University Hospital model uses fire exit alleyways. An outdoor decontamination facility can prevent entry of contaminants into the HCF and obviates dedicating space with room ventilation and vapor isolation. An outdoor facility is also more suitable for the influx of mass casualties. Outdoor decontamination, however, must offer protection from inclement weather and have adequate lighting for night operations.

Because clothing will be removed before decontamination, privacy must be protected to ensure compliance with full decontamination. The sexes should be separated, with a visual barrier between shower lines. The need for protection of privacy was demonstrated by a successful lawsuit against a fire department whose personnel decontaminated 2 women without ensuring adequate privacy.[57]

Another important consideration is rapid patient progression through the decontamination process. Traditional HAZMAT decontamination is passive (using 2 responders to clean each patient), which is time consuming and unnecessary for the majority of ambulatory patients in the nonmedical decontamination area. Promoting patient self-decontamination will significantly decrease the required number of health care workers. Of course, decontamination assistance for some patients in the nonmedical decontamination area and full passive decontamination in the medical decontamination area must still be available.

Decontamination facilities should contain multiple shower stations that are designed to allow patients to progress at various rates without compromising overall flow. Patients whose clinical condition deteriorates in the decontamination line can impede the progress of others. Plans must include means for sidetracking these patients into an area separate from the main decontamination sites, where treatment can be initiated.

Decontamination can be accomplished by using a sequential copious warm water rinse, a hypoallergenic liquid soap wash, another warm water rinse, and then a final rinse after walking past other in-use showers. Incapacitated patients will require soap and water cleansing by staff, with attention to washing and rinsing the patient's back and the nonabsorbent backboard. The water temperature must be adjustable. Excessively warm water should be avoided, as this may promote peripheral vasodilatation and toxin absorption. Stiff brushes or abrasives should also be avoided as they may enhance dermal absorption of the toxin and can produce skin lesions that may be mistaken for chemical injuries.[58,59] Sponges and disposable towels are affordable and effective alternatives.

Secondary Triage

Persons with major or moderate casualties would be referred to treatment areas designated for such cases. Those with minor or no apparent injuries should be sent to a holding area for further evaluation, observation, and eventual treatment if needed.

Holding Area

Large spaces such as cafeterias or auditoriums can be used for observation of large numbers of patients with minor or no apparent injuries and illnesses by physicians and nurses. At this time, HCF staff should also provide information on the agent involved, potential short- and long-term effects, recommended treatment, stress reactions, and possible avenues to further assistance. It is essential to provide important information in writing because the memory of patients may be impaired by the psychological stress of dealing with an exposure. All potentially exposed individuals should also be enrolled in a long-term surveillance program to monitor possible health effects.

Logistics for Treatment

Specific therapies for chemical and biological agent casualties vary according to the etiologic agent and are described elsewhere.[15,16,60,61] Mass casualties requiring specific chemical antidotes, vaccinations, or antibiotics will quickly deplete available supplies. In most cases, current hospital stocks of medications would be inadequate to meet the needs of even a few of these patients.[62] Several efforts are under way to address this problem, including a federal initiative to stockpile antibiotics and vaccines.[63] Other concerns have not yet been adequately addressed. After a smallpox release, for example, postexposure vaccination might be indicated, but smallpox vaccine is no longer produced and current stocks are limited.[16,64]

Otherwise straightforward medical problems, including eye injuries, bronchospasm, and burns, may also need mass intervention. Ventilators and other critical care supplies may be needed in large quantities. This problem could be resolved in part through mutual aid agreements between HCFs. Such an agreement established in the Washington, DC, area provides for pooling of resources (including personnel, supplies, and equipment), and sharing of information.[65] Contingency plans of this type may be vital to saving lives, since time constraints prevent reliance on resupply support from state and federal agencies during the initial crucial period of an event.

Epidemiological Considerations

Health care facility involvement will extend beyond the treatment of patients who are acutely ill or exposed. A comprehensive community response will include epidemiological analysis undertaken by local and national public health organizations to identify all potential exposed individuals. This should be done during the brief interval when early intervention can save lives and containment can reduce secondary transmission of contagious agents. Such

©2000 American Medical Association. All rights reserved.

Reprinted with permission from: *JAMA*; January 12, 2000, Vol 283, No.2

analysis will require participation by HCFs.

Information Resources

Health care facility personnel must identify sources of expert information on chemical and biological agents to ensure ready access to such information. Ideally, a repository or data bank could be established at the community or national level. This would allow for the distribution of uniform information.

Other resources include medical management handbooks developed by the US Army's chemical and biological defense medical laboratories.[54,60,61] Some civilian-based protocols, such as pediatric recommendations, have also been established; these are currently being revised by the US Public Health Service.[66] Consensus statements organized by the Working Group on Civilian Biodefense also provide useful guidance.[15,16] Consultation is also available 24 hours a day by remote access through the National Response Center at (800) 424-8802.

Public Information

Prompt attention must be given to information issued to the public through the news media and bulletins. Media inquiries must be carefully handled, and the content of these communications should be discussed with appropriate emergency management authorities to prevent the release of conflicting or erroneous reports.

Postincident Actions

Following the event, HCF management should conduct an incident review with hospital personnel involved in the emergency response. The purpose of such a review is to determine, in a nonpejorative manner, the sequence of events and to disseminate the rationale behind controversial decisions. Exposure risks and necessary countermeasures should be discussed to alleviate some of the psychological impact of incident stress. The incident critique, which will take place later, is a technical review designed to evaluate and improve the response plan. The

staff should also have access to formalized stress debriefing at a later date.

Because injuries and illnesses sustained during the response would be covered under employee compensation insurance, all staff members involved should be registered in a health surveillance program. This will ensure that medical issues will receive proper attention, and demonstrate the HCFs commitment to employee health. In view of the possible delayed or chronic effects of some chemical agents, surveillance could continue for years. Assistance for this type of surveillance is available through the Agency for Toxic Substances and Disease Registry, which the US Department of Health and Human Services has identified as the lead agency for the registration of personnel exposed to chemical or biological warfare agents.[67]

It will be essential to clean the decontamination facilities and process the possessions of contaminated patients, as well as dispose of solid waste. Cleanup will be guided by the specific agent involved and the law enforcement investigation. If no adequate, financially viable method is available to inactivate a highly toxic, persistent agent such as the nerve gas VX, assistance may be required from other local, state, or federal entities.[68]

CONTROVERSIES AND RESEARCH REQUIRED

Personal Protective Equipment

One major question concerns the optimal approach to PPE. To simplify guidelines and reduce confusion about the variety of choices, PPE recommendations could be standardized. This measure would ease financial disincentives as well as training requirements. Although published research on adequacy of PPE is limited, the consensus emerging among researchers and medical planners is that level C protection (using a full-face mask with powered or nonpowered canister filtration system) is adequate for HCF workers.[21,68,69] A few reports recommend a higher level of protection, level B, which includes a mask supplied by an exter-

nal air source (hose-supplied air with an escape cylinder or a self-contained air tank).[70] However, these reports do not mention whether higher levels of protection produce a quantified increase in safety, nor do they discuss the possible disadvantages such as additional cost, weight, and training requirements.

Choosing a specific material to provide chemical barrier protection for HCF personnel is difficult. Many types of chemically resistant suits are available. They vary in cost and each has unique properties.[71] Industrywide testing is based on permeation rates of pure substances directly applied to the material, but such data may not be relevant to the exposure in the HCF response model.[72] Health care workers remote from the impact site or incident scene will be exposed only to the agent that remains on the skin and clothing of those exposed, so concentrations of substances encountered during decontamination at the HCF will be more dilute than concentrations used for the testing PPE materials.[68] Less expensive barrier materials may therefore be adequate.

Decontamination Solution

Another controversial concept concerns patient decontamination. Should decontamination be simplified by establishing a universal process for all incidents, as suggested by Cox?[71] Some authors have already published universal decontamination protocols for chemical exposures.[50] There is little argument that soap and water will be effective for most agents. In the past, an agent neutralizer such as a 0.5% solution of hypochlorite was recommended. It inactivates biological agents (except mycotoxins) and, at a slower rate, chemical agents such as mustard and organophosphates.[13,60,61] The studies indicate, however, that 15 to 20 minutes of contact time is necessary for hydrolysis or oxidation and, thus, for the inactivation of chemical agents.[60] Furthermore, dilute bleach can cause tissue damage in open wounds, exposed nerve tissue, and the eyes.[13,73] The lack of clear safety and efficacy data for bleach decontamination suggests that

©2000 American Medical Association. All rights reserved.

Reprinted with permission from: *JAMA*; January 12, 2000, Vol 283, No.2

it should be avoided, especially if soap and water are immediately available. There may be rare exceptions to a universal decontamination process. For instance, pure metals and strong corrosives require dry decontamination (ie, gentle brushing or vacuuming of larger particles) before water is applied.[68,74]

Agent Detectors

Yet another controversial issue is what role agent detectors should play in an HCF response plan. Agent detectors and monitors are used in the military and HAZMAT/EMS arenas. In the HCF environment, however, they would only complicate and lengthen the decontamination process. Much of the monitoring and detection equipment for chemical and biological agents is expensive and training intensive. Even handheld assays require attention to standard protocols. Moreover, some agent detectors can give false-positive readings when perfume, diesel vapors, or nonthreatening contaminants are present.[75] In some cases, cool air, the presence of a nonmilitarized agent, or other factors can produce false-negative results. Detection can also be time consuming. If an HCF is operating without any means of detection, HCF personnel must consider that most biological agents and some selected chemical toxins (eg, mustard) have delayed clinical manifestations. Contingency plans must include the capability to treat potentially exposed persons, if indicated, while confirmatory tests are under way.

Decontamination Wastewater

Questions have also been raised about the potential environmental impact of releasing decontamination wastewater into the water treatment system. To date, the Environmental Protection Agency has not published an official statement on this issue in relation to HCF planning. The decision not to contain wastewater can be justified for most agents in a life-threatening mass casualty situation. Biological agents may pose only a temporary risk to the environment or to the people in the area because of rapid environmental degradation or difficult

reaerosolization.[10,13] On the other hand, a large-scale chemical incident usually results in significant environmental pollution; the amount of agent borne by patients presenting to HCFs will constitute only a small fraction of the total environmental burden. Some authors suggest that as much as 75% to 90% of the hazardous agent may be removed by disrobing.[70,71,75] The remaining skin contaminant may be minuscule and can be diluted further during washing and passing into public wastewater systems. The installation of a large-volume wastewater containment system is a prohibitively expensive undertaking. Even if installed, the final disposition of wastewater containing hazardous materials can be a catastrophic financial burden. If the facility design does not provide wastewater containment, appropriate water authorities should be notified at the time of the event.

Unanswered Questions

These and other pressing questions must be investigated if research is to help improve response strategies:

• What are the actual risks to first responders, clinicians, and other health care workers from reaerosolizing biological agents on contaminated clothing, skin, or environmental surfaces?

• What is the minimum adequate amount of washing/rinsing time required for adequate decontamination from most agents?

• What are the specific limitations of level C and level B PPE for HCF personnel caring for exposed patients removed from a site where a chemical or a biological agent has been released?

• What are the ideal avenues through which HCFs can disseminate information during an event of this type or magnitude?

• What equipment and training requirements can HCFs realistically support for this preparedness? Should public policy provide funding for HCF preparedness?

• Does every HCF in a defined area need this preparedness capability?

• Are there specific chemical and biological agents (in the amounts carried

by contaminated patients presenting to HCFs) that cannot be safely washed into public water runoff?

CONCLUSION

The threat of a large-scale incident involving intentional release of chemical or biological agents in the United States is significant, but currently, no practical models exist for HCF response to a suddenly recognized event requiring the decontamination of mass casualties. The time has come to establish a forum of experts to address the questions presented in this article and elsewhere and to reach a consensus on how to develop and disseminate comprehensive guidelines for HCFs. These solutions should be fully integrated into the community response plan for chemical or biological terrorism.

Precedence for this consensus approach may be found in the method used by the Federal Emergency Management Agency for the creation of the National Urban Search and Rescue System.[76] Above all, the process must be an operationally oriented cooperative effort and remain uninfluenced by financial gain and unproved technologies.

The threat posed by chemical and biological terrorism must be kept in proper perspective. Disaster preparedness plans must maintain readiness for these events as well as the terrorist use of conventional explosives.[77,78] Accidental HAZMAT exposures remain even more likely. Robust, effective HCF preparedness integrated with local community planning will help address the more conventional threats.

Disclaimer: The opinions and findings in this article are those of the authors and should not be construed as official policies or positions of the US Department of the Army, US Department of the Air Force, US Public Health Service, or US government.

REFERENCES

1. US Congress, Office of Technology Assessment. *Proliferation of Weapons of Mass Destruction: Assessing the Risks.* Washington, DC: US Government Printing Office; 1993. Publication OTA-ISC-559.
2. *The Emergency Regarding Weapons of Mass Destruction.* Congressional Record; November 8, 1995: S16818-16820. Executive order 12938.
3. Flanagin A, Lederberg J. The threat of biological weapons. *JAMA.* 1996;275:1714-1715.
4. Christen H, Maniscalco P. *The EMS Incident Man-*

©2000 American Medical Association. All rights reserved.

agement System. Upper Saddle River, NJ: Prentice-Hall Inc; 1998:1-15.

5. Nozaki H, Aikawa N, Shinozawa Y, et al. Sarin gas poisoning in the Tokyo subway. *Lancet*. 1995;345: 980-981.

6. Sidell F, Urbanetti J, Smith W, Hurst C. Vesicants. In: Zatchuk R, ed. *Textbook of Military Medicine*. Washington, DC: US Dept of Army, Surgeon General, and the Borden Institute; 1997:197-228.

7. Carmeli A, Liberman N, Mevorach L. Anxiety-related somatic reactions during missile attacks. *Isr J Med Sci*. 1991;27:677-680.

8. Nozaki H, Hori S, Shinozawa Y, et al. Secondary exposure of medical staff to sarin vapor in the emergency room. *Intensive Care Med*. 1995;21:1032-1035.

9. Merritt N, Anderson M. Malathion overdose. *J Emerg Nurs*. 1989;15:463-465.

10. Birenzvige A. *Inhalation Hazard from Reaerosolized Biological Agents: A Review*. Aberdeen, Md: US Army Chemical Research, Development and Engineering Center; 1992. Report TR-413.

11. Association for Professionals in Infection Control and Epidemiology Bioterrorism Task Force and Centers for Disease Control and Prevention Bioterrorism Working Group. *Bioterrorism Readiness Plan: A Template for Healthcare Facilities*. April 13, 1999. Available at: http://www.apic.org/html/resc/biomain.html. Accessed November 12, 1999.

12. Keim M, Kaufmann A. Principles for emergency response to bioterrorism. *Ann Emerg Med*. 1999;34: 177-182.

13. Hurst C. Decontamination. In: Zatchuk R, ed. *Textbook of Military Medicine*. Washington, DC: US Dept of Army, Surgeon General, and the Borden Institute; 1997:351-359.

14. Franz D, Jahrling P, Friedlander A, et al. Clinical recognition and management of patients exposed to biological warfare agents. *JAMA*. 1997;278:399-411.

15. Inglesby TV, Henderson DA, Bartlett JG, et al, for the Working Group on Civilian Biodefense. Anthrax as a biological weapon. *JAMA*. 1999;281:1735-1745.

16. Henderson DA, Inglesby TV, Bartlett JG, et al, for the Working Group on Civilian Biodefense. Smallpox as a biological weapon. *JAMA*. 1999;281:2127-2137.

17. US Army Soldier Biological and Chemical Command. *Biological Warfare Improved Response Program*. March 10, 1999. Available at: http://dp.sbccom.army.mil/fs/index.html. Accessed November 29, 1999.

18. Hall H, Dhara V, Price-Green P, Kaye W. Surveillance for emergency events involving hazardous substances—United States, 1990-1992. *MMWR Morb Mortal Wkly Rep*. 1994;43(SS-2):1-6.

19. Binder S. Deaths, injuries and evacuations from acute hazardous material releases. *Am J Public Health*. 1989;79:1042-1044.

20. US Department of Health and Human Services. *Managing Hazardous Materials Incidents*. Washington, DC: Agency for Toxic Substances and Disease Registry; 1992.

21. Centers for Disease Control and Prevention. CDC recommendations for civilian communities near chemical weapons depots. 60 *Federal Register* 33307-33318 (1995).

22. Carnes S, Watson A. Disposing of the US chemical weapons stockpile. *JAMA*. 1989;262:653-659.

23. Memorandum 35 from President Richard M. Nixon regarding national security decision; November 25, 1969.

24. Memorandum 44 from President Richard M. Nixon regarding national security decision; February 20, 1970.

25. Fullerton C, Ursano R. Health care delivery in the high stress environment of chemical and biological warfare. *Mil Med*. 1994;159:524-528.

26. Bleich A, Shmuel K, Margalit C, et al. Israeli psychological casualties of the Persian Gulf War. *Isr J Med Sci*. 1991;27:673-676.

27. Okumura T, Takusa N, Ishimatsu S, et al. Report on 640 victims of the Tokyo subway sarin attack. *Ann Emerg Med*. 1996;28:129-135.

28. Lillibridge S, Liddle J, Leffingwell S, Sidell F. *Report of the American Medical Delegation to Japan*. Atlanta, Ga: Centers for Disease Control and Prevention; 1995.

29. Haynes V, Coates J. Motive unclear for 2 charged in germ plot. *Chicago Tribune*. February 22, 1998:E98.

30. *United States v Wheeler*, 98 F3d 330 (8th Cir 1996).

31. Torok TJ, Tauxe RV, Wise RP, et al. Large community outbreak of salmonellosis caused by intentional contamination of restaurant salad bars. *JAMA*. 1997;278:389-395.

32. Horowitz S. B'nai B'rith package contained common bacteria. *Washington Post*. April 29, 1997:B2.

33. Bioterrorism alleging use of anthrax and interim guidelines for management—United States, 1998. *MMWR Morb Mortal Wkly Rep* 1999;48:69-74.

34. Cone D, Davidson S. Hazardous materials preparedness in the emergency department. *Prehosp Emerg Care*. 1997;1:85-90.

35. Landesman L, Leonard R. SARA three years later. *J Prehosp Disaster Med*. 1993;8:39-44.

36. Sorokin E. Mystery mail sickens, briefly shuts Fairfax ER. *Fairfax Journal*. May 2, 1997:A11.

37. Waldron R, Danielson R, Schultz H, et al. Radiation decontamination unit for the community hospital. *AJR Am J Roentgenol*. 1981;136:977-981.

38. General Description and Discussion of the Levels of Protection and Protective Gear, 29 USC §1910.120B (1989).

39. El Sanadi N, Grove C, Takacs M, Daly S, Ellenberger D. A hospital-based, hazardous materials decontamination and treatment unit. *J Prehosp Disaster Med*. 1993;8:337-340.

40. Cancio LC. Chemical casualty decontamination by medical platoons in the 82d Airborne Division. *Mil Med*. 1993;158:1-5.

41. Rivkind A, Barach P, Israeli A, Berdugo M, Richter E. Emergency preparedness and response in Israel during the Gulf War. *Ann Emerg Med*. 1997;30:513-521.

42. Karsenty E, Shemer J, Alschech I, et al. Medical aspects of the Iraqi missile attacks on Israel. *Isr J Med Sci*. 1991;27:603-607.

43. Fehr S. Strike team proposed for quick response to terrorist attack. *Washington Post*. Nov 7, 1995:B3.

44. Nunn-Lugar-Domenici Amendment to the FY 97 Defense Authorization Act, Pub L No. 104-201, Title XIV: Defense Against Weapons of Mass Destruction, Subtitle A: Domestic Preparedness. US Congress; June 27, 1996.

45. *Report to Congress: Response to Threats of Terrorist Use of Weapons of Mass Destruction*. Washington, DC: US Dept of Defense; January 31, 1997.

46. Domestic Preparedness Program, Defense Against Weapons of Mass Destruction. *Technician-Hospital Provider Course Manual*. Aberdeen, Md: US Army CB-DCOM, Domestic Preparedness Office; 1997.

47. Graham B. Anti-terrorism plans termed inadequate. *Washington Post*. October 3, 1998:A9.

48. Hauer JM. Preparing for terrorism involving weapons of mass destruction. Presented at: US Capitol Police Board; February 26, 1998; Washington, DC.

49. HAZ/MAT DQE involved in national preparedness. *HAZ/MAT DQE News*. 1998;6:2.

50. Burgess J, Kirk M, Borron S, Cisek J. Emergency department hazardous materials protocol for contaminated patients. *Ann Emerg Med*. 1999;34:205-212.

51. Londorf D. Hospital application of the incident management system. *J Prehosp Disaster Med*. 1995; 10:184-188.

52. Access to PPE. In: *Chemical and Biological Terrorism; Research and Development to Improve Civilian Medical Response*. Washington, DC: National Academy Press; 1999:35-36.

53. Protective measures and handling of casualties. In: *Treatment of Chemical Agent Casualties and Conventional Military Chemical Injuries*. Washington, DC: US Government Printing Office; 1990. FM 8-285, NAVMED P-5041, AFM 160-11.

54. Eitzen E, Pavlin J, Cieslak T, et al, eds. *Medical Management of Biological Casualties Handbook*. 3rd ed. Fort Detrick, Md: US Army Medical Research Institute of Infectious Disease; 1998:appendix B.

55. PPE specifically for biologic agents. In: *Chemical and Biological Terrorism; Research and Development to Improve Civilian Medical Response*. Washington, DC: National Academy Press; 1999: 41-42.

56. Adler J. Missile attacks on Israel during the Gulf War. Handout prepared for: National Disaster Medical System Conference on Lifesaving Intervention; May 4-7, 1997; Tampa, Fla.

57. Gong E, Dauber W. Policewomen win settlement. *Seattle Times*. July 11, 1996:B1.

58. Stokes J, Banderet L. Psychological aspects of chemical defense and warfare. *Mil Psychol*. 1997;9: 395-415.

59. Sidell F. What to do in case of the unthinkable chemical warfare attack or accident. *Postgrad Med*. 1990;88:70-84.

60. *Medical Management of Chemical Casualties Handbook*. Aberdeen, Md: US Army Medical Research Institute of Chemical Defense; 1995.

61. *Medical Management of Biological Casualties Handbook*. Fort Detrick, Md: US Army Medical Research Institute of Infectious Diseases; 1996.

62. Woolf A, Chrisanthus K. On-site availability of selected antidotes. *Am J Emerg Med*. 1997;15:62-66.

63. Graham B. Clinton to order reserves of germ weapon antidotes. *Washington Post*. May 21, 1998:A1.

64. McClain D. Smallpox. In: Zatchuk R, ed. *Textbook of Military Medicine*. Washington, DC: US Dept of Army, Surgeon General, and the Borden Institute; 1997:539-559.

65. *Hospital Mutual Aid Emergency Preparedness Plan*. Washington, DC: District of Columbia Hospital Association; 1996.

66. *Metropolitan Medical Strike Team Field Operations Guide*. Rockville, Md: United States Public Health Service, Office of Emergency Preparedness; 1997.

67. *Health and Medical Services Support Plan for the Federal Response to Acts of Chemical/Biological (C/B) Terrorism*. Washington, DC: US Dept of Health and Human Services; 1996.

68. Sullivan J, Krieger G. *Hazardous Materials Toxicology*. Baltimore, Md: Williams & Wilkins; 1992.

69. Shapira Y, Bar Y, Berkenstadt H, Atsmon J, Danon Y. Outline of hospital organization for a chemical warfare attack. *Isr J Med Sci*. 1991;27:616-622.

70. Levitin H, Siegelson H. Hazardous materials. *Emerg Med Clin*. 1996;14:327-348.

71. Cox R. Decontamination and management of hazardous materials exposure victims in the emergency department. *Ann Emerg Med*. 1994;23:761-770.

72. Noll G, Hildebrand M, Yvorra J. Personal protective clothing and equipment. In: Daly P, ed. *Hazardous Materials*. Stillwater: Fire Protection Publications, Oklahoma State University; 1995:285-322.

73. Gold M, Bongiovanni R, Scharf B, Gresham V, Woodward C. Hypochlorite solution as a decontaminant in sulfur mustard contaminated skin defects in the euthymic hairless guinea pig. *Drug Chem Toxicol*. 1994;17:499-527.

74. Borak J, Callan M, Abbott W. *Hazardous Materials Exposures*. Englewood Cliffs, NJ: Brady Publications; 1991:145.

75. Sullivan F, Wang R, Jenouri I. Principles and protocols for prevention, evaluation, and management of exposure to hazardous materials. *Emerg Med Rep*. 1998;19:21-32.

76. Barbera J, Macintyre A. Urban search and rescue. *Emerg Med Clin North Am*. 1996;14:399-412.

77. Frykberg E, Tepas J. Terrorist bombings. *Ann Surg*. 1988;208:569-576.

78. Mallonee S, Shariat S, Stennies G, et al. Physical injuries and fatalities resulting from the Oklahoma City bombing. *JAMA*. 1996;276:382-390.

©2000 American Medical Association. All rights reserved.

Reprinted with permission from: *JAMA*; January 12, 2000, Vol 283, No.2